Praise for *Complete Gluten-Free Cookbook*, *The Best Gluten-Free Family Cookbook* and *125 Best Gluten-Free Recipes*

"My soon to be 5-year-old Hannah said 'Yummm, this is delicious' about the Morning Glory Muffins, which is quite a compliment from a young celiac. I liked the use of the various flours for nutrients and the fact that there is not a lot of oil in the recipe."

— *Angela Drew, mother, Victoria, British Columbia*

"I made the Pumpkin Chocolate Chip Cookies for a Halloween party. One of my friends follows a gluten-free diet, and they were a hit! Everyone loved them. I took some over to my parents' house, and only after they told me how much they enjoyed the cookies did I tell them they were gluten-free. I recommend your three gluten-free cookbooks to my friends and family all the time!"

— *Alisa Bar-Dayan, RD, Hospital for Sick Children, Toronto, Ontario*

"I love and completely agree with your approach of emphasizing whole grains and nutritious ingredients. You've *proved* that a large percentage of starch in a GF flour blend is not necessary. Your recipes taste delicious, and I believe the hearty flavor of the whole grains actually makes them tastier than the counterpart made with a traditional rice/starch GF flour mix. My favorite bread recipe is the Ancient Grains Bread. I make this regularly, and my kids (non-celiacs, age 6 and 8) actually prefer it to wheat bread. The Honey Walnut Bread is wonderful too."

— *C. Coffey, GIG Support Group, Rochester, New York*

"I would like to thank you both for attending the Celiac Convention in Victoria. I attended your 'lectures' and learned a lot. I purchased your book *Complete Gluten-Free Cookbook*. I have purchased all of the flours and made the Make-Your-Own Muffin Mix. I then made the Pineapple Nut Muffins and froze the rest of the muffin mix. I am most impressed! I have made many muffins, but none turned out as good as these ones. I have to be egg-free, so I was a bit skeptical about using the ground flaxseed as a replacement, but never had a problem with it. Thank you both for creating a cookbook for both gluten-free and egg-free. I am so glad I attended the convention. I live in Victoria, so I am already blessed with beauty around me, but you both made my life more beautiful."

— *K. Hilder, Victoria, British Columbia*

"I have to tell you that your cookbooks have restored my confidence. My husband was diagnosed six years ago with celiac disease, and two of our then four children were also diagnosed over the next year and a half. I am not celiac myself, and I still have three kids who seem to be fine, so we have a split household and I still try to cater to both. I considered myself a pretty good baker, but did I ever struggle with gluten-free baking. I had failure after failure, so I quit baking. Every once in a while, I would gather up the courage to try again. Then my mom gave me *125 Best Gluten-Free Recipes* for Christmas one year, and I have had more success with your recipes than any other! We love the White Cake recipe (cake is one thing my husband really misses) and for Christmas I now always make your Poultry Stuffing Bread from *Best Gluten-Free Family Cookbook*! Thanks so much for what you do!"

— *K. Bauer, Texas*

"You can imagine my joy when I tried your Brown Bread recipe and had immediate success. My husband's reaction was, 'You've arrived.' Since then, I've had even better results by adding the flaxseed egg replacer. I like the simplicity of the recipe, especially being able to add the yeast to the flour. Another thing about your *Complete Gluten-Free Cookbook* that I really like is the Gluten-Free Pantry section. The use and storage instructions are really helpful, and the information blocks in the sidebars are very interesting. Thanks for your gluten-free cookbooks. They are a godsend."

— *E. Hodges, Steinbach, Manitoba*

"If you are gluten intolerant or wheat sensitive, *Best Gluten-Free Family Cookbook* is a 'must-have' cookbook. I have tried quite a few of the recipes. In almost all cases, the results were a superior, tasty product. In fact, my family, who are not gluten intolerant, prefer the muffin and waffle recipes over traditional wheat products. As a final bonus, the authors have incorporated higher fiber and nutrient-dense grains to guard against nutritional deficiencies."

— *D. Mccullough, Kansas*

"I always enjoy seeing you, and your knowledge, expertise and attention to detail always make me feel confident that whatever I make from your cookbooks will turn out perfectly. Just wanted to let you know that this week I have made both your lasagna and the Peppered Zucchini Loaf, and the reaction was *wow*. The aroma of lasagna was so wonderful that we had a *very* difficult time waiting for dinnertime to enjoy it. But it was definitely worth the wait. We, somewhat reluctantly, portioned the remainder and froze it, as it will come in very handy on evenings when we need something quick.

"When looking for ways to use zucchini from the garden, I stumbled across the Peppered Zucchini Loaf in *125 Best*, and was I ever glad I did! What a fabulous taste! We were both so taken with it that we are serving it when we have our friends over for dinner tomorrow evening.

"Thanks to you both for all your awesome recipes that make GF dining a delight. No one using your recipes could ever say GF food was boring, and most don't realize that they are eating GF. I can honestly say that I have never had one of your recipes turn out bad."

— *S. Green, London, Ontario*

"Since both grandchildren have celiac disease, we had to find some gluten-free recipes that didn't make them feel deprived. Try the Chocolate Chip Bars. They were greedily gobbled up by both gluten-free and 'regular' eaters, to great delight. They also keep very well, so make a double batch. I heartily recommend *Best Gluten-Free Family Cookbook*. And there are some lovely color pictures if you need some inspiration. Gluten-free does not mean 'taste-free,' especially with this book for a guide."

— *K. Toutolmin, California*

"Your cookbooks have been amazing and inspiring! Everything I have tried is delicious, and my family appreciates it too. I was diagnosed with celiac disease last year, and I was very disappointed until my daughter purchased your books for us. Since I was about 13 years old, I have always had a passion for being in the kitchen, whether to cook or to bake. When I found out I could no longer enjoy the same cooking or foods anymore, I didn't know if I could obey these rules. After receiving your cookbooks, I began to read and learn, and I went shopping for the various types of flours, etc. Since I've tried baking your bread recipes, I will never buy a frozen gluten-free bread again! Your recipes (not just the bread) are wonderful. Pizza is great. My son, Marc, approves, and he was giving me a hard time about the gluten-free diet. I feel it is a healthier way of life, and for this reason, I *only* cook and bake gluten-free for the whole family, rather than just for myself. My health has since improved dramatically."

— *A. Simonetta, Richmond Hill, Ontario*

"I love *125 Best Gluten-Free Recipes*! The Pineapple-Carrot Cake is amazing. I made it for my boyfriend's birthday — and any time I can find an excuse to make it. It is so moist and yummy… even people without celiac say it is the best carrot cake they have had! I am always making the pizza crust too! I haven't tried many of the other recipes, but those two definitely make the book worth the purchase for me!"

— *R. Okalice, Spokane, Washington*

"I made the Mock Pumpernickel Loaf. I can honestly tell you this is the best loaf ever. My husband, who is not a celiac, tried a piece and said it reminds him of bread we could buy in England, which was a malt loaf. I have never found any bread here that remotely resembled it. Thank you so much for the great recipes and for your help."

— *J. McArthur, Western Canada*

"I had the pleasure of meeting you both at the Celiac Conference in May. I purchased two copies of your latest book, one for myself and one for a friend. We both love your recipes and are so pleased with the reliable products each recipe produces. Last week, I made your Ciabatta (*125 Best Gluten-Free Recipes*, page 38) and we all love it. In fact, I have made three more since then, two of those today. My daughter and I (both celiac) now look forward to lunch — both making it and eating it. Thank you so much for all the time and effort you put into your recipes. Recently, I was asked to bring an appetizer to a neighborhood party. I made Pear Pizza using your Plain Pizza Crust recipe (*125 Best Gluten-Free Recipes*, page 48). It was a tremendous hit. One lady asked me specifically about the crust. She commented that it was so delicious, yet different from other pizza crusts. I love it when wheat eaters like my GF product as much as a wheat product — or in this case even *better*!"

— *C. Sullivan, Ottawa, Ontario*

"Donna and Heather's cookbooks are a great addition to the Specialty Food Shop! I do not hesitate to recommend them to customers looking for quality gluten-free cookbooks that offer appetizing and nutritious recipes."

— *Cristina Cicco, RD, Hospital for Sick Children,*
Toronto, Ontario

250 Gluten-Free favorites

250 Gluten-Free favorites

Includes Dairy-Free, Egg-Free and White Sugar–Free Recipes

Donna Washburn & Heather Butt

Robert ROSE

For complete cataloguing information, see page 401.

Disclaimer
The recipes in this book have been carefully tested by our kitchen and our tasters. To the best of our knowledge, they are safe and nutritious for ordinary use and users. For those people with food or other allergies, or who have special food requirements or health issues, please read the suggested contents of each recipe carefully and determine whether or not they may create a problem for you. All recipes are used at the risk of the consumer.

We cannot be responsible for any hazards, loss or damage that may occur as a result of any recipe use.

For those with special needs, allergies, requirements or health problems, in the event of any doubt, please contact your medical adviser prior to the use of any recipe.

Design and Production: Daniella Zanchetta/PageWave Graphics Inc.
Editor: Sue Sumeraj
Recipe Editor and Tester: Jennifer MacKenzie
Nutrient Analysis: Magda Fahmy
Proofreader: Sheila Wawanash
Indexer: Gillian Watts
Photography: Colin Erricson
Food Styling: Kathryn Robertson
Prop Styling: Charlene Erricson

Cover image: Lemon Pepper Thins (page 92), Sun-Dried Tomato Green Onion Cornbread (page 239) and Rosemary Breadsticks (page 187)

We acknowledge the financial support of the Government of Canada through the Book Publishing Industry Development Program (BPIDP) for our publishing activities.

Published by Robert Rose Inc.
120 Eglinton Avenue East, Suite 800, Toronto, Ontario, Canada M4P 1E2
Tel: (416) 322-6552 Fax: (416) 322-6936

Printed and bound in Canada

2 3 4 5 6 7 8 9 CPL 17 16 15 14 13 12 11 10

We want to dedicate this book to our mothers,
both of whom were career women — caring teachers
by profession. By example, they instilled in us the important
values of honesty, integrity and a strong desire to challenge
ourselves to continue to grow in our lifelong search for knowledge.
Without them, our friendship would never have developed
and this book would never have been written.

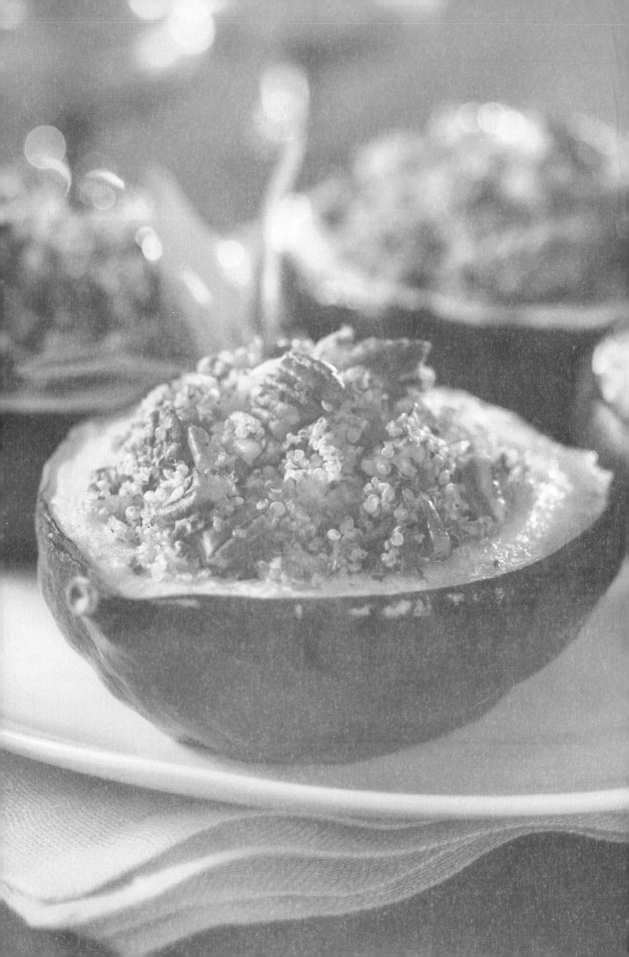

Contents

Acknowledgments

THIS BOOK HAS had the support and assistance of many from its inception to the final reality. We want to thank those who helped us along the way.

Our thanks to the following for supplying products for recipe development: Doug Yuen of Dainty Foods for an assortment of rice, brown rice flour and rice bran; George Birinyi Jr. of Grain Process Enterprises Ltd. for potato and tapioca starches, grape skin flour, sorghum flour, amaranth flour, whole bean flour, chickpea flour, pea flour and quinoa grain and flour; Amy Rempel and Chuck Cundari of Canbrands Specialty Foods for Pane Riso Foods (formerly Kingsmill) Egg Replacer®; Raj Sukul of Maplegrove Food & Beverage Co. Ltd. for the Pastato pasta and bouillon cubes; Ivan Shih of Rizopia Food Products Inc. for a variety of white, brown and wild rice pastas; Howard Selig of Valley Flaxflour Ltd. for flax flour and flaxseed, both brown and golden; Heartland's Finest for the bean flour pasta; Margaret Hudson of Burnbrae Farms Ltd. for Naturegg Simply Whites and Break Free liquid eggs; Egg Farmers of Ontario for whole shell eggs; Michel Dion of Lallamand Inc. for Eagle Instaferm® yeast; Beth Armour and Tracy Perry of Cream Hill Estates Ltd. for oat flour and rolled oats; Beth Armour of Cream Hill Estates Ltd. for permission to share recipes originally developed by her; Seaton Smith Family of Gluten-Free Oats® Company for old-fashioned rolled oats; FarmPure Foods Inc. for Only Oats™, oat bran, flour, flakes and steel-cut pearls; CanolaInfo and Canbra Foods Ltd. for Canola Harvest canola oil, HiLo spray and baking/waffle spray; Dorothy Long of CanolaInfo for permission to share recipes originally developed for them; Omega Nutrition for pumpkin flour, sunflower flour, Nutriflax, pumpkin seed butter, balsamic vinegar, apple cider vinegar and extra virgin olive oil; Best Cooking Pulses for organic pea fiber, whole yellow pea flour and chickpea flour; Northern Quinoa Corp. for quinoa flour; Workinesh Spice Blends, Inc. for providing teff flour; and Tortilla Factory for teff tortillas.

Thank you to the many manufacturers of bread machines who continue to supply the latest models to our test kitchen: Salton/Toastmaster Inc., Breadman, Cuisinart, Oster, Black & Decker and Zojirushi. Also thank you to Jarden Consumer Solutions for the Sunbeam stand mixer and Hamilton Beach Brands for the food processor.

A huge thank you to the members of our focus group, who faithfully and tirelessly tasted and tested gluten-free recipes and products from the beginning to end of recipe development. Your comments, suggestions and critical analysis were invaluable and helped make this a better book. A very special thanks to Craig Butt for the nutritional analysis charts, and to Orla McDougall and the members of the Brockville chapter of the Canadian Celiac Association, Cathy Maggio-Howley and her family and Deanna Jennett for their assistance.

We want to express our appreciation to photographer Colin Erricson, food stylist Kathy Robertson and prop stylist Charlene Erricson. Thank you for making the photographs of our gluten-free recipes look delicious. Once again, we enjoyed baking for the photo shoot.

Bob Dees, our publisher, and Marian Jarkovich, Sales and Marketing Manager, National Retail Accounts, at Robert Rose Inc. deserve special thanks for their ongoing support.

To Andrew Smith, Daniella Zanchetta and Joseph Gisini of PageWave Graphics Inc., thank you for working through this cookbook's design, layout and production. Thank you to Sue Sumeraj, our editor.

Thank you to our families, Heather's husband, our sons, daughters-in-law and grandchildren. You helped bring balance to our lives when we became too focused on our work.

And finally, to you who must follow a gluten-free diet, we sincerely hope these recipes help make your life easier and more enjoyable. We developed them with you in mind.

— Donna and Heather

Introduction

HERE WE ARE on the road again. It is May and we are on our way back from the Canadian Celiac Association Conference in beautiful Victoria, British Columbia. We are driving through the rugged country of Northern Ontario, and around the corner is another magnificent view. We never cease to marvel at the crystal clear lakes, the miles of trees and the early morning fog. As we traveled across the Prairies, whichever one of us wasn't behind the wheel proofed recipes, and together we planned our talk to the Rochester Support Group in Upper New York State the day after we returned. The miles just flew. If you ever get an opportunity to drive across Canada, take advantage of it. Plan lots of time and enjoy the changing scenery. In early May, we had snow in the Rockies, gorgeous flowers in sunny British Columbia and modern grain elevators off in the distance in the Prairies.

During our many miles on the road, we planned what to take to Texas and Omaha, to the CSA and GIG conferences later in the year. We reminisced about past conferences and wondered which of the many celiac friends we have made over the years would be there. We hoped many. So many of you hold such precious memories for us!

As we stopped at restaurants along the way, we wondered what you would order from the menu and tried to pick out items we felt were safely gluten-free. What a challenging task! They were few and far between at some stops. We understood why you need to carry safe foods in the car with you. We picked out several snacks that would be delicious, and as we tasted them wrote notes on the backs of napkins and planned how we would develop gluten-free recipes for them in this book. Our favorites included Asian Slaw with Lime Sesame Dressing (page 106), Roasted Garlic Caesar Dressing (page 80) and Maple Pecan Cheesecake (page 302).

While we were in Victoria, Donna met Joan Segee, who asked us to develop a recipe for her. She promised to send us an original copy to modify. We had recently developed a Welsh Cakes recipe for a friend from London, Ontario. She actually brought us the wheat version she'd had as a child so we could taste the original. We sent her our GF version, and she was ecstatic. Shortly after we arrived home, Joan sent us two recipes from the Maritimes, Ginger Marble Cake and Gingerbread Cookies. We developed gluten-free versions of each and sent the recipes to her for her approval. We have already made the cake for friends, and it has become one of our favorites. You will find these and other recipes in the Favorites by Request chapter.

When in Victoria, we spoke about bread machine baking and advanced baking techniques. You will find two chapters on bread baking in this book. The new machines are quite different, so we have given very detailed directions for using the new Gluten-Free cycles, as well as the Dough and Bake cycles. Bread machines continue to be a challenge!

Keep in touch with us. We appreciate your emails and letters, as they give us much-appreciated feedback. We know it takes time in your busy lives to write. Your questions and comments are important to us.

Donna J. Washburn, P.H.Ec., and Heather L. Butt, P.H.Ec.
Quality Professional Services
1104 Burnside Drive
Brockville, Ontario K6V 5T1

Phone/fax: (613) 923-2116
Email: bread@ripnet.com
Website: www.bestbreadrecipes.com

Understanding Whole Grains

"A whole grain is the entire seed, including the naturally occurring nutrients of an edible plant. The size, shape and color of the seed, also referred to as the 'kernel,' vary with the species. A grain is considered a whole grain when it contains all three seed parts: bran, germ and endosperm."

— *The Whole Grains Council (www.wholegrainscouncil.org)*

What Is Meant by "Whole Grain"?

As the quote above explains, a whole grain consists of three parts: the bran, the germ and the endosperm. The **bran**, or outer coating, is made up of several layers. It is rich in insoluble fiber and contains antioxidants and B vitamins. Just beneath the bran layers is a small structure called the **germ**. The germ is rich in healthy oils, B vitamins, minerals including magnesium and iron, and some protein. The **endosperm** is the largest portion of the grain. It contains starch, protein, soluble fiber and small amounts of vitamins and minerals.

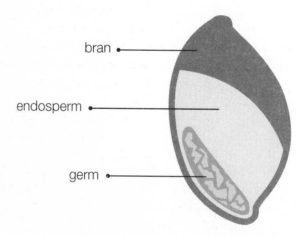

bran

endosperm

germ

Whole grains contain all three parts, whereas refined grains (white rice, defatted soy, degerminated cornmeal) have the bran and germ removed, leaving only the endosperm. Refined grains are not as nutritious as whole grains. Some refined grains may be enriched (some of the nutrients that were removed are added back), but few GF grains, flours or products such as cereals and pasta are enriched. It is very important to read labels every time when purchasing products made commercially with GF flours.

Whole grains can be eaten whole, cracked, ground or milled into flour.

They can be the basis of commercial pastas, cereals and baked products. A whole grain that has been processed (cracked, crushed, ground, milled, rolled, extruded and/or cooked) still contains approximately the same nutrients found in the original grain seed.

Flour is the ground form of a grain. It can be milled from the whole grain or may be a refined and processed grain.

Many gluten-free flours are whole grains.

These include:

- amaranth
- buckwheat
- corn, including whole cornmeal
- millet
- Montina™ (Indian rice grass)
- GF oats, including oatmeal
- quinoa
- rice, both brown and colored
- wild rice
- sorghum
- teff

(Approved and endorsed by the Whole Grains Council, May 2004, www.wholegrainscouncil.org)

Amaranth

Amaranth seeds (also known as whole-grain amaranth) are off-white, golden, tan or light brown in color and are about the size of poppy seeds. The flavor ranges from mild, slightly sweet and nutty, to a more robust, peppery whole-grain taste. Stews and soups can be thickened by adding a small amount of amaranth seeds. Use amaranth seeds raw in crackers, granola, breading, crusts, toppings for casseroles and sweets with molasses or honey. The seeds can be cooked with other whole grains, or added to stir-fries, soups or stews. You can also enjoy them as a breakfast cereal. Be careful not to overcook them, as they become very gummy.

Amaranth flour is very fine and has a light cream color and a pleasant, nutty taste. Because of its high moisture content, use it in combination with other flours. It produces baked goods that are moist and dense, but added starch helps to lighten the texture. The grain of the bread is more open, the texture not as silky and the crumb color slightly darker than wheat flour breads. Amaranth flour tends to form a crust on the outside of a product during baking, sealing the outside before the product is completely cooked on the inside, so use the smallest amount of liquid you can and allow for slightly longer baking times than you might otherwise. Products baked with amaranth flour tend to brown quickly and may need to be tented with foil during the last third of the baking time. Make sure you check to make sure the internal temperature of the baked product reaches 200°F (100°C), as it may look baked on the outside before the center is done. We enjoy amaranth flour in yeast breads, muffins, cookies, pancakes, flatbreads and donuts. Amaranth flour is one of our favorites for thickening gravy, soups and stews, as it results in a dull finish and holds well.

Further Information

- www.nuworldamaranth.com
- www.lesliebeck.com

Buckwheat

Buckwheat groats are the hulled, white to cream-colored, triangular-shaped kernels of the buckwheat (saracen corn) plant. Soft in texture and bitter in flavor, they are available whole or cracked into coarse, medium or fine grinds.

Finely cracked groats (grits) may be labeled "cream of buckwheat." They cook quickly and are served like rice, or are combined with rice to dilute their intense flavor. In Russia, buckwheat groats are served as a hot porridge for breakfast. They are also used to thicken gravy and sauces or added to casseroles, stews, salads and side dishes.

Kasha is roasted or toasted buckwheat groats. The groats darken to brown, the bitter flavor disappears and the nutty, earthy flavor becomes stronger. Kasha is used in dishes ranging from pilafs to meat mixtures.

Buckwheat flakes (oatmeal-style buckwheat) are rolled flakes made from buckwheat groats treated with hot steam. These small, brittle flakes look like small rolled oats, but have a slightly sweeter flavor and a slightly browner color. Those who can't tolerate oatmeal can substitute buckwheat flakes.

Buckwheat flour is very fine, with a unique, strong, musty, slightly sour, slightly nutty flavor. For light buckwheat flour, the hull is removed before the groats are ground. Dark buckwheat flour is made of unhulled groats; it is grayish, with tiny black specks of hull, and has a strong, earthy taste. Buckwheat flour tends to make baked goods heavier and give them a distinctive, stronger taste. It is usually blended with other flours. Buckwheat flour is used in pancake mixes, waffles, Russian blinis, Japanese soba noodles (which contain wheat), crêpes, muffins, dumplings, unleavened chapati and pastries. It can be used as a meat extender in a sausage meat mixture or combined with other GF flours to make breads and quick breads.

> Bees use the nectar in buckwheat flowers to make a dark, strong-flavored honey. Buckwheat is sometimes planted just for the honey.

- www.whfoods.com
- www.recipetips.com
- www.innvista.com

Some people have
difficulty digesting
buckwheat.

Corn

Cornmeal is milled from corn. It has larger granules than regular flour
and can be yellow, white, red or blue. Although these varieties are slightly
different in texture and flavor, one can be substituted for the other. The
coarser the grind, the more granular the texture of the finished product
and the more intense the corn flavor. Cornmeal can be used to make
cornbread, spoon bread, polenta or muffins, or can be cooked and served
as a hot cereal. It can also be used as a coating for fried foods or as a meat
extender. Cornmeal is sometimes used to dust a greased pan, which helps
keep the product from sticking to the pan and gives the crust extra crunch
and a hint of flavor.

Degerminated cornmeal is ground between massive steel rollers. The
fiber and corn germ are separated out, leaving a less nutritious and less
flavorful grain. When you're looking for whole-grain cornmeal, avoid
products that are labeled "degerminated."

Corn flour is more finely ground than cornmeal. Baked goods made
using corn flour have a lighter texture than those made with cornmeal.
Cornbread made with corn flour is richer and less crumbly.

Further Information

- www.momsretro.com/recipe_
  tips-corn.html

Corn flour and cornstarch
are not interchangeable
in recipes.

Millet

Millet grain is not a true grain but is closely related to corn and sorghum.
It is yellow or white, small and round, with a mild, delicate, corn-like
flavor and a texture much like that of brown rice. Millet takes on the
flavor of whatever it is cooked with. It can be used in pilafs or casseroles,
as a stuffing for vegetables or meat, or in Asian dishes that call for rice,
quinoa or buckwheat. We like to add dry millet grain to yeast breads,
biscuits and muffins, for a crunchy texture.

Millet grits are coarsely ground millet grain; **millet meal** is more
finely ground and has a slightly sweet flavor, similar to that of corn.

Millet flour is made from finely ground millet grain. It can be
substituted for rice flour in small amounts in most recipes and adds
a lovely cream color to baked goods. Millet flour is used in flatbreads

or is mixed with other GF flours for baking. It produces light, dry, delicate breads with a thin, buttery, smooth crust. A small amount can be substituted for other GF flours, but results may vary.

Further Information
- www.chetday.com/millet.html

Montina™

Montina is the registered trade name for flour milled from the seed of a native North American grass called Indian rice grass (which is not related to rice, despite its name). In 2001, the Amazing Grains Grower Cooperative of Montana was formed to grow and market Montina. It is now available in almost every state in the U.S., but is not available in Canada.

Forms of Montina
- **Montina Pure Baking Flour Supplement** is 100% Indian rice grass and is used in combination with other GF flours. It is a light brown-gray color and has a nutty but slightly sweet flavor. Substitute Montina Pure Baking Flour Supplement for 15% to 20% of any other GF flour in a recipe.
- **Montina All-Purpose Flour Blend** is a combination of white rice flour, tapioca flour and Montina Pure. Montina All-Purpose Flour Blend can be used cup for cup (mL for mL) to replace any GF flour or wheat flour. It doesn't need to be mixed with another GF flour, but xanthan gum or guar gum must be added. It can be used to make muffins, breads and pancakes and to thicken gravies, soups and stews.

Further Information
- www.amazinggrains.com

Oats

Oat groats, the whole-grain form of oats, are the oat kernel with the hull removed. They look like brown rice: long and thin, with a smooth, shiny surface. Groats have a sweet, nutty taste with a slight hint of pecan flavor. Combine them with other grains, such as rice, cook and serve instead of potatoes or plain rice or in a pilaf.

Rolled oats (oat flakes or oatmeal) result when groats are steamed and then rolled to flatten. Some rolled oats are also roasted to provide more flavor. These large, separate flakes are also called old-fashioned, thick-cut or porridge oats; they take longer to cook than quick-cooking oats (which are cut into smaller pieces to reduce the cooking time), but they also retain more flavor and nutrition. This is what most people think of as "oatmeal."

Rolled oats can be eaten as a hot breakfast cereal, added to muesli, breads and scones, used to thicken soups and stews or added as a filler or extender to meatloaf and casseroles. Popular uses in North America are in cookies and granolas.

Oat flour is made from finely ground groats, which contain much of the bran. Depending on how it is ground, the flour can be almost as nutritious as the whole grain itself (it is heat during grinding that causes nutrient loss). The high oil content provides a sweet, nutty flavor. Oat flour makes baked items moist and more crumbly, but the products stay fresh longer than items baked with wheat flour. Use it in quick breads, yeast breads, cookies and cakes or to thicken soups, stews, sauces and gravies.

> To make your own oat flour, process rolled oats in a blender or food processor until finely ground.

Oat bran is the outer layer of the oat groat, the part of the grain that contains soluble fiber, which is known to lower cholesterol. Light tan in color, it provides a distinctive texture and a rich, nutty flavor. When used in baked goods such as muffins, pancakes, scones, breads and cookies, it increases their fiber content. It can also be added to breakfast cereals or eaten alone as a hot cereal. Breads may be dusted with oat bran before they are baked, to create a flavorful topping. Oat bran can also be used as a meat extender, as a thickener for gravies, sauces and stews, or as a coating (alone or mixed with a dry rub) for meat or fish.

Further Information

- www.creamhillestates.com
- www.glutenfreeoats.com
- www.onlyoats.ca
- www.bobsredmill.com
- www.innvista.com

> The North American celiac organizations have each taken an individual position on the use of oats in the gluten-free diet, but all agree on the need to consult your doctor before adding oats to your diet. Look for oats labeled "pure," "uncontaminated" or "gluten-free."

Quinoa

Quinoa seeds are small and flat, with a pointed oval shape. The color can range from cream or pale yellow to pink, orange, purple and black. Quinoa seeds have a delicate, almost bland flavor. Cooked quinoa has a fluffy consistency and is excellent as a hot cereal, in casseroles, soups and stews or in stir-fries. Serve as the base for salad or tabbouleh. Quinoa can replace rice as a side dish or be cooked in combination with rice as a pilaf. For information on cooking quinoa, see the Techniques Glossary, page 398. As quinoa cooks, the outer germ around each grain twists outward, forming a small white spiraled tail that is attached to the kernel. The grain itself is soft and delicate, while the tail is crunchy; this creates an interesting texture combination and a pleasant crunch.

Quinoa flakes are whole quinoa kernels rolled flat into flakes of $\frac{1}{8}$ to $\frac{1}{4}$ inch (0.25 to 0.5 cm) in diameter. Add quinoa flakes to cookie recipes or use them to replace GF oatmeal or buckwheat flakes in toppings for fruit crisps.

Quinoa flour is finely ground and tan-colored, with a strong, slightly nutty flavor. Because of its strong flavor, use it in small amounts. Baked products made with quinoa flour have a tender, moist crumb and keep well. We enjoy quinoa flour in pancakes, bread, muffins and crackers.

Further Information

- www.quinoa.com
- www.quinoa.net

Rice

Long-grain white rice is refined, with the bran and germ removed, and is milled until white. It is sometimes called "polished white rice." Once cooked, it has a soft, fluffy texture with separate kernels that are four to five times longer than they are wide.

Medium-grain white rice has a shorter, wider kernel (two to three times longer than its width) than long-grain. **Short-grain white rice** has a short, plump, almost round kernel. Both are moister and more tender than long-grain, with a greater tendency to cling together.

Brown rice is the whole, unpolished grain, with the bran and germ intact, and is available in long-, medium- and short-grain. It gets its light brown color, nutty flavor and chewy texture from the bran layers.

Parboiled rice is a convenient "in-between" rice. The rice is soaked and partially steamed in the husk before the outer bran layer is removed, locking in some of the extra nutrients found in brown rice and giving the uncooked rice a slightly amber color. It has a mild, nutty flavor similar to brown rice. Parboiled rice is often sold under the brand names Conditioned™ or "Converted."

Precooked white or brown rice has been completely cooked and dehydrated after milling. It is often sold in "boil in the bag" packages. It is convenient when you're short on time, but is more expensive.

Arborio rice can be medium- or short-grain. The translucent, plump, creamy kernels have an opaque white dot at the center. They have the ability to absorb large quantities of liquid and, when stirred frequently during cooking, develop a creamy texture with a chewy center.

Basmati rice is available in both brown and white. It swells only lengthwise when cooked, resulting in long, thin grains (double the length of regular long-grain rice). It has a pungent odor and a strong flavor similar to roasted nuts. The dry, firm grains stay separate.

> Rinsing rice or cooking it in excess water, then draining, results in a loss of water-soluble vitamins and minerals.

Cooking Rice

Combine rice and liquid in a saucepan and bring to a boil. Reduce heat, cover and simmer for the specified time. After rice begins to simmer, do not remove the cover and peek. Peeking allows the steam to escape and the rice to become too dry. If rice is not quite tender or liquid is not absorbed after the specified cooking time, replace the lid and cook for 2 to 4 minutes longer. Remove from heat and let stand, covered, for 5 to 10 minutes or until all liquid is absorbed. Fluff with a fork.

A serving of cooked rice is considered to be $\frac{1}{2}$ cup (125 mL).

Uncooked rice (1 cup/250 mL)	Liquid*	Cooking time	Yield	Use
White (long-grain)	1¾ to 2 cups (425 to 500 mL)	15 to 20 minutes	3 to 4 cups (750 mL to 1 L)	Casseroles, Asian-style dishes, fried rice, pilafs, rice salads
White (medium- or short-grain)	1½ to 1¾ cups (375 to 425 mL)	15 to 20 minutes	3 cups (750 mL)	Dishes where stickier rice is preferred, such as risotto, sushi or rice pudding
Brown	2 to 2½ cups (500 to 625 mL)	45 to 50 minutes	3 to 4 cups (750 mL to 1 L)	Any rice dish, but especially rice salads and pilafs
Parboiled	2 to 2½ cups (500 to 625 mL)	20 to 25 minutes	3 to 4 cups (750 mL to 1 L)	Any dish that calls for rice
Precooked	Check package directions	Check package directions	Check package directions	
Arborio**	1½ cups (375 mL)	12 to 14 minutes	3 cups (750 mL)	Rice puddings, risottos
Basmati***	2 cups (500 mL)	12 to 14 minutes	2 cups (500 mL)	Indian and Middle Eastern dishes, such as curries and pilafs
Jasmine***	1½ to 2 cups (375 to 500 mL)	12 to 15 minutes	2 cups (500 mL)	Asian dishes, such as stir-fries or red or green curries
Wild rice***	6 cups (1.5 L)	35 minutes uncovered, then 10 minutes covered	3 cups (750 mL)	Dishes containing almonds, hazelnuts, wild mushrooms, oranges and pine nuts

* Liquid can be water, GF stock or reconstituted GF stock powder

** This information applies to steamed rice. If making risotto, extra liquid and time will be required; see individual recipes. Do not rinse Arborio rice before cooking.

*** Rinse basmati, jasmine and wild rice well before cooking.

Jasmine rice is a long-grain white rice. When cooked, its soft, moist kernels cling together. Its fragrance adds an authentic touch to Asian dishes.

Wild rice is not actually rice at all but a marsh grass seed with long, shiny black or dark brown grains. Because of its rich, roasted, smoky, nutty flavor and chewy texture, it complements wild game, poultry and berries.

Further Information

- www.daintyrice.ca
- www.usarice.com
- www.purcellmountainfarms.com
- www.sunrice.com
- www.wildfoods.ca

Rice Flours

Brown rice flour is milled from the whole grain. It has a grainy texture and provides more fiber and nutrients than white rice flour. It is only a shade darker than white rice flour and has a mild, nutty flavor. Brown rice flour results in a product with a grainy texture and a fine, dry crumb. Use it in recipes calling for rice flour.

Rice bran and **rice polish** are the two outer parts of the rice kernel, removed during milling for white rice flour. Rice bran is the outermost layer. When bran and polish are added in small amounts to recipes, the fiber content is increased. They are interchangeable in recipes.

Sweet rice flour (glutinous rice flour, mochiko flour, sticky rice flour, mochi flour, sushi rice flour) is made from short-grain rice. It contains more starch than brown or white rice flour. There are two grades: one is beige, grainy and sandy-textured; the other is white, starchy, sticky and less expensive. The latter works better in recipes. It is often used to bread foods before frying or to thicken Asian dishes. We use it to dust baking pans or our fingers for easier handling of sticky dough.

Wild rice flour is gray-brown to black and has a nutty flavor and an interesting texture. It can be added to pancakes, muffins, scones and cookies or used to thicken casseroles, sauces, gravies and stews. Try it in fish, chicken and tempura batters.

Further Information

- www.bobsredmill.com
- www.wildfoods.ca

Sorghum

Sorghum grains (also known as milo) are white ovals smaller than peppercorns, with a hearty, chewy texture and a slightly sweet, nutty, earthy taste. They can be extruded, steam-flaked, popped, or puffed and micronized. Sorghum grains are used to make porridges, tortillas and rice substitute. They can be used in place of barley in soups. They are also sold popped, just like popcorn.

> Sorghum should not be used as a sprouting grain, as the young shoots are very poisonous.

Sorghum flour ranges in color from a gray-tan to eggshell white, and the grinds vary from coarse (stone-ground) to very fine. Because its flavor is neutral, it absorbs other flavors well. The most wheat-like of all GF flours, it is the best general-purpose flour, giving baked items a warm, creamy color. Sorghum flour adds protein to home-baked goods such as scones, cakes, cookies, breads, muffins, pizza dough, waffles, cereals, energy bars, salty snack foods, pastas and chapati (an unleavened Indian flatbread).

> The protein and starch in sorghum endosperm are more slowly digested than those in other grains, making it beneficial for people with diabetes. Some sorghum varieties are so rich in antioxidants, which protect against cell damage, that they are comparable to blueberries (known for their high antioxidant levels).

Other sorghum products include: puffed sorghum (used in snacks, granola, cereals, granola bars, baked products and dry snack cakes, and added to soups as a GF substitute for couscous, bulgur and pearled barley); cracked sorghum (used in legume and/or vegetable mixtures); sorghum syrup, a molasses-like sweetener that is not as popular today as it once was; sorghum grits, which are similar in texture to cream of wheat porridge; and sorghum beer.

> Rather than using a standard mix of flours in our recipes, we like to vary the proportions of flours and starches so that each recipe has a unique flavor and texture. We love the results we get when we use a mixture of sorghum flour and bean flour with strong flavors such as pumpkin, chocolate, molasses, dates and rhubarb.

Further Information

- www.csaceliacs.org
- www.innvista.com
- www.recipetips.com
- www.sorghumgrowers.com

Teff

Teff grain is the smallest grain in the world, tinier than a poppy seed and only twice the size of the period at the end of this sentence. The seeds can be white, ivory or brown. Brown teff has a subtle hazelnut, almost chocolate-like flavor; white teff has a chestnut-like flavor; ivory teff has a mild, slightly molasses-like sweetness and nutty taste. The darker varieties are earthier-tasting. The grain can be sprouted to use in salads and sandwiches. Raw teff grain can substitute for some of the seeds, nuts or other small grains in recipes. Due to its small size, use only ½ cup (125 mL) of teff to replace 1 cup (250 mL) of sesame seeds. Teff grain is a good thickener for soups, stews and gravies.

Use teff grain in stir-fry dishes and casseroles and to make grain burgers. Cook it to make breakfast porridge, a polenta-like side dish, stuffing or pilaf. It can be cooked alone or in combination with other grains and vegetables. It combines well with brown rice, millet, kasha (toasted buckwheat groats) and cornmeal. Cooked teff can be seasoned with cinnamon, ginger, garlic, cardamom, chiles, basil or cilantro. Ethiopians use teff as the main ingredient in their staple bread, injera.

> Due to a low glycemic index, teff is digested slowly, which makes it beneficial for diabetics and athletes.

> A hundred and fifty teff seeds weigh as much as one kernel of wheat; seven grains will fit onto the head of a pin.

Teff flour milled from brown teff has a sweet, nutty flavor, while flour from white teff is milder. Teff flour has excellent baking qualities. Use it in breads, quick breads, pancakes, waffles, pie crusts, gingerbread, crackers and cookies. Teff flour is also a good thickener for soups, sauces, stews, gravies and puddings.

Further Information

- www.hort.purdue.edu/newcrop/cropfactsheets/teff.html
- www.innvista.com
- www.recipetips.com
- www.teffco.com

> Like rice, teff cooks quickly. Cook it just long enough to open the grain. For extra flavor, toast the grains first.

Storing Whole Grains and Whole-Grain Flours

Whole grain or whole-grain flour	Room temperature*	Refrigerator	Freezer	Additional information
Amaranth seeds	1 month	6 months	1 year	Refrigerate cooked seeds for up to 3 days or freeze for up to 6 months.
Amaranth flour		6 months	1 year	
Buckwheat groats	1 year			
Kasha		6 months	1 year	
Buckwheat flakes	2 years			
Buckwheat flour		2 months	6 months	
Cornmeal/corn flour	1 month	6 months	1 year	
Degerminated cornmeal	6 months			
Millet grain, grits, meal and flour		6 months	1 year	
Montina™	2 years			
Oat groats and rolled oats	2 months		6 months	
Oat flour	3 months		6 months	
Oat bran		6 months	1 year	
Quinoa seeds	1 month	6 months	1 year	Refrigerate cooked quinoa for up to 3 days or freeze for up to 6 months.
Quinoa flakes	2 months			
Quinoa flour		6 months	1 year	
White rice	2 years			Refrigerate cooked rice for up to 7 days or freeze for up to 6 months.
Brown rice**		6 months		Refrigerate cooked rice for up to 7 days or freeze for up to 6 months.
Rice flours	1 year		1 year	
Rice bran and rice polish		6 months	1 year	
Sorghum grains and flour	1 month	6 months	1 year	
Teff grain and flour	1 month	6 months	1 year	Refrigerate cooked teff grain for up to 3 days or freeze for up to 6 months.

* All gluten-free grains and flours should be stored in airtight containers in a cool, dry, dark place.

** The bran layers in brown rice contain oil that could become rancid; thus, brown rice must be refrigerated.

How Much Should I Eat?

The U.S. Department of Agriculture's MyPyramid (www.mypyramid.gov), revised in 2005, recommends that adults eat a total of 6 ounce (175 g) equivalents of grains a day (based on a 2,000-calorie diet). At least 3 ounces (90 g) of this should include whole-grain cereals, breads, crackers, rice or pasta. One ounce (30 g) equals 1 slice of bread, 1 cup (250 mL) of breakfast cereal or ½ cup (125 mL) of cooked rice, cereal or pasta, all of which can be considered one ounce (30 g) equivalent.

Canada's Food Guide (www.hc-sc.gc.ca), revised in 2007, recommends that children and adults eat 3 to 8 servings from the grain products group each day. The recommended number of servings depends on age and sex. For example, females between 19 and 50 should eat 6 to 7 servings; males in the same age range should eat 8 servings. Of these servings, health experts suggest that at least half should be whole-grain products, especially those low in fat, sugar and salt. One serving is 1 slice of bread, 1 ounce (30 g) of cold cereal, ¾ cup (175 mL) of hot cereal or ½ cup (125 mL) of pasta or rice.

Suggestions for Including Whole Grains in a GF Diet

- Eat a variety of whole grains, such as teff, brown rice, quinoa, wild rice and pure, uncontaminated oats.
- Bake whole-grain breads using a combination of whole grains.
- Choose whole-grain flours to bake muffins, breads and desserts.
- Add whole grains such as millet grain and amaranth seeds to whole-grain flours when preparing baked goods.
- Use whole grains to prepare your own granola or snacks.
- Prepare pilafs, stir-fries, salads and stuffings with wild rice, brown rice, quinoa and oat groats, or a combination of these.
- Buy GF cereals made from whole grains. The first ingredient listed should be a whole grain such as oats, amaranth, brown rice, wild rice or quinoa.
- Select GF pasta made from whole grains, including quinoa or wild rice. Some GF pastas are enriched with nutrients lost during processing.
- Look for a label that states "100% whole grain," not just "whole grain" — the latter may contain only a small proportion of whole grains.
- Get in the habit of reading the Nutrition Facts table, as well as ingredient lists, to become familiar with the amounts of nutrients in specific products.

Other Gluten-Free Baking Ingredients

Fats

Fats are either saturated or unsaturated.

Saturated fats are solid at room temperature. They come mainly from animal sources and include butter, cheese, whole milk, cream, ice cream, egg yolks, lard, suet, drippings and fatty meats. Some plant fats, such as coconut oil, palm oil and other tropical oils, are also high in saturated fat; these are semisolid at room temperature.

> Cholesterol is made in our bodies, but we also get it from meat, poultry, seafood, eggs, dairy, lard and butter.

Unsaturated fats come mainly from vegetable sources and are liquid at room temperature. There are two types: monounsaturated and polyunsaturated.

- **Monounsaturated fats** are found in fruit, seed and nut oils, including avocado, olive, sesame seed, peanut and canola oils. They can start to solidify in the refrigerator, but become liquid again at room temperature.

- **Polyunsaturated fats** are found in vegetable, seed and nut oils, including corn, sunflower, safflower, soybean, cottonseed and sesame seed oils. Omega-3 and omega-6 fatty acids are also polyunsaturated fats. Natural sources of omega-3 fats include seafood and certain plants (see box, below). Omega-6 fats are found in vegetable oils.

> - Fish, including salmon, mackerel, albacore tuna, sardines, rainbow trout, herring and anchovies, are particularly good sources of omega-3 fatty acids.
> - Plant sources of omega-3s include flaxseed, flax oil and walnut oil. Small amounts are found in canola and soybean oil and some soft, non-hydrogenated margarine.
> - Many foods, including some eggs, milk, bread and soy beverages, are now enriched with omega-3 fats.

Trans fats are produced during hydrogenation, which is the process that adds hydrogen to liquid oils, changing them into solid fats such as shortening or margarine. In the process, any health benefits the oils may have had are destroyed, and trans fats behave like saturated fats in the body. Soft margarine sold in tubs has some hydrogen added to the oil and is "partially hydrogenated"; solid or stick margarine has more added and is a fully hydrogenated product. In addition, many fast foods and processed foods have a high trans fat content.

> "Smoke point" is the temperature at which a heated oil or fat begins to smoke.

For health reasons, the majority of your fat intake should be from monounsaturated oils and soft, non-hydrogenated margarines. Wherever you can in cooking and baking, use vegetable oils or soft margarine instead of butter, lard, shortening or hard margarine.

Flaxseed

Whole flaxseed (also known as linseed) refers to the unbroken seed. The seeds are small, flat and tear-shaped. They range in color from dark reddish-brown to golden and have a nutty flavor and a crisp, yet chewy texture.

Cracked flaxseed is not sold in stores but can be prepared at home: use a coffee grinder to crack the outer coating of the seed slightly, resulting in pieces of different sizes and textures. Cracked flaxseed is easier to digest than whole flaxseed. For extra crunch, add slightly cracked flaxseed to yeast breads and quick breads or sprinkle it on salads and hot or cold cereals. Add just before serving, as it becomes sticky.

Ground flaxseed is sold as flax flour, milled flaxseed or sprouted flax flour. All forms of ground flaxseed are interchangeable in recipes. You can prepare your own by grinding whole flaxseed to a gold to medium brown powder with slightly darker flecks. Replace up to $\frac{1}{3}$ cup (75 mL) of vegetable oil in recipes with 1 cup (250 mL) of ground flaxseed. You can add up to 1 tbsp (15 mL) ground flaxseed to the batter for cookies, cakes or pancakes without decreasing the other flours or starches. If you add more, the amount of liquid and other flours may have to be adjusted.

> Use a coffee grinder or food processor to crack or grind whole flaxseed to the consistency you want for your recipe. For optimum freshness, grind it as you need it. Refrigerate any extra.

Further Information

- www.flaxcouncil.ca
- www.flaxflour.com
- www.saskflax.com

> Ground Salba can be substituted for ground flaxseed. Grind Salba seeds even finer than flaxseed, or the product might be slightly gritty.

Legume Flours

Legumes (also called pulses) include peas, beans, lentils and peanuts. Besides using dried legumes in our recipes, we also use their flours.

- **Fava bean flour** is made from earthy-flavored fava beans.
- **Chickpea flour** (garbanzo bean flour, gram, besan, chana dal) has a mild, nut-like taste, with a hint of lemon. It adds a rich, sweet flavor to baked foods. It is used in East Indian cuisine and to thicken soups and gravies.

> Legume flours combine well with other GF flours.

- **Garfava flour** (sold as garbanzo-fava bean flour in Canada) is a blend of garbanzo bean (chickpea) flour and fava bean flour. It has a nutty taste.
- **Whole bean flour** is made from Romano beans (also called cranberry beans or speckled sugar beans). The dried beans are cooked (heat-treated, micronized) to help reduce flatulence, then stone-ground to a uniform, fine, dark, strong-tasting flour. When one of our recipes calls for whole bean flour, use this one; however, if it's not available, any bean or pea flour can be substituted.
- **White (navy) bean flour** is made from small, white round or oval beans. The white flour has a mild flavor and a powdery texture. Use it to thicken sauces, gravies and soups.

> All legume flours are a shade of yellow and have a very fine texture. They complement recipes made with molasses, brown sugar, chocolate, pumpkin, applesauce and rhubarb.

- **Pinto bean flour** has a slightly pink tinge, although the pinto beans it is made from have a spotty beige and brown color.
- **Pea flours** are produced from dried field peas with the bran (hull) removed. Green pea flour has a sweeter flavor than yellow pea flour. Pea flours keep baked products softer longer and improve dough made in a bread machine. They can be used as a natural colorant in baked goods, homemade noodles and other foods. Pea flours complement recipes made with banana, peanut butter and strong spices such as cloves.
- **Pea fiber**, ground from yellow pea hulls, is a fine-textured, light-yellow-colored, bland-tasting powder. It increases the volume of doughs and can replace fat in a recipe because of its ability to bind with water. It is a source of insoluble dietary fiber and increases the fiber content of products made with it. Use it in breads, cakes, cookies, tortillas, pasta, soups and fiber drinks.

> All types of bean flours (except soy flour) can be used interchangeably with pea flours in our recipes.

- **Soy flour** (soya flour), made from soybeans, is powdery fine, with a pungent, nutty, slightly bitter flavor that is enhanced by the flavors of accompanying flours. Soy flour is available in full-fat (natural), low-fat and defatted versions. The higher the fat content, the deeper the color. Full-fat soy flour contains the natural oils found in the soybean; defatted soy flour has had the oils removed during processing. Soy flour has a strong odor when wet that disappears with baking.

  Soy is one of the top 10 allergens in Canada and one of the top 8 in the U.S.

  It adds rich color, fine texture, a pleasant nutty flavor, tenderness and moistness to baked goods. Products containing soy flour bake faster and tend to brown quickly, so the baking time may need to be shortened or the oven temperature lowered. Tenting baked goods with foil partway through the baking time also helps.

  Soy flour can also be used to thicken sauces and gravies, to add a nutty flavor and extra protein to pancake batter and to enrich pasta and breakfast cereals. Added to fried foods such as donuts, soy flour reduces the amount of fat absorbed by the dough.

  Studies have shown that 15% of celiacs cannot tolerate soybeans or soy products.

Further Information
- www.farmbuilt.com
- www.foodprocessing.com
- www.thumboilseed.com/soy-flour.htm
- www.soyfoods.org
- www.bestcookingpulses.com

Nut Flours and Meals

Nut flours and meals are made from very finely ground nuts such as almonds, hazelnuts and pecans. They are not as smooth or as fine as grain flours. Nut flours can be purchased, or you can grind them yourself (see the Techniques Glossary, page 398). Grind the nuts when you're ready to prepare the recipe. We like to toast them first, for a nuttier flavor (see page 398). Toasting also dries nut flour, helping to prevent clumping.

- **Almond flour**, or **meal**, is made from blanched almonds and is creamy white. Sugar or flour is sometimes added during grinding to absorb the oil from the almonds and prevent clumping, so check purchased almond flour to be sure it is gluten-free. Combine almond flour with rice flour or amaranth flour when a white, delicate-flavored product is desired.

- **Hazelnut flour** is a creamy color with dark brown to black flecks. It has a full, rich flavor that is sweet and nutty. We enjoy it in pastry and anything with orange or chocolate.

- **Pecan meal** is a warm brown, similar in color to ground flaxseed. It complements recipes made with maple, pumpkin and dried fruits such apricots and dates.

> Nut meals and flours are interchangeable in recipes.

Further Information
- www.bluediamond.com
- www.diamondnuts.com

Starches

Starches, which are complex carbohydrates, have two purposes in gluten-free cooking: to lighten baked products and to thicken liquids for sauces or gravies.

Baking with Starches

- **Arrowroot** (arrowroot starch, arrowroot powder, arrowroot starch flour) is a fine, white, tasteless starchy powder with a mild aroma. Arrowroot is more expensive and may be more difficult to find than other starches. When mixed with GF flours to make breads, cookies and pastries, arrowroot helps the baked goods bind better and lightens the finished product.
- **Cornstarch** (corn flour, maize, *crème de maïs*) is a fine, silky, white, tasteless starchy powder. When mixed with GF flours to make breads, cookies and pastries, cornstarch helps the baked goods bind better and lightens the finished product.
- **Potato flour** is made from the whole potato, including the skin. Because it has been cooked, it absorbs large amounts of water. Potato flour is much denser and heavier than potato starch and has a definite potato flavor. Potato flour is not used like other flours in baking as it would absorb too much liquid and make the product gummy, but small amounts can be used in breads, puddings and cakes to hold the product together. We rarely use potato flour (with the exception of our Banana Raisin Sticky Buns, page 362), but we frequently use potato starch.

> Potato starch is often confused with potato flour, but one cannot be substituted for the other.

- **Potato starch** (potato starch flour) is made from only the starch of potatoes, and is therefore less expensive than potato flour. It is a very fine, silky, white powder with a bland taste. It lumps easily and must be sifted frequently. When combined with other GF flours, it

> A permitted ingredient for Passover (unlike cornstarch and other grain-based foods), potato starch is often found with kosher products in supermarkets

adds moistness to baked goods and gives them a light and airy texture. It also causes breads to rise higher.

- **Tapioca starch** (tapioca flour, tapioca starch flour, cassava flour, yucca starch, manioc, manihot or *almidon de yucca*) is powdery fine, white and mildly sweet. Tapioca starch lightens baked goods and gives them a slightly sweet, chewy texture.

Thickening with Starches

All starches can be used to thicken soups, gravies, sauces, stews and meat dishes.

- **Arrowroot** thickens liquids almost immediately at a lower temperature than either cornstarch or wheat flour, which means it's less likely to burn, but it loses its thickening ability if it's boiled even a little bit too long, so always add it at the end of the cooking process. Due to its greater thickening ability, use only half as much arrowroot as wheat flour. Its consistency does not hold as long after cooking. Use arrowroot as a thickener for acidic liquids such as Chinese dishes, stir-fries, clear glazes for fruit pies and clear fruit sauces. It should not be used to thicken dairy-based sauces, as it turns them slimy.

  > Sauces thickened with arrowroot can be frozen and defrosted.

- **Cornstarch** doesn't thicken well when mixed with acidic liquids such as lemon juice. Use cornstarch to thicken cream fillings, custards and puddings and in clear glazes for fruit pies and clear fruit sauces. To avoid lumps, cornstarch must be dissolved in an equal amount of cold water before it is added to hot liquids. (Mixing it with a granular solid, such as granulated sugar, also disperses it into a liquid.) Cornstarch has twice the thickening power of wheat flour. It helps prevent eggs from curdling in custards and causes heat to be transmitted more evenly throughout. Sauces made with cornstarch turn spongy when frozen.

- **Potato flour** mixes well in cold water, cooks quickly without lumps and turns transparent after heating. Potato flour is always used in very small quantities. It thickens quickly when heated with water, and at a lower temperature than cornstarch, so it can be added to sauces at the last minute.

- **Potato starch** should be mixed with twice the amount of cold water before it is added to hot liquids, for the best thickening results. Liquids thickened with potato starch should never be boiled, or the thickening ability will be lost. Sauce thickened using potato starch becomes watery again when cooled.

- **Tapioca starch** gives a transparent high gloss to fruits and makes a perfectly smooth filling. It's the perfect product to use with high-acid fruits. In addition to sauces, it is used to thicken glazes, puddings, custards and juicy fruit pie fillings.

  > If you plan to freeze a dish, use tapioca starch, as it remains stable when frozen.

Further Information

- www.glutenfreemall.com
- www.recipetips.com
- www.foodsubs.com
- www.jodelibakery.netfirms.com

Sugars

Most sugar is made from either sugarcane or sugar beets and varies in color, flavor, sweetness and crystal size (coarse, medium, fine, extra-fine, superfine). It can be either refined or raw.

> In this book, recipes labeled "white sugar–free" contain no white (granulated) sugar as an added ingredient but may contain another type of sugar, including brown sugar, honey, molasses, corn syrup or maple syrup. And some of the ingredients we call for, such as dried cranberries, may contain white sugar added during processing. There is much discussion about the type of sugar we use today. Nutritionally, the important point is not the kind of sugar but the quantity we consume. Excess sugar is the problem.

White (Granulated) Sugar

White (granulated) sugar is highly refined and is sold in various crystal sizes:

- **Coarse sanding sugar** has large crystals that sparkle when light is reflected through them. It is used to decorate cookies and other desserts.
- The most common size is sold as white sugar or granulated sugar; it's what we often simply call sugar. The finer grades are made by sieving white sugar.
- **Fruit sugar** is slightly finer than regular white sugar. It is used in gelatin, pudding and powdered drink mixes.
- **Superfine sugar** (also known as bar sugar, berry sugar in B.C. and castor sugar in Britain) is finer than granulated sugar but not as fine as confectioner's sugar. The tiny crystals dissolve instantly and completely. It is used to make caramel, fine-textured cakes, drinks and meringues.
- **Confectioner's sugar** (also called icing sugar, powdered sugar and fondant) is simply white sugar that has been ground to a fine powder, then sifted. It usually contains 3% cornstarch as an anticaking agent, to prevent clumping. It is used in icings, confections and whipped cream. Canadian icing sugar may contain wheat starch, so check the label. Always sift confectioner's sugar just before using.

> White sugar (granulated sugar) is dried to prevent clumping.

Brown Sugar

Brown sugar (brilliant yellow, golden yellow, light yellow, yellow, dark brown) is from late stages of refining. The crystals are brown and fine and contain moisture and varying amounts of molasses. The darker the color, the higher the molasses content, the stronger the flavor and the higher the moisture. Light brown sugar is used for baking and to make butterscotch, condiments and glazes. Dark brown sugar is used to make gingerbread, mincemeat and baked beans.

> Brown sugar should be stored in an airtight container so it doesn't lose moisture and become hard. If it does harden, put a slice of bread, a piece of apple or a damp paper towel in the container to provide moisture until the sugar softens.
>
> If you need to use hardened brown sugar immediately, heat the required amount in a 250°F (120°C) oven for a few minutes, or microwave it on Low (10%) for 1 to 2 minutes per cup (250 mL).

Raw Sugars

Raw sugars are the products of the first stage of the sugarcane refining process. There are slight differences among them.

- **Demerara sugar** has large crystals that are light to golden brown in color. It is very moist and adds a crunchy texture when sprinkled on hot and cold cereals, cakes, cookies, fruit and desserts. It is also used as a sweetener for tea or coffee.
- **Muscovado sugar** (Barbados sugar) is coarser and moister than regular brown sugar. It ranges in color from light to very dark brown, and has a strong molasses flavor.
- **Turbinado sugar** (plantation sugar) is a specialty raw brown sugar that has been steam-cleaned. It has a mild caramel flavor and is golden in color. It is used to sweeten tea and other beverages.

Liquid Sugars

- **Molasses** is a by-product of the sugarcane and sugar beet refining process. In the United States, molasses is sold in three varieties: light, dark and blackstrap. In Canada, the varieties are called fancy molasses, cooking molasses and blackstrap molasses. Light (fancy) molasses is, as you would expect, the lightest in both color and flavor; it is used in baked goods and main dishes. Cooking (dark) molasses is a combination of light and blackstrap; it is used in dishes where a more pronounced molasses flavor is desired. Blackstrap molasses is very dark and bitter, but it contains minerals, vitamins and trace elements lost in the refining of the other grades; it is used in baked goods.

- **Treacle,** most commonly used in the U.K., is a syrup made during the refining of sugarcane. There are two kinds: light treacle (also called golden syrup) and dark treacle. Dark treacle is similar to molasses, while light treacle has a lighter flavor.

- **Corn syrup** is made from cornstarch. It keeps foods moist and prevents them from spoiling quickly. It is common for corn syrup to be flavored with vanilla extract. You will find corn syrup in numerous commercial products and in home-baked items such as frosting and fudge.

- **High-fructose corn syrup (HCFS)** is manufactured from cornstarch. It has a higher sugar content than white (granulated) sugar and is an ingredient in most processed foods, including soft drinks, cereals, ketchup, crackers and many more. It is used to improve taste and keep foods and beverages fresher longer.

- **Maple syrup** is made by boiling the sap of the sugar maple tree to concentrate the flavor. Forty gallons (150 L) of sap yield 1 gallon (4 L) of maple syrup. If made properly, it never freezes because of its low moisture and high sugar content. It can be stored in the refrigerator for up to 2 months or in the freezer for up to 1 year. If it crystallizes, heat it gently by standing the container in a bowl of warm water until the crystals dissolve, or microwave it on High for 90 seconds per cup (250 mL).

- **Honey** is a natural sugar made by bees. The flavor depends on the variety of flower it is made from; common flavors include clover, orange blossom and lavender. The color indicates the strength of flavor and ranges from near white to deep golden yellow to deep brown or black. The texture ranges from thin to heavy. Honey has a natural emulsifying quality, so it is a good addition to oil-and-vinegar salad dressings.

  Honey can trigger allergic reactions in some individuals. Children under 12 months of age should not eat honey because of a rare but serious risk of botulism.

  Store honey in a cool location, away from direct sunlight, in a tightly covered container. It will last indefinitely. If cloudiness develops and hard crystals form over time, simply warm the honey gently by placing the jar in a pan of hot water and stirring the honey. If honey is overheated, the sugars will caramelize and the flavor and color may change.

  Before measuring honey, coat the measuring cup with vegetable spray — the honey will flow more easily and rapidly.

Xanthan Gum

Xanthan gum is a natural carbohydrate produced from the fermentation of glucose. It helps prevent baked goods from crumbling, gives them greater volume, improves their texture and extends their shelf life. It also helps prevent pastry fillings from "weeping," so your crust won't get soggy. Do not omit xanthan gum from a recipe.

Xanthan gum can be purchased at health food stores, online or where you purchase other gluten-free ingredients. Before working with xanthan gum, be sure to wipe counters and containers with a dry cloth; when it comes in contact with water, it becomes slippery, slimy and almost impossible to wipe up.

Guar gum is gluten-free, but it may act as a laxative in some people. It can be substituted for xanthan gum in equal proportions.

Storing Other Gluten-Free Baking Ingredients

Ingredient	Room temperature*	Refrigerator	Freezer	Additional information
Baking powder and baking soda	6 months			
Flaxseed, whole	1 year			
Flaxseed, cracked or ground		6 months	1 year	For optimum freshness, grind only as needed.
Hemp seeds, hulled		Once open, use within 1 year		Purchase hemp seeds and hemp seed flour only from stores that sell refrigerated products.
Legumes, canned	5 years			
Legumes, dried	1 year			
Legumes, cooked		Lentils and split peas: 4 days Beans: 5 days	6 months	
Legume flours		6 months	1 year	
Nut flours and meals**		3 months	1 year	Store away from foods with strong odors, such as fish and onions.
Nuts, unshelled**	6 months		1 year	
Salba seeds		6 months		Prepare ground Salba and Salba gel as needed.
Seeds (pumpkin, poppy, sesame and sunflower)**		6 months	1 year	
Soybeans, dried	1 year			
Soy flour, full-fat		6 months	1 year	
Soy flour, defatted	1 year			
Starches	Indefinitely			
Xanthan gum and guar gum	6 months		Indefinitely	
Yeast (instant and bread machine)	2 months		12 months	Open before expiry date.

* All gluten-free baking ingredients should be stored in airtight containers in a cool, dry, dark place.
** Because of their high oil content, seeds, nuts and nut flours tend to become rancid quickly. Purchase in small quantities and taste before using.

Nutrient Content of Gluten-Free Flours and Starches

Gluten-free flour (per 1 cup/250 mL)	Protein (g)	Fat (g)	Carbohydrates (g)	Fiber (g)	Calcium (mg)	Iron (mg)
Whole-grain flours						
Amaranth flour	17	8	80	18	51	9
Brown rice flour	11	4	124	7	17	3
Oat flour	21	9	78	12	50	7
Quinoa flour	13	8	84	6	61	9
Sorghum flour	12	4	88	8	35	6
Teff flour	16	4	88	16	201	7
Other flours and starches						
Almond flour	24	56	24	12	750	5
Cornstarch	0	0	117	1	3	1
Flax flour	24	45	38	36	332	8
Garfava flour	35	6	72	12	104	8
Soy flour (low-fat)	47	6	38	18	241	9

Sources: USDA, Case Nutrition Consulting Inc., Bob's Red Mill, Nu-World Amaranth, Northern Quinoa Corp., Twin Valley Mills and Nutrition Data.

Protein helps us maintain and repair body tissues. Complete proteins (meat, fish, poultry, milk and milk products and eggs) provide all the amino acids necessary for a healthy body; incomplete proteins (grains, legumes, vegetables) lack some of the essential amino acids. However, the body has the ability to use amino acids from a variety of sources to form complete proteins. Here are some suggested combinations: beans and rice, cereals and milk, nuts and grains; whole-grain breads and legumes. All grains are not created equal: some contain more and higher levels of essential amino acids than others. It is therefore important to bake with a variety of nutritious grains.

Fat provides the essential fatty acids that the body cannot produce. It protects the organs and muscles with padding and insulation. Although fats are necessary for a healthy diet, they have two and a half times as many calories per gram as protein and carbohydrates, so the amount of fat consumed should be controlled.

Carbohydrates are the primary source of energy for the body. They provide fuel as the body breaks down complex carbohydrates into simple sugars.

Fiber is found only in plants and plays a significant role in keeping us healthy. Insoluble fiber aids in digestion, while soluble fiber can lower cholesterol. Sources of insoluble fiber include rice bran, brown rice, almond meal and legumes. Sources of soluble fiber include flaxseed and pears. Oat bran, whole-grain oats and soybeans contain both types. When increasing fiber in the diet, do so gradually.

Calcium helps the body build strong bones and teeth. It is also required for blood clotting and nerve and muscle function.

Iron is necessary for the formation of hemoglobin in red blood cells. It also helps the immune system function.

Current Changes in Product Labeling

Over the past few years, there have been many much-needed changes in allergen labels on products. This has been of enormous assistance to celiacs and others concerned about food allergies and intolerances. Much more is happening, so keep an eye out for updates.

United States

In 2006, the Food Allergen Labeling and Consumer Protection Act (FALCPA) took effect. Today, packaged food bound for U.S. sales has to identify which (if any) of the top eight food allergens — milk, eggs, fish, shellfish, tree nuts, peanuts, wheat and soybeans — are contained in the ingredients. U.S. law also identifies as a major food allergen any ingredient that contains protein derived from any of these eight foods.

The U.S. has thereby dealt with whole ingredients, but what about cross-contamination in manufacturing? What about processes that may cause a little bit of those top eight allergens to make their way into a product? This may not be a concern for some, but it's a huge issue for those who are highly sensitive.

Further Information
- www.fns.usda.gov/fdd/facts/nutrition/foodallergenfactsheet.pdf
- www.fda.gov/Food/LabelingNutrition/FoodAllergensLabeling/ GuidanceComplianceRegulatoryInformation/ucm106890.htm

Canada

In Canada, the Food and Drug Regulations (FDR) currently require that a complete and accurate list of ingredients appear on the label of most prepackaged foods. However, certain components of ingredients are exempt from mandatory declaration at this time. For example, when flavorings, flour, seasonings and margarine are used as ingredients in other foods included in the product, these components do not need to be specified. As a result, a prepackaged food product may be unsafe for consumers with food allergies if some of the component ingredients not declared on the label are priority food allergens, gluten sources or added sulphites.

Health Canada, the Canadian Food Inspection Agency (CFIA), allergy associations and the medical community have identified those substances most frequently associated with food allergies and allergic-like reactions. These priority allergens must be listed in plain English and/or French (e.g., "milk" instead of "casein") on packaging, and the components of ingredients will have to be specified if they are priority allergens.

The following foods, and proteins derived from these foods, are considered priority food allergens: tree nuts, peanuts, sesame seeds, wheat and gluten, eggs, milk, soybeans, shellfish, fish and added sulphites (over 10 ppm).

Manufacturers will have to declare food allergens, gluten sources and added sulphites by name at the end of the list of ingredients in a statement called Allergy and Intolerance Information, even if the allergens and gluten sources have already been declared in the ingredients list.

Health Canada is publishing its proposed food allergen labeling regulatory amendments in *Canada Gazette, Part I*. Once the final regulations are published in *Canada Gazette, Part II*, manufacturers and importers will have one year to adopt the new labeling changes. It could be early 2011 before the regulations are in place.

Further Information

- www.hc-sc.gc.ca/fn-an/label-etiquet/allergen/index-eng.php
- www.inspection.gc.ca/english/fssa/labeti/alerg/allerge.shtml

---

Under the proposed regulations, the gluten source will need to be declared when a food contains gluten protein or modified gluten protein from barley, oats, rye, triticale or wheat, including kamut or spelt.

Dairy-Free, Lactose-Free, Egg-Free

Dairy-Free Recipes

Many children with autism spectrum have been known to do better on a gluten-free, casein-free diet (casein is the milk protein in dairy products). We have therefore included many dairy-free recipes in this book.

We have identified recipes that are dairy-free by the label "dairy-free" near the recipe title.

Dairy products are defined as those containing milk or milk proteins, including butter, cheese, cream cheese, sour cream, yogurt, cream and ice cream, as well as products with ingredients such as whey, lactose, casein or caseinate (note that this is not a complete list). Hidden sources include many processed foods.

Remember that dairy products are the main source of calcium in the diet; do not eliminate them unless you have a medical need to do so.

Further Information
- www.godairyfree.org
- www.autismcanada.org/glutensugar.htm

Lactose Intolerance

The inability to digest lactose is called lactose intolerance or lactase deficiency. Lactose is a natural sugar found in milk and milk products. Lactase, an enzyme made within the digestive tract, is needed to digest lactose into two simpler sugars the body can use. When not enough lactase is made, lactose is not broken down and abdominal pain, bloating and diarrhea result. The symptoms vary among individuals.

We have identified recipes that are lactose-free by the label "lactose-free" near the recipe title.

Sources of Lactose

Lactose is found in cow's milk and goat's milk — whether non-fat or whole, in liquid or in powdered form — and products made from milk, including cottage cheese, cream, yogurt, buttermilk, butter, sour cream and ice cream.

Hidden sources may include sausages and wieners, commercial baking mixes, snacks and cookies, and other commercially prepared products. Lactose itself is not listed on food labels, but look for lactic acid, lactalbumin, lactate, calcium compounds or casein.

A Lactose-Free Diet

All milk products do not contain the same amount of lactose. The processes that turn milk into yogurt and hard cheese (including Parmesan, mozzarella, Swiss and aged Cheddar) lower the lactose level, and these items may be digestible even for those with lactose intolerance. Look for yogurt containing an active or live culture.

> Parve foods do not contain dairy products. Other kosher products may or may not have dairy in them — read the label.

Lactose-Free Milk Substitutes

- **Soy beverage** (fortified soy beverage, soy milk) has a sweet, nutty flavor and is more easily digested than cow's milk but should not be used as a substitute for infant formulas. Fresh soy beverage is sold plain and flavored and in full-fat, reduced-fat and fat-free forms. Keep it refrigerated in its original container and use before the best-before date. It needs to be shaken well every time it is used, as it settles. Soy beverage sold in an aseptic (shelf-stable) package can be kept at room temperature for up to 1 year; after opening, it needs to be refrigerated and should be used within 1 week. Freezing is not recommend (it can be frozen, but upon defrosting it tends to separate).

  Because of soy beverage's bland flavor, baked goods made with it may need more seasonings. Soy beverage can be used to replace milk cup for cup (mL for mL) in milkshakes, puddings, soups and creamy sauces. Use soy beverage instead of evaporated milk to make lower-fat custards, cream sauces and pumpkin pies.

  Soy beverage is a good source of protein and, unlike cow's milk, contains fiber, is low in saturated fat and is cholesterol-free. It is a good source of isoflavones (though not as good a source as soybeans themselves or tofu). Since eliminating milk and milk products from the diet also eliminates a major source of calcium, look for a soy beverage that is fortified with calcium and vitamins A, D_2, B_{12} and riboflavin.

> To make lactose-free buttermilk, add 1 tsp (5 mL) lemon juice or vinegar to 1 cup (250 mL) soy beverage or lactose-free milk products and let stand for 5 minutes.

- **Coconut milk, rice milk and almond milk** are non-soy-based lactose-free milk products.

Lactose-Free Yogurt Substitutes

Yogurt containing an active bacterial culture is more easily digested than other dairy products. However, if you can't tolerate dairy yogurt, soy yogurt has a similar texture and consistency. It is available plain and in a variety of flavors. Soy yogurt must be refrigerated and used before the best-before date. We found it held well, and we were able to use some and store the rest for later. It did not become thin and watery. Enjoy it in both dips and baking.

Lactose-Free Fat Substitutes

We found a variety of buttery spreads and lactose-free margarines that worked well in baking. Read the label carefully, though, as several buttery spreads contain lactose. These spreads soften quickly, directly out of the refrigerator, so they do not need to be brought to room temperature before use in baking. Be careful not to cream them too long with a mixer, or they could become watery.

Some products labeled "nondairy," such as powdered coffee creamer and whipped toppings, may include ingredients that are derived from milk and therefore contain lactose.

Further Information

- www.neilsondairy.com
- www.sonice.ca
- www.sunrise-soya.com

Egg-Free Baking

Eggs have several different roles in baking — they are used for leavening or lightness, and as a binder to help hold baked goods together. Here are some of the ways you can adjust recipes to be egg-free.

We have identified recipes that are egg-free by the label "egg-free" near the recipe title.

Ground Flaxseed Gel

Ground flaxseed can replace eggs in many baking recipes. The ground flaxseed you use can be flax flour, milled flaxseed, sprouted flax flour or grind-your-own flaxseed. When you combine it with warm water and let it stand for at least 5 minutes, it forms a thick gel, about the consistency of a raw egg white.

In many baking recipes, each egg can be replaced with 2 tbsp (25 mL) ground flaxseed and $\frac{1}{4}$ cup (50 mL) warm tap water. However, this may need to be adjusted to create a product similar to the original. We like to add the gel with the liquid ingredients while the mixer is running. When using a bread machine, we add the gel to the bread pan with the other liquids.

Baked goods made with ground flaxseed tend to brown more quickly than those made with eggs and sometimes need to be tented with foil to prevent burning. However, many require an extra couple of minutes of baking time to reach the internal temperature of 200°F (100°C). The baked product rises slightly higher, browns more and is lighter in texture, with a slightly nuttier taste. It does not become dry and crumbly but stays moist when frozen.

Ground Salba® Gel

Salba® seeds are flat and oval, similar to sesame seeds in size and shape. They range from off-white to deep brown. Grind the seeds as needed in a coffee grinder. Make sure they are finely ground, or the product might be slightly gritty. To make the gel, combine 1 part ground Salba® with 4 parts warm tap water. This gel can be substituted for eggs in baking recipes. For each egg, use 1 tbsp (15 mL) ground Salba® and 1/4 cup (50 mL) warm water.

Commercial Egg Replacer

Egg replacer is a white powder containing a combination of baking powder and starches. It is added with the dry ingredients so that it is well mixed in before it touches the liquids. The oil or other fat in the recipe may have to be increased slightly.

Further Information

- www.ener-g.com
- www.glutenfree.com
- www.kingsmill.com
- www.pioneerthinking.com

> The egg substitutes sold in most supermarkets contain egg products and should not be confused with commercial egg replacer.

Using an Instant-Read Thermometer

When we bake gluten-free, it is important to use a thermometer to test foods for doneness, as it is more difficult to tell when they are baked: the outside of the bread or cake may look browned enough when the inside is still raw. The indicators you may be used to looking for when baking with wheat may not be reliable, as gluten-free foods often have a different appearance. A thermometer is the only accurate way to be sure the food is done.

Purchasing

The best thermometer for this purpose is a bimetallic stemmed thermometer often called an instant-read or chef's thermometer. It has a round head at the top, a long metal stem and a pointed end that senses the temperature. There are both digital and dial versions available. Check the temperature range to be sure it covers the temperatures you need. Instant-read thermometers are widely available in department stores, some grocery stores, specialty shops and box stores, and can also be purchased online.

Use

To test baked goods for doneness, insert the thermometer into the center of the product. Gluten-free baked goods, whether breads, cakes or muffins, are baked when they reach 200°F (100°C). Do not leave the thermometer in the product during baking, as the plastic cover will melt, ruining the thermometer.

To test for doneness in meats, insert the metal stem halfway or at least 2 inches (5 cm) into the product, making sure you do not touch the pan, bone or fat. (Some of the newer thermometers only need to be inserted to a depth of ¾ inch/2 cm, so check the manufacturer's instructions.) With thin cuts, it may be necessary to insert the stem horizontally. Meatballs can be stacked.

Clean the probe thoroughly after each use and store the thermometer in the plastic sleeve that came with it. Some of the more expensive ones (but not all) are dishwasher-safe. Read the manufacturer's instructions.

How to Calibrate Your Thermometer

It is important to make sure your thermometer is reading temperatures accurately, so you'll want to test it periodically. There are two ways of doing this and either will work, though we prefer the boiling-water method.

- **Boiling-water method:** Bring a pot of water to a boil. Insert the thermometer probe into the boiling water, making sure it doesn't touch the pot. It should read 212°F or 100°C. (Be careful not to burn yourself on the steam; we hold the thermometer with needle-nose pliers.)
- **Ice-water method:** Fill a container with crushed ice and cold water (mostly ice; just use water to fill the gaps). Insert the thermometer probe into the center of the ice water, making sure it doesn't touch the container. It should read 32°F or 0°C.

If the temperature reading is not exact, hold the calibration nut (found right under the round head) with a wrench and rotate the head until it reads the correct number of degrees.

Speaking Our Language: Are We All on the Same Page?

- "GF" means "gluten-free," such as GF sour cream, GF mayonnaise, etc., when both gluten-free and gluten-containing products are available. We recommend that you read package labels every time you purchase a GF product. Manufacturers frequently change the ingredients.

Keeping the following points in mind as you prepare our recipes will help you get the same great results we did:

- We selected specific GF flour combinations for individual recipes based on the desired texture and flavor of the final product. Unless mentioned as a variation, we have not tested other GF flours in the recipes. Substituting other flours may adversely affect the results.

- GF recipes can be temperamental. Even an extra tablespoon (15 mL) of water in a baked product can cause the recipe to fail. Use a graduated, clear, liquid measuring cup for all liquids. Place it on a flat surface and read it at eye level.

- Select either metric or imperial measures and stick to that for the whole recipe; do not mix.

- Select the correct dry measures (e.g., $\frac{1}{2}$ cup and $\frac{1}{4}$ cup when the recipe calls for $\frac{3}{4}$ cup, or 125 mL and 50 mL for 175 mL). For accuracy and perfect products, use the "spoon lightly, heap and level once" method of measuring. For small amounts, use measuring spoons, not kitchen cutlery. (Long-handled, narrow measuring spoons made especially to fit spice jars are accurate and fun to use.)

- We used large eggs, liquid honey, light (fancy) molasses, bread machine (instant) yeast, fruit juice (not fruit drinks) and salted butter. Expect different results if you make substitutions.

- We tested with 2%, 1% or nonfat milk, yogurt and sour cream, but our recipes will work with other fat levels.

- Unless otherwise stated in the recipe, eggs and dairy products are used cold from the refrigerator.

- All foods that require washing are washed before preparation. Foods such as onions, garlic and bananas are peeled, but fresh peaches and apples are not (unless specified).

- If the preparation method (chopped, melted, diced, sliced) is listed before the food, it means that you prepare the food before measuring. If it is listed after the food, measure first, then prepare. Examples are "melted butter" vs. "butter, melted"; "ground flaxseed" vs. "flaxseed, ground"; and "cooked brown rice" vs. "brown rice, cooked."

- If in doubt about a food term, a piece of equipment or a specific recipe technique, refer to the glossaries, located on pages 387 to 399.

Brunch

Heather's Granola

**Makes 14 cups (3.5 L)
(½ cup/125 mL per
serving)**

*We've updated
this everything
cereal recipe from a
Mennonite cookbook
of the '70s for today's
lifestyle. It can be
different every time
you make it! Use
any amount, in any
combination, from
the lists of ingredients
at right.*

• Preheat oven to 300°F (150°C)
• 10- by 10- by 2¼-inch (25 by 25 by 6 cm) casserole dish

7 cups	GF large-flake oat flakes	1.75 L
4 cups	dry ingredients	1 L
2 cups	liquid ingredients	500 mL
3 cups	dried fruit	750 mL

1. In the casserole dish, combine oat flakes and dry ingredients. Set aside.

2. In a 4-cup (1 L) liquid measuring cup, combine liquid ingredients. Pour over oat mixture and stir until combined.

3. Bake in preheated oven for 40 to 50 minutes, stirring every 10 minutes, until toasted and light golden brown. Let cool completely. Stir in dried fruit.

4. Store in an airtight container in the refrigerator for up to 4 weeks.

Dry Ingredients
Quinoa flakes, rice or oat bran, ground flaxseed, flaked coconut, nuts, seeds (pumpkin, flax, sesame, poppy, sunflower)

Liquid Ingredients
Fruit juices, liquid honey, light (fancy) molasses, pure maple syrup, corn syrup, vegetable oil, peanut butter, tahini, frozen orange juice concentrate

Dried Fruit
Cranberries, raisins, coarsely chopped or snipped apricots, mango, papaya, apple, dates, figs

Nutritional value per serving	
Calories	271
Fat, total	12 g
Fat, saturated	2 g
Cholesterol	0 mg
Sodium	7 mg
Carbohydrate	36 g
Fiber	5 g
Protein	7 g
Calcium	69 mg
Iron	4 mg

Tips

To use brown sugar as part of the liquid ingredients, add 2 tbsp (25 mL) water for every ¼ cup (50 mL) packed brown sugar.

If you like smaller pieces of fruit in your granola, halve or quarter the larger pieces.

One example of a combination of 4 cups (1 L) dry ingredients includes:

½ cup	oat bran	125 mL
½ cup	ground flaxseed	125 mL
½ cup	cracked flaxseed	125 mL
½ cup	pumpkin seeds	125 mL
½ cup	sunflower seeds	125 mL
½ cup	coarsely chopped pecans	125 mL
½ cup	coarsely chopped walnuts	125 mL
¼ cup	poppy seeds	50 mL
¼ cup	sesame seeds	50 mL

One example of a combination of 2 cups (500 mL) liquid ingredients includes:

1 cup	cranberry juice	250 mL
⅓ cup	pure maple syrup	75 mL
⅓ cup	extra virgin olive oil	75 mL
⅓ cup	frozen orange juice concentrate, thawed	75 mL

One example of a combination of 3 cups (750 mL) dry fruit includes:

½ cup	dried apricots, quartered	125 mL
½ cup	coarsely chopped dried apples	125 mL
½ cup	dried cranberries	125 mL
½ cup	coarsely chopped dates	125 mL
½ cup	raisins	125 mL
¼ cup	coarsely chopped mango	50 mL
¼ cup	coarsely chopped papaya	50 mL

Variation

Replace half of the GF oat flakes with any GF flaked grain, including buckwheat or amaranth flakes.

Carrot Orange Bars

**Makes 16 bars
(1 per serving)**

*These breakfast bars
are packed with
carrots and high
in beta-carotene.
Excellent for breakfast
on the go!*

Tip

Layer bars between sheets
of parchment or waxed
paper in an airtight
container and store at
room temperature for
up to 5 days or freeze
for up to 3 months.

- **9-inch (23 cm) square baking pan, lightly greased**

1 cup	sorghum flour	250 mL
¼ cup	quinoa flour	50 mL
2 tbsp	tapioca starch	25 mL
½ cup	packed brown sugar	125 mL
1½ tsp	xanthan gum	7 mL
1 tsp	GF baking powder	5 mL
½ tsp	baking soda	2 mL
½ tsp	salt	2 mL
1 tsp	ground cinnamon	5 mL
1	egg	1
1 tbsp	grated orange zest	15 mL
⅓ cup	freshly squeezed orange juice	75 mL
¼ cup	vegetable oil	50 mL
1½ cups	grated carrots	375 mL

1. In a large bowl or plastic bag, combine sorghum flour, quinoa flour, tapioca starch, brown sugar, xanthan gum, baking powder, baking soda, salt and cinnamon. Mix well and set aside.

2. In a separate bowl, using an electric mixer, beat egg, orange zest, orange juice and oil until combined. Add dry ingredients and mix just until combined. Fold in carrots.

3. Spoon batter into prepared pan. Using a moistened rubber spatula, spread to edges and smooth top. Let stand for 30 minutes. Meanwhile, preheat oven to 350°F (180°C).

4. Bake for 25 to 30 minutes or until a tester inserted in the center comes out clean. Let cool completely in pan on a wire rack. Cut into bars.

Variation

Make 12 muffins by spooning batter evenly into a lightly greased 12-cup muffin tin. Let stand as directed and bake in a 350°F (180°C) oven for 18 to 20 minutes.

Nutritional value per serving

Calories	110
Fat, total	4 g
Fat, saturated	0 g
Cholesterol	12 mg
Sodium	123 mg
Carbohydrate	17 g
Fiber	1 g
Protein	2 g
Calcium	30 mg
Iron	1 mg

Betty's Good-for-You Breakfast Bars

**Makes 30 bars
(1 per serving)**

Betty Barfield of Fort Worth, Texas, won first prize in the Gluten Intolerance Group recipe contest. She kindly gave us permission to publish her winning recipe for you.

Tip

Place bars in an airtight container and refrigerate for up to 3 days or freeze for up to 1 month.

Nutritional value per serving

Calories	159
Fat, total	5 g
Fat, saturated	2 g
Cholesterol	8 mg
Sodium	101 mg
Carbohydrate	27 g
Fiber	2 g
Protein	3 g
Calcium	24 mg
Iron	1 mg

- **Preheat oven to 350°F (180°C)**
- **15- by 10-inch (40 by 25 cm) jelly roll pan, lightly greased**

3 cups	large-flake GF oats	750 mL
1 cup	brown rice flour	250 mL
1/2 cup	packed brown sugar	125 mL
1 tsp	baking soda	5 mL
1/4 tsp	salt	1 mL
1 tsp	ground cinnamon	5 mL
1/2 tsp	ground nutmeg	2 mL
1/4 cup	dried blueberries	50 mL
1/4 cup	dried cranberries	50 mL
1/4 cup	chopped dates	50 mL
1/4 cup	raisins	50 mL
2 tbsp	ground flaxseed	25 mL
2 tbsp	Salba®	25 mL
2 tbsp	sesame seeds	25 mL
3	egg whites	3
3/4 cup	liquid honey	175 mL
1/2 cup	butter, melted	125 mL
1 tsp	vanilla extract	5 mL

1. In a very large bowl, combine oats, brown rice flour, brown sugar, baking soda, salt, cinnamon, nutmeg, blueberries, cranberries, dates, raisins, flaxseed, Salba® and sesame seeds. Set aside.

2. In a separate bowl, whisk together egg whites, honey, butter and vanilla. Add to the dry ingredients and stir until thoroughly combined. With wet fingers, press mixture evenly into prepared pan.

3. Bake in preheated oven for 20 minutes or until lightly browned and firm to the touch. Let cool completely in pan on a wire rack. Cut into bars.

Variations

Substitute chopped dried mango, papaya or figs for any or all of the dried fruit.

Substitute ground flaxseed or ground hemp seed for the Salba®.

Add 2 tbsp (25 mL) unsweetened shredded coconut and/or 1/4 cup (50 mL) finely chopped almonds, pecans, hazelnuts or walnuts.

Streusel-Topped Walnut Brunch Cake

Makes 9 to 12 servings

A holiday brunch isn't complete without a coffee cake served fresh from the oven!

Tips

Do not cover or store coffee cake until completely cooled.

Coffee cakes get stale more quickly if refrigerated. Store in an airtight container at room temperature for up to 2 days.

- 9-inch (23 cm) square baking pan, lightly greased and bottom lined with parchment paper

Walnut Crumb Topping

½ cup	coarsely chopped walnuts	125 mL
¼ cup	packed brown sugar	50 mL
1 tsp	ground cinnamon	5 mL

Brunch Cake

1 cup	sorghum flour	250 mL
½ cup	amaranth flour	125 mL
½ cup	tapioca starch	125 mL
1½ tsp	xanthan gum	7 mL
2 tsp	GF baking powder	10 mL
1 tsp	baking soda	5 mL
¼ tsp	salt	1 mL
2	eggs	2
1¼ cups	plain yogurt or sour cream	300 mL
½ cup	white (granulated) sugar	125 mL
¼ cup	vegetable oil	50 mL
1 tsp	vanilla extract	5 mL

1. *Topping:* In a small bowl, combine walnuts, brown sugar and cinnamon. Set aside.

2. *Cake:* In a large bowl or plastic bag, combine sorghum flour, amaranth flour, tapioca starch, xanthan gum, baking powder, baking soda and salt. Mix well and set aside.

3. In a separate bowl, using an electric mixer, beat eggs, yogurt, sugar, oil and vanilla. Add dry ingredients and mix until combined.

4. Spoon batter into prepared pan. Using a moistened rubber spatula, spread to edges and smooth top. Sprinkle with topping. Let stand for 30 minutes. Meanwhile, preheat oven to 350°F (180°C).

5. Bake for 25 to 30 minutes or until a tester inserted in the center comes out clean. Let cool in pan on a wire rack for 10 minutes. Remove from pan and let cool completely on rack.

Nutritional value per serving	
Calories	230
Fat, total	10 g
Fat, saturated	0 g
Cholesterol	33 mg
Sodium	185 mg
Carbohydrate	32 g
Fiber	2 g
Protein	5 g
Calcium	109 mg
Iron	2 mg

Bacon, Tomato and Cheese Crustless Quiche

Makes 4 servings

Hate making pastry but crave quiche? This one has all the flavor of a traditional quiche, minus the calories, extra time and work.

Tip

Quiche can be stored in an airtight container in the refrigerator for up to 2 days. Reheat in the microwave on Medium (50%) until warm. Let stand for 5 minutes before cutting.

- Preheat oven to 325°F (160°C)
- 10-inch (25 cm) quiche dish or deep-dish pie plate, lightly greased

1½ cups	shredded Swiss cheese	375 mL
½	onion, finely chopped	½
2 to 3	plum (Roma) tomatoes, thickly sliced	2 to 3
1 tbsp	chopped fresh basil	15 mL
6	slices GF bacon, cooked crisp and cut in half	6
4	eggs	4
1 cup	evaporated milk	250 mL
2 tbsp	Dijon mustard	25 mL
¼ tsp	salt	1 mL
Pinch	freshly ground black pepper	Pinch

1. Sprinkle cheese and onion in prepared dish. Top with tomatoes, basil and bacon. Set aside.

2. In a bowl, whisk together eggs, evaporated milk, mustard, salt and pepper. Pour over ingredients in dish.

3. Bake in preheated oven for 25 to 30 minutes or until egg mixture is just set and a tester inserted in the center comes out clean. Let stand for 5 minutes. Cut into wedges. Serve hot, warm or at room temperature.

Variations

Add 1 cup (250 mL) cooked broccoli florets, sliced zucchini or mushrooms.

Make in a 9-inch (23 cm) square baking pan and cut into small squares to serve as an hors d'oeuvre.

Substitute ¼ tsp (1 mL) dry mustard for the Dijon mustard.

Substitute fresh oregano or thyme for the basil.

Nutritional value per serving

Calories	519
Fat, total	39 g
Fat, saturated	18 g
Cholesterol	259 mg
Sodium	1,436 mg
Carbohydrate	14 g
Fiber	1 g
Protein	27 g
Calcium	627 mg
Iron	2 mg

Vegetable Quiche with Oat Groat Crust

White sugar–free

Makes 6 servings

Beth Armour of Cream Hill Estates developed this recipe and has given us permission to include it for you. It's a good way to use up leftover vegetables from dinner, or you can plan to cook extras just to make this quiche.

Tips

For the vegetables, you can use any combination you like; just keep the total to 1 cup (250 mL) cooked vegetables. We like a mixture of bite-size pieces of broccoli, spinach, tomatoes and red, yellow or orange bell peppers. For a more intense flavor, try using roasted vegetables.

This is an ideal time to use liquid eggs. Use 1¼ cups (300 mL) to replace the 5 eggs.

Nutritional value per serving

Calories	284
Fat, total	15 g
Fat, saturated	8 g
Cholesterol	218 mg
Sodium	349 mg
Carbohydrate	18 g
Fiber	2 g
Protein	19 g
Calcium	378 mg
Iron	3 mg

• **Preheat oven to 350°F (180°C)**

1	Oat Groat Crust (see recipe, opposite)	1
5	eggs	5
2 tbsp	milk	25 mL
½ tsp	salt	2 mL
1⅔ cups	shredded Swiss cheese (about 7 oz/210 g)	400 mL
1 cup	cooked vegetables (see tip, at left)	250 mL
¼ cup	chopped fresh rosemary	50 mL

1. Bake crust in preheated oven for 5 minutes.

2. Meanwhile, in a large bowl, using an electric mixer, beat eggs, milk and salt until combined. Stir in cheese, vegetables and rosemary. Spoon into partially baked crust.

3. Bake for 25 to 30 minutes or until center bubbles up. Let cool for 10 minutes before serving.

**Makes 1 crust
(1/6 crust per serving)**

Tips

Be sure to press the oat groat mixture evenly into the bottom and up the sides of the quiche dish. Don't let it get too thick where the sides meet the bottom. Use the back of a dessert spoon for easier spreading.

Crust can be covered and refrigerated for up to 2 days or frozen for up to 3 weeks.

Use this crust as the base of a meat pie.

Oat Groat Crust

- 9-inch (23 cm) quiche dish or deep-dish pie plate, lightly greased

2 cups	water	500 mL
1 cup	whole oat groats	250 mL
1	egg, lightly beaten	1

1. In a saucepan, bring water to a boil over high heat. Add oat groats and return to a boil. Remove from heat, cover and let stand for 30 minutes.

2. Bring groats mixture to a simmer over medium-low heat. Simmer for 20 to 25 minutes or until softened but still firm. Remove from heat, drain and let stand for 10 minutes.

3. Add egg and stir until well coated. Press mixture into bottom and up sides of prepared dish.

4. Bake according to recipe directions.

Nutritional value per serving	
Calories	81
Fat, total	2 g
Fat, saturated	1 g
Cholesterol	31 mg
Sodium	9 mg
Carbohydrate	12 g
Fiber	2 g
Protein	3 g
Calcium	14 mg
Iron	2 mg

Seafood Frittata

Makes 6 to 8 servings or 12 to 16 appetizer wedges

A frittata can be described as a Spanish-Italian omelet or a crustless quiche. We cleaned out the refrigerator to prepare this quick and easy any-time-of-day meal.

Tips

Store in an airtight container in the refrigerator for up to 2 days. If desired, reheat individual portions in the microwave on Medium (50%) until just hot.

To ovenproof a nonstick skillet with a non-metal handle, wrap the handle in a double layer of foil, shiny side out, and turn it so it's not directly under the broiler.

- Preheat broiler
- 9- to 10-inch (23 to 25 cm) ovenproof nonstick or cast-iron skillet, sides and bottom lightly greased

2 tbsp	extra virgin olive oil	25 mL
1 cup	sliced cremini mushrooms	250 mL
2	green onions, coarsely chopped	2
1/2	red bell pepper, cut into 1/2-inch (1 cm) squares	1/2
8	egg whites	8
4	eggs	4
1/2 cup	snipped fresh tarragon	125 mL
2 tbsp	snipped fresh parsley	25 mL
1/2 tsp	salt	2 mL
1/8 tsp	freshly ground white pepper	0.5 mL
1 tsp	Dijon mustard	5 mL
2 cups	broccoli florets, cooked	500 mL
1 cup	shredded Cheddar cheese	250 mL
1/2 cup	shredded Asiago cheese	125 mL
1/2 cup	crumbled feta cheese	125 mL
1 cup	shredded cooked crabmeat (1/2-inch/1 cm pieces)	250 mL
12	medium shrimp, peeled, deveined, cooked and halved	12
4	sea scallops, cooked and quartered	4

1. In an ovenproof skillet, heat oil over medium heat. Sauté mushrooms, green onions and red pepper for 5 minutes or until softened. Remove skillet from heat and reduce heat to medium-low.

2. In a large bowl, whisk together egg whites, eggs, tarragon, parsley, salt, pepper and mustard. Stir in broccoli, Cheddar, Asiago and feta. Fold in crabmeat, shrimp and scallops.

3. Pour egg mixture into skillet and return to heat. Cook for 12 to 15 minutes, lifting the edges to allow uncooked egg to run to bottom of skillet, until bottom and sides are firm but top is still moist.

Nutritional value per serving	
Calories	243
Fat, total	15 g
Fat, saturated	7 g
Cholesterol	158 mg
Sodium	547 mg
Carbohydrate	6 g
Fiber	2 g
Protein	22 g
Calcium	284 mg
Iron	1 mg

Tips

See the Techniques Glossary, page 395, for instructions on cleaning a cast-iron skillet.

To prevent a cast-iron skillet from rusting, set it on a warm stove element to dry completely before storing. Be careful: the handle gets hot.

4. Place under preheated boiler, 3 inches (7.5 cm) from the element, and broil for 2 to 5 minutes or until golden brown and set. Cut into wedges and serve hot or at room temperature.

Variations

Substitute any cheeses you like, keeping the total quantity at 2 cups (500 mL). Other cheeses we'd suggest include Swiss, Emmental and Romano.

Vary the seafood to your liking. Use about $2\frac{1}{2}$ to 3 cups (625 to 750 mL) total volume.

Christmas Morning Strata

Makes 6 servings

Busy enough on Christmas morning? Assemble this the night before. All you need to add is fresh fruit, and breakfast is ready.

Tips

Choose portobello, cremini or button mushrooms, or a mixture.

Try Swiss, aged Cheddar, Monterey Jack or a Tex-Mex mixture for the cheese.

- 8-inch (20 cm) square baking pan, lightly greased

1 tbsp	butter	15 mL
1	small onion, chopped	1
8 oz	mushrooms (see tip, at left), sliced	250 g
4 oz	GF ham, cut into ½-inch (1 cm) cubes	125 g
2 tbsp	chopped fresh parsley	25 mL
1 tbsp	chopped fresh basil	15 mL
3 cups	cubed GF bread (½-inch/1 cm cubes)	750 mL
2 cups	shredded cheese (see tip, at left)	500 mL
4	eggs	4
1 cup	milk	250 mL
1 tbsp	Dijon mustard	15 mL

1. In a large skillet, melt butter over medium heat. Sauté onion and mushrooms for 4 to 6 minutes or until tender. Remove from heat and stir in ham, parsley and basil.

2. Arrange half the bread cubes in prepared pan. Top with half the ham mixture and half the cheese. Repeat layers.

3. In a small bowl, whisk together eggs, milk and mustard until blended. Pour over strata. Cover with foil and refrigerate overnight.

4. Preheat oven to 350°F (180°C). Bake, covered with foil, for 20 minutes. Remove foil and bake for 30 to 35 minutes or until center is set and top is golden.

Variations

Use GF salami or GF prosciutto instead of the GF ham.

Try rosemary, dill or marjoram in place of the basil.

Nutritional value per serving	
Calories	480
Fat, total	22 g
Fat, saturated	11 g
Cholesterol	181 mg
Sodium	1,040 mg
Carbohydrate	45 g
Fiber	2 g
Protein	25 g
Calcium	470 mg
Iron	5 mg

French Toast

**Makes 2 servings
(1 slice per serving)**

Quick, easy, traditional breakfast fare. And it makes good use of leftover bread.

Tips

We like to use Multigrain Bread (page 204 or 232) or Historic Grains Bread (page 202 or 230) for this recipe. Ancient Grains Bread (from our *Complete Gluten-Free Cookbook*) and Cinnamon Raisin Bread (from *The Best Gluten-Free Family Cookbook*) also make delicious French toast.

Sprinkle with ground cinnamon and GF confectioner's (icing) sugar just before serving.

Nutritional value per serving	
Calories	273
Fat, total	13 g
Fat, saturated	5 g
Cholesterol	228 mg
Sodium	373 mg
Carbohydrate	28 g
Fiber	2 g
Protein	10 g
Calcium	63 mg
Iron	3 mg

• **8-inch (20 cm) skillet**

2	eggs	2
2 tbsp	milk	25 mL
2	slices GF bread	2
1 tsp	butter	5 mL
	Maple syrup, honey, yogurt or fresh fruit	

1. In a shallow bowl or pie plate, whisk together eggs and milk. Add bread slices and let soak for 1 minute. Turn and soak for 1 minute.

2. In the skillet, melt butter over medium heat. Add soaked bread and cook for 2 minutes or until bottom is deep golden. Turn and cook for 2 minutes or until bottom is golden. Serve immediately with your choice of topping.

Buttermilk Waffles

A breakfast treat for a lazy Sunday morning! Make ahead and freeze for weekday use.

Tips

Recipe can be doubled or tripled.

Store extra waffles between layers of waxed paper in an airtight container in the refrigerator for up to 3 days or in a plastic freezer bag in the freezer for up to 1 month. Reheat from frozen in the toaster.

Resist the temptation to add extra liquid — the batter should be thick.

Beat the batter until smooth — no need to leave it lumpy.

- Waffle maker, lightly greased, then preheated

½ cup	amaranth flour	125 mL
½ cup	sorghum flour	125 mL
¼ cup	tapioca starch	50 mL
2 tbsp	white (granulated) sugar	25 mL
½ tsp	xanthan gum	2 mL
2¼ tsp	GF baking powder	11 mL
¾ tsp	baking soda	4 mL
Pinch	salt	Pinch
2	eggs, separated	2
¾ cup	buttermilk	175 mL
2 tbsp	vegetable oil	25 mL

1. In a large bowl or plastic bag, combine amaranth flour, sorghum flour, tapioca starch, sugar, xanthan gum, baking powder, baking soda and salt. Mix well and set aside.

2. In a small bowl, using an electric mixer, preferably with wire whisk attachment, beat egg whites until stiff but not dry.

3. In a separate bowl, using an electric mixer, beat egg yolks, buttermilk and oil until combined. Add dry ingredients and beat until smooth. Fold in beaten egg whites.

4. Pour in enough batter to fill preheated waffle maker two-thirds full. Close lid and cook for 6 to 8 minutes or until no longer steaming. Repeat with remaining batter, greasing waffle maker between waffles as necessary.

Variation
Add fresh fruit, nuts or seeds to the batter.

Nutritional value per serving	
Calories	188
Fat, total	7 g
Fat, saturated	1 g
Cholesterol	63 mg
Sodium	260 mg
Carbohydrate	26 g
Fiber	2 g
Protein	6 g
Calcium	142 mg
Iron	3 mg

Chocolate Orange Waffles

Fudgy chocolate and orange are two flavors that just naturally go together. These waffles are irresistible to children — and adults too!

Tips

Recipe can be doubled or tripled.

Store extra waffles between layers of waxed paper in an airtight container in the refrigerator for up to 3 days, or in a plastic freezer bag in the freezer for up to 1 month. Reheat from frozen in the toaster.

Top with fresh strawberries and drizzle with chocolate syrup. For a gourmet touch, dust with GF confectioner's (icing) sugar pressed through a sieve.

Nutritional value per serving	
Calories	247
Fat, total	10 g
Fat, saturated	2 g
Cholesterol	50 mg
Sodium	241 mg
Carbohydrate	38 g
Fiber	3 g
Protein	7 g
Calcium	166 mg
Iron	2 mg

• Waffle maker, lightly greased, then preheated

⅔ cup	sorghum flour	150 mL
¼ cup	whole bean flour	50 mL
2 tbsp	tapioca starch	25 mL
¾ cup	white (granulated) sugar	175 mL
½ cup	unsweetened cocoa powder, sifted	125 mL
½ tsp	xanthan gum	2 mL
2¼ tsp	GF baking powder	11 mL
¾ tsp	baking soda	4 mL
¼ tsp	salt	1 mL
2 tbsp	grated orange zest	25 mL
2	eggs, separated	2
1½ cups	plain yogurt	375 mL
¼ cup	vegetable oil	50 mL

1. In a large bowl or plastic bag, combine sorghum flour, whole bean flour, tapioca starch, sugar, cocoa powder, xanthan gum, baking powder, baking soda, salt and orange zest. Mix well and set aside.

2. In a small bowl, using an electric mixer, preferably with wire whisk attachment, beat egg whites until stiff but not dry.

3. In a separate bowl, using an electric mixer, beat egg yolks, yogurt and oil until combined. Add dry ingredients and beat until smooth. Fold in beaten egg whites.

4. Pour in enough batter to fill preheated waffle maker two-thirds full. Close lid and cook for 7 to 9 minutes or until no longer steaming. Repeat with remaining batter, greasing waffle maker between waffles as necessary.

Banana Pecan Waffles

**Makes six 4½-inch
(11 cm) waffles
(1 per serving)**

*Donna's grandkids
love these for breakfast
when they visit on
the weekends. Make
ahead and freeze for
weekday use.*

Tips

Recipe can be doubled or
tripled.

Store extra waffles between
layers of waxed paper in
an airtight container in
the refrigerator for up
to 3 days, or in a plastic
freezer bag in the freezer
for up to 1 month. Reheat
from frozen in the toaster.

Resist the temptation to
add extra liquid — the
batter should be thick.

Beat the batter until
smooth — no need to leave
it lumpy.

Nutritional value per serving

Calories	282
Fat, total	14 g
Fat, saturated	2 g
Cholesterol	62 mg
Sodium	229 mg
Carbohydrate	36 g
Fiber	4 g
Protein	6 g
Calcium	106 mg
Iron	2 mg

- **Waffle maker, lightly greased, then preheated**

¾ cup	sorghum flour	175 mL
¼ cup	quinoa flour	50 mL
¼ cup	tapioca starch	50 mL
2 tbsp	white (granulated) sugar	25 mL
½ tsp	xanthan gum	2 mL
2¼ tsp	GF baking powder	11 mL
¾ tsp	baking soda	4 mL
Pinch	salt	Pinch
½ cup	chopped pecans	125 mL
2	eggs, separated	2
1 cup	mashed bananas	125 mL
2 tbsp	vegetable oil	25 mL

1. In a large bowl or plastic bag, combine sorghum flour, quinoa flour, tapioca starch, sugar, xanthan gum, baking powder, baking soda, salt and pecans. Mix well and set aside.

2. In a small bowl, using an electric mixer, preferably with wire whisk attachment, beat egg whites until stiff but not dry.

3. In a separate bowl, using an electric mixer, beat egg yolks, bananas and oil until combined. Add dry ingredients and beat until smooth. Fold in beaten egg whites.

4. Pour in enough batter to fill preheated waffle maker two-thirds full. Close lid and cook for 5 to 7 minutes or until no longer steaming. Repeat with remaining batter, greasing waffle maker between waffles as necessary.

Variation

Increase the sugar to ¼ cup (50 mL) to turn these into dessert waffles, and serve with fresh fruit and or chocolate sauce.

Buckwheat Pancakes

*Looking for a more
flavorful, nutritious
pancake? Here it is.*

Tip

For information on how to
know when your griddle
is hot enough, see the
Techniques Glossary,
page 396.

• Griddle or nonstick skillet, lightly greased

1/3 cup	buckwheat flour	75 mL
1/3 cup	brown rice flour	75 mL
2 tbsp	tapioca starch	25 mL
2 tsp	white (granulated) sugar	10 mL
1/2 tsp	xanthan gum	2 mL
2 tsp	GF baking powder	10 mL
1 tsp	baking soda	5 mL
1/4 tsp	salt	1 mL
1	egg	1
1 cup	buttermilk	250 mL
1 tbsp	vegetable oil	15 mL

1. In a bowl or plastic bag, combine buckwheat flour, brown rice flour, tapioca starch, sugar, xanthan gum, baking powder, baking soda and salt. Mix well and set aside.

2. In a bowl, using an electric mixer, beat egg, buttermilk and oil until combined. Add dry ingredients and beat until almost smooth.

3. Heat prepared griddle or skillet over medium-high heat. For each pancake, pour 1/4 cup (50 mL) batter onto prepared griddle and cook for about 3 minutes or until the bottom is deep golden and the top surface wrinkles around the edges. Turn and cook for 30 to 60 seconds longer or until bottom is golden. Repeat with remaining batter, greasing griddle between batches as necessary. Serve immediately.

Variation

Sprinkle each pancake with 1 to 2 tbsp (15 to 25 mL) fresh or thawed frozen blueberries before turning to cook the second side.

Nutritional value per serving

Calories	89
Fat, total	3 g
Fat, saturated	1 g
Cholesterol	24 mg
Sodium	272 mg
Carbohydrate	14 g
Fiber	1 g
Protein	3 g
Calcium	94 mg
Iron	1 mg

Russian Blini

These little yeast-leavened buckwheat pancakes are traditionally served with sour cream, caviar and smoked salmon. They make a wonderful treat for Thanksgiving or Christmas.

Tip

For fluffier blini, warm egg whites to room temperature before beating. See the Techniques Glossary, page 396.

• Griddle, cast-iron skillet or nonstick skillet, lightly greased

1/3 cup	milk	75 mL
1 tbsp	white (granulated) sugar	15 mL
1/2 tsp	bread machine or instant yeast	2 mL
1	egg yolk	1
1 tsp	vegetable oil	5 mL
1/3 cup	amaranth flour	75 mL
2 tbsp	buckwheat flour	25 mL
1/2 tsp	salt	2 mL
2	egg whites	2
Pinch	cream of tartar	Pinch

1. In a small microwave-safe bowl, microwave milk on Medium (50%) for 45 seconds or until body temperature. Stir in sugar and yeast.

2. In another bowl, whisk together egg yolk and oil. Whisk in milk mixture, amaranth flour, buckwheat flour and salt until smooth. Cover and set in a pan of warm water for 1¼ hours.

3. Preheat oven to 250°F (120°C).

4. In a clean bowl, using an electric mixer, preferably with whisk attachment, beat egg whites and cream of tartar until stiff but not dry. Using a spatula, fold gently into batter.

Nutritional value per serving	
Calories	27
Fat, total	1 g
Fat, saturated	0 g
Cholesterol	14 mg
Sodium	84 mg
Carbohydrate	4 g
Fiber	0 g
Protein	1 g
Calcium	12 mg
Iron	1 mg

Tips

For information on cleaning, seasoning and preheating a cast-iron skillet, see the Techniques Glossary, page 395.

To prevent a cast-iron skillet from rusting, set it on a warm stove element to dry completely before storing. Be careful: the handle gets hot.

5. Heat prepared griddle or skillet over medium-high heat. For each blini, spoon 2 tbsp (25 mL) batter onto prepared griddle, spreading batter with the back of the spoon for thinner blini. Cook for about 2 minutes or until the bottom is deep golden and bubbles appear on the top surface. Turn and cook for 30 to 60 seconds longer or until bottom is golden. Transfer to a plate and keep warm in oven. Repeat with remaining batter, greasing griddle between batches as necessary. Serve immediately.

Variations

For a stronger buckwheat flavor, increase the buckwheat flour to 3 tbsp (45 mL) and decrease the amaranth flour to 1/4 cup (50 mL).

Add fresh or thawed frozen blueberries to the batter.

Soy-Free, Corn-Free Pancakes

This recipe is a request from folks who can't tolerate either soy or corn.

Tips

For information on how to know when your griddle is hot enough, see the Techniques Glossary, page 396.

If pancakes stick to the griddle, leave them for a few more seconds, then try again — they often loosen when they're ready to be turned.

Nutritional value per serving

Calories	139
Fat, total	5 g
Fat, saturated	1 g
Cholesterol	48 mg
Sodium	34 mg
Carbohydrate	20 g
Fiber	2 g
Protein	4 g
Calcium	94 mg
Iron	1 mg

• Griddle or nonstick skillet, lightly greased

½ cup	sorghum flour	125 mL
¼ cup	brown rice flour	50 mL
¼ cup	whole bean flour	50 mL
¼ cup	potato starch	50 mL
2 tbsp	white (granulated) sugar	25 mL
½ tsp	xanthan gum	2 mL
2 tsp	GF baking powder	10 mL
2	eggs	2
1	egg white	1
¾ cup	milk	175 mL
2 tbsp	vegetable oil	25 mL

1. In a bowl or plastic bag, combine sorghum flour, brown rice flour, whole bean flour, potato starch, sugar, xanthan gum and baking powder. Mix well and set aside.

2. In a bowl, using an electric mixer, beat eggs, egg white, milk and oil until combined. Add dry ingredients and beat until almost smooth.

3. Heat prepared griddle or skillet over medium-high heat. For each pancake, pour ¼ cup (50 mL) batter onto prepared griddle and cook for about 3 minutes or until the bottom is deep golden and the top surface wrinkles around the edges. Turn and cook for 1 to 2 minutes longer or until bottom is golden. Repeat with remaining batter, greasing griddle between batches as necessary. Serve immediately.

Variations

To make Banana Pancakes, substitute mashed banana for half the milk.

If you like thinner pancakes, add an extra 2 tbsp (25 mL) milk.

Pineapple Strawberry Smoothie

Makes 2 to 3 servings

Try our smooth, thick, refreshing smoothie for breakfast on the move. A great way to increase your calcium and fiber!

Tip

Freezing the fruit overnight makes for a thicker, creamier smoothie; if you'd prefer to skip this step, add 1 cup (250 mL) ice cubes.

1 cup	fat-free GF strawberry yogurt	250 mL
1 cup	fresh pineapple pieces, frozen	250 mL
1 cup	fresh strawberries, frozen	250 mL
¼ cup	milk	50 mL

1. In a blender or food processor, purée yogurt, pineapple, strawberries and milk until smooth. Serve immediately.

Nutritional value per serving	
Calories	132
Fat, total	0 g
Fat, saturated	0 g
Cholesterol	3 mg
Sodium	55 mg
Carbohydrate	29 g
Fiber	2 g
Protein	5 g
Calcium	142 mg
Iron	1 mg

Banana Blueberry Smoothie

Makes 2 servings

This smoothie is a great way to increase your fruit servings in a day.

Tips

To freeze bananas for a smoothie — or any time they ripen before you're ready to use them — peel, slice, wrap in parchment paper and freeze for at least 2 hours or place in an airtight container and freeze for up to 3 weeks.

1½ cups	freshly squeezed orange juice	375 mL
2	bananas, cut into 1-inch (2.5 cm) pieces and frozen	2
1 cup	fresh blueberries, frozen	250 mL

1. In a blender or food processor, purée orange juice, bananas and blueberries until smooth. Serve immediately.

Variation
Substitute 1 cup (250 mL) chopped fresh mango, frozen, for the blueberries.

Nutritional value per serving	
Calories	229
Fat, total	1 g
Fat, saturated	0 g
Cholesterol	0 mg
Sodium	4 mg
Carbohydrate	56 g
Fiber	5 g
Protein	3 g
Calcium	34 mg
Iron	1 mg

Dips, Dressings and Sauces

Spicy Hummus

**Makes about 2⅓ cups
(575 mL)
(2 tbsp/25 mL per
serving)**

*Take this ever-popular
dip along to your next
potluck. Our version is
moderately spicy, but
you can adjust it to
your preferred heat.*

Tips

A chipotle is a dried
smoked jalapeño pepper.
They're commonly
available canned in adobo
sauce, a Mexican sauce
made of ground chiles,
herbs and vinegar.

If you only have a 14-oz
(398 mL) can of chickpeas,
you may not need all of the
yogurt. Add just enough to
make a thick dip.

Serve with vegetable
crudités, Sesame Crispbread
(page 93) or Sun-Dried
Tomato Lavosh (page 94).

1 cup	fat-free plain yogurt	250 mL
2	cloves garlic, minced	2
1	chipotle pepper in adobo sauce, chopped	1
1	can (14 to 19 oz/398 to 540 mL) chickpeas, drained and rinsed	1
2 tbsp	freshly squeezed lemon juice	25 mL
1 tbsp	extra virgin olive oil	15 mL
1 tbsp	sesame oil	15 mL
1 tsp	ground cumin	5 mL
¼ tsp	salt	1 mL

1. Line a large sieve with a double layer of cheesecloth and set over a large bowl. Place yogurt in sieve and refrigerate for 2 hours, until reduced to about ½ cup (125 mL), or overnight.

2. In a food processor, purée yogurt, garlic, chipotle, chickpeas, lemon juice, olive oil, sesame oil, cumin and salt for 2 to 3 minutes or until smooth.

3. Serve immediately or transfer to an airtight container and refrigerate for up to 3 days.

Variations

Substitute ¼ cup (50 mL) finely chopped fresh basil or cilantro for the cumin.

For a milder flavor, omit the chipotle or use a fresh jalapeño pepper, seeded and chopped. Add extra chipotle to increase the heat.

Nutritional value per serving

Calories	46
Fat, total	2 g
Fat, saturated	0 g
Cholesterol	1 mg
Sodium	105 mg
Carbohydrate	6 g
Fiber	1 g
Protein	2 g
Calcium	28 mg
Iron	0 mg

Greek Pesto

**Makes about 1 cup
(250 mL)
(2 tbsp/25 mL per
serving)**

Heather's brother-in-law enjoys this Greek version of an Italian favorite.

Tips

Make lots of pesto during the summer, when herbs are plentiful, and freeze in small quantities for up to 3 months.

To keep basil fresh, trim bottom of stalks and stand in a glass of water at room temperature. Cover the leaves with a plastic bag. Change the water frequently.

The pesto can darken on the top and the edges during storage in the refrigerator.

Spread pesto on a partially baked pizza crust and add your favorite toppings. We enjoy spinach, mushrooms and extra feta.

Nutritional value per serving	
Calories	156
Fat, total	15 g
Fat, saturated	4 g
Cholesterol	13 mg
Sodium	227 mg
Carbohydrate	3 g
Fiber	1 g
Protein	3 g
Calcium	110 mg
Iron	1 mg

8	cloves garlic, minced	8
4 cups	packed fresh basil leaves	1 L
1 cup	crumbled feta cheese	250 mL
½ cup	kalamata olives, pitted	125 mL
½ cup	extra virgin olive oil	125 mL
	Salt and freshly ground black pepper	

1. In a food processor, combine garlic, basil, feta, olives and oil; process until nearly smooth. Season to taste with salt and pepper.

2. Use immediately or transfer to an airtight container and refrigerate for up to 3 days.

Variation

For a milder pesto, add a coarsely chopped green bell pepper.

Sun-Dried Tomato Pesto

**Makes about 2½ cups
(625 mL)
(2 tbsp/25 mL per
serving)**

*What a good way to
use the extra basil and
parsley from your herb
garden.*

Tips

Drain sun-dried tomatoes
well to avoid adding extra
oil.

One 9½-oz (270 mL) jar
of oil-packed sun-dried
tomatoes yields 1 cup
(250 mL) drained.

2	cloves garlic	2
2 cups	drained oil-packed sun-dried tomatoes	500 mL
1 cup	freshly grated Parmesan cheese	250 mL
¼ cup	packed fresh basil leaves	50 mL
¼ cup	packed fresh parsley leaves	50 mL
¼ cup	walnuts	50 mL
¼ cup	extra virgin olive oil	50 mL
	Freshly ground black pepper	

1. In a food processor, combine garlic, sun-dried tomatoes, Parmesan, basil, parsley, walnuts and oil; pulse until almost smooth and quite thick. Season to taste with pepper.
2. Use immediately or transfer to an airtight container and store in the refrigerator for up to 1 month.

Variations

Substitute pine nuts, pistachios or hazelnuts for the walnuts.

If you want to use the pesto as a base for pizza toppings, thin it with a small amount of extra virgin olive oil or GF beef broth.

Nutritional value per serving

Calories	65
Fat, total	5 g
Fat, saturated	1 g
Cholesterol	3 mg
Sodium	98 mg
Carbohydrate	2 g
Fiber	1 g
Protein	2 g
Calcium	61 mg
Iron	0 mg

Roasted Garlic Dip

**Makes about 2 cups
(500 mL)
(2 tbsp/25 mL per
serving)**

*Roasting garlic takes
the bitter bite out of it,
so go ahead and enjoy.*

Tips

If you can only find smaller
cans of black beans, use
2 cups (500 mL) drained
rinsed beans.

For information about
roasting garlic, see the
Techniques Glossary,
page 396.

2 tsp	extra virgin olive oil	10 mL
1	onion, finely chopped	1
1	can (19 oz/540 mL) black beans, drained and rinsed	1
1	bulb garlic, roasted and cloves squeezed out	1
2 tbsp	snipped fresh sage	25 mL
1 tbsp	balsamic vinegar	15 mL
1 tsp	freshly squeezed lemon juice	5 mL
½ tsp	salt	2 mL
¼ tsp	freshly ground black pepper	1 mL

1. In a skillet, heat oil over medium heat. Sauté onion for 2 to 3 minutes or until tender.

2. In a food processor, combine onion, beans, roasted garlic cloves, sage, vinegar, lemon juice, salt and pepper; pulse, scraping down sides occasionally, until smooth.

3. Transfer to an airtight container and refrigerate for at least 2 hours to allow flavors to develop and blend. Store in the refrigerator for up to 2 weeks.

Variation

Choose any variety of canned beans, such as chickpeas (garbanzo beans), white beans or pinto beans.

Nutritional value per serving

Calories	25
Fat, total	1 g
Fat, saturated	0 g
Cholesterol	0 mg
Sodium	169 mg
Carbohydrate	5 g
Fiber	2 g
Protein	1 g
Calcium	14 mg
Iron	0 mg

Yogurt Dill Dip

**Makes about ⅔ cup (150 mL)
(2 tbsp/25 mL per serving)**

Serve with Crispy Calamari (page 100) or fresh fish, or use as a dip with raw vegetables.

Tip

Dill is easy to grow and easily self-seeds each year.

2	cloves garlic, minced	2
1 tbsp	snipped fresh dill	15 mL
1 tsp	grated lemon zest	5 mL
¼ tsp	salt	1 mL
½ cup	plain yogurt	125 mL
2 tbsp	GF mayonnaise	25 mL

1. In a small bowl, combine garlic, dill, lemon zest, salt, yogurt and mayonnaise.

2. Cover and refrigerate for at least 2 hours to allow flavors to develop and blend. Store in an airtight container in the refrigerator for up to 2 weeks.

Variation

Substitute 1 tsp (5 mL) dried dillweed for the fresh.

Nutritional value per serving	
Calories	31
Fat, total	2 g
Fat, saturated	1 g
Cholesterol	3 mg
Sodium	151 mg
Carbohydrate	2 g
Fiber	0 g
Protein	1 g
Calcium	40 mg
Iron	0 mg

Raspberry Vinaigrette

Makes about ¾ cup (175 mL) (1½ tbsp/22 mL per serving)

Spinach and raspberry vinaigrette are a natural go-together. You'll discover lots of other good uses for this dressing too.

Tips

To dress 8 cups (2 L) of greens, or 4 servings, you'll need about 6 tbsp (90 mL) dressing.

For better flavor, let vinaigrette stand at room temperature for at least 30 minutes before serving.

To thicken a blended low-oil vinaigrette, add an ice cube and shake well.

½ cup	frozen unsweetened raspberry juice concentrate, thawed	125 mL
1 tbsp	raspberry-flavored vinegar	15 mL
1 tsp	grated orange zest	5 mL
¼ tsp	salt	1 mL
¼ tsp	freshly ground black pepper	1 mL
3 tbsp	vegetable oil	45 mL

1. In a small bowl, whisk together raspberry juice concentrate, vinegar, orange zest, salt and pepper. Gradually whisk in oil.

2. Set aside for at least 1 hour or cover and refrigerate overnight to let flavors develop and blend. Store in an airtight container in the refrigerator for up to 3 weeks.

Variation

For a milder flavor, substitute white wine vinegar for the raspberry-flavored vinegar.

Nutritional value per serving

Calories	84
Fat, total	5 g
Fat, saturated	0 g
Cholesterol	0 mg
Sodium	83 mg
Carbohydrate	9 g
Fiber	0 g
Protein	1 g
Calcium	14 mg
Iron	0 mg

Basil Vinaigrette

**Makes about 1 cup
(250 mL)
(2 tbsp/25 mL per
serving)**

*This lower-fat
vinaigrette is still high
in flavor.*

Tips

For better flavor, let
vinaigrette stand at room
temperature for at least
30 minutes before serving.

For a creamier texture,
mix the vinaigrette in a
blender.

2 tbsp	snipped fresh parsley	25 mL
2 tbsp	snipped fresh chives	25 mL
2 tbsp	snipped fresh basil	25 mL
½ tsp	freshly ground black pepper	2 mL
¼ tsp	salt	1 mL
¼ cup	white or red wine vinegar	50 mL
1 tbsp	honey Dijon mustard	15 mL
½ cup	extra virgin olive oil	125 mL

1. In a small bowl, whisk together parsley, chives, basil,
   pepper, salt, vinegar and mustard. Gradually whisk
   in oil.

2. Set aside for at least 1 hour or cover and refrigerate
   overnight to let flavors develop and blend. Store in an
   airtight container in the refrigerator for up to 3 weeks.

Variations

Substitute the tops of green onion for the chives.

To turn this into tarragon vinaigrette, substitute tarragon-
flavored vinegar for the wine vinegar and fresh tarragon for
the basil.

Nutritional value per serving	
Calories	105
Fat, total	11 g
Fat, saturated	2 g
Cholesterol	0 mg
Sodium	78 mg
Carbohydrate	1 g
Fiber	0 g
Protein	0 g
Calcium	4 mg
Iron	0 mg

Poppy Seed Dressing

⅓ cup	white (granulated) sugar	75 mL
1 tbsp	poppy seeds	15 mL
1 cup	GF mayonnaise	250 mL
¼ cup	milk	50 mL
2 tbsp	cider vinegar	25 mL

Whether or not you like poppy seeds, you'll love this creamy dressing.

Tip

To enhance the flavor of the dressing, let it stand at room temperature for up to 30 minutes before serving.

1. In a blender or food processor, combine sugar, poppy seeds, mayonnaise, milk and vinegar; process until smooth.

2. Transfer to a bowl and set aside for at least 1 hour or cover and refrigerate overnight to let flavors develop and blend. Store in an airtight container in the refrigerator for up to 3 weeks.

Variation

Substitute ½ cup (125 mL) GF sour cream or drained plain yogurt for half the mayonnaise.

Nutritional value per serving	
Calories	76
Fat, total	6 g
Fat, saturated	1 g
Cholesterol	6 mg
Sodium	130 mg
Carbohydrate	6 g
Fiber	0 g
Protein	0 g
Calcium	15 mg
Iron	0 mg

Roasted Garlic Caesar Dressing

**Makes about 1½ cups
(375 mL)
(2 tbsp/25 mL per
serving)**

*We tried a salad with
this dressing in a
restaurant on our way
to the Canadian Celiac
Association Conference
in Victoria, British
Columbia. Garlic
becomes sweet with
roasting and adds a
subtle flavor to the
dressing.*

Tips

For information on roasting
garlic, see the Techniques
Glossary, page 396.

Try drizzling this
dressing over cold cooked
asparagus.

1	head garlic, roasted and cloves mashed	1
1 tbsp	white (granulated) sugar	15 mL
⅛ tsp	freshly ground black pepper	0.5 mL
¾ cup	extra virgin olive oil	175 mL
¼ cup	freshly squeezed lemon juice	50 mL
2 tbsp	Dijon mustard	25 mL

1. In a small bowl, whisk together garlic, sugar, pepper, oil, lemon juice and mustard. Cover and refrigerate overnight to let flavors develop and blend.

2. Remove dressing from refrigerator and let stand at room temperature at least 30 minutes before serving. Stir or shake well before serving.

3. Store in an airtight container in the refrigerator for up to 3 weeks.

Variation

The dressing will solidify in the refrigerator due to the olive oil. You could use another kind of vegetable oil to replace some or all of the olive oil, if you prefer.

Nutritional value per serving

Calories	110
Fat, total	11 g
Fat, saturated	2 g
Cholesterol	0 mg
Sodium	51 mg
Carbohydrate	2 g
Fiber	0 g
Protein	0 g
Calcium	6 mg
Iron	0 mg

Whole-Grain Croutons

Makes 4 dozen croutons (6 per serving)

Here's a healthy version of croutons to top off a salad.

Tip

Use an electric knife or a knife with a serrated edge to cube bread slices.

- Preheat oven to 375°F (190°C)
- Rimmed baking sheet

4	slices day-old Historic Grains Bread (page 202 or 230), cut into 1-inch (2.5 cm) cubes	4
1 tbsp	extra virgin olive oil	15 mL
2 tbsp	dried tarragon	25 mL

1. In a bowl, toss bread cubes with olive oil and tarragon. Spread in a single layer on baking sheet. Bake in preheated oven, turning often, for 10 to 15 minutes or until crisp and golden. Let cool completely on baking sheet.

2. Use immediately or store in an airtight container at room temperature for up to 3 weeks.

Variation

Use any other leftover day-old GF bread.

Nutritional value per serving

Calories	103
Fat, total	4 g
Fat, saturated	1 g
Cholesterol	13 mg
Sodium	107 mg
Carbohydrate	14 g
Fiber	2 g
Protein	3 g
Calcium	32 mg
Iron	2 mg

Blue Cheese Croutons

**Makes about 2 cups
(500 mL)
(¼ cup/50 mL per
serving)**

*Add tang to any soup
or salad with these
delightful cheesy
croutons.*

Tips

Two slices of bread
will yield about 2 cups
(500 mL) bread cubes.

The baking time depends
on how dry the bread
cubes are.

- **Preheat oven to 375°F (190°C)**
- **Rimmed baking sheet**

2 cups	cubed GF bread	500 mL
2 tbsp	crumbled GF blue cheese	25 mL
1 tbsp	finely snipped fresh parsley	15 mL
2 tbsp	red wine vinegar	25 mL
1 tbsp	extra virgin olive oil	15 mL
1 tbsp	Dijon mustard	15 mL

1. Spread bread cubes in a single layer on baking sheet. Bake in preheated oven, turning often, for 15 minutes or until crisp.

2. Meanwhile, in a bowl, whisk together blue cheese, parsley, vinegar, oil and mustard. Add warm croutons and toss to coat.

3. Return to baking sheet and bake, turning often, for 10 to 15 minutes or until deep golden and crisp. Let cool completely on baking sheet.

4. Use immediately or store in an airtight container in the refrigerator for up to 2 days.

Variation
Substitute finely chopped walnuts for the parsley.

Nutritional value per serving	
Calories	39
Fat, total	2 g
Fat, saturated	0 g
Cholesterol	1 mg
Sodium	104 mg
Carbohydrate	4 g
Fiber	0 g
Protein	1 g
Calcium	12 mg
Iron	0 mg

Cream Sauce

**Makes about 1 cup
(250 mL)
(¼ cup/50 mL per
serving)**

*A smooth, creamy
sauce is a great
starting point for
many flavorful dishes.
You can use the thin
sauce in cream soups;
the medium sauce in
cheese sauce (as on
page 84), vegetable
sauce, casseroles and
pot pie; and the thick
sauce in croquettes,
soufflés and puddings.*

Tips

The shortest cooking
time is for thin sauce; the
longest, for thick.

Use a 4-cup (1 L)
microwave-safe measuring
cup to prepare the sauce.

Thin Cream Sauce

1 tbsp	butter	15 mL
1 tbsp	amaranth flour	15 mL
1 cup	milk	250 mL
	Salt and freshly ground black pepper	

Medium Cream Sauce

2 tbsp	butter	25 mL
2 tbsp	amaranth flour	25 mL
1 cup	milk	250 mL
	Salt and freshly ground black pepper	

Thick Cream Sauce

3 tbsp	butter	45 mL
3 tbsp	amaranth flour	45 mL
1 cup	milk	250 mL
	Salt and freshly ground black pepper	

1. In a microwave-safe bowl, microwave butter on High
for 1 to 3 minutes or until melted. Stir in amaranth
flour and microwave on High for 1 to 3 minutes or
until mixture is the consistency of dry sand. Stir in milk
and microwave on High for 3 to 5 minutes, stirring
occasionally, until mixture comes to a boil and has
thickened. Season to taste with salt and pepper.

Thin Cream Sauce • Nutritional value per serving	
Calories	58
Fat, total	4 g
Fat, saturated	2 g
Cholesterol	10 mg
Sodium	59 mg
Carbohydrate	4 g
Fiber	0 g
Protein	2 g
Calcium	78 mg
Iron	1 mg

Medium Cream Sauce • Nutritional value per serving	
Calories	90
Fat, total	7 g
Fat, saturated	4 g
Cholesterol	18 mg
Sodium	88 mg
Carbohydrate	5 g
Fiber	0 g
Protein	3 g
Calcium	82 mg
Iron	1 mg

Thick Cream Sauce • Nutritional value per serving	
Calories	122
Fat, total	9 g
Fat, saturated	6 g
Cholesterol	25 mg
Sodium	117 mg
Carbohydrate	6 g
Fiber	0 g
Protein	3 g
Calcium	85 mg
Iron	1 mg

Cheese Sauce

Egg-free
White sugar–free

**Makes about 2 cups
(500 mL)
(1/4 cup/50 mL per
serving)**

*Use this sauce to make
macaroni and cheese,
to serve over cooked
vegetables or as the
base for a cheese
soufflé. It can easily
be halved or doubled.*

Tip

Add the cheese as soon
as you remove the cream
sauce from the microwave;
otherwise, it won't all melt.

1/2 cup	shredded sharp (old) Cheddar cheese	125 mL
1/4 cup	shredded Swiss cheese	50 mL
2 tbsp	freshly grated Parmesan cheese	25 mL
2 cups	hot Medium Cream Sauce (page 83)	500 mL

1. In a small bowl, combine Cheddar, Swiss and Parmesan. Add to hot cream sauce and stir until cheese is melted.

Variation

Substitute Asiago, Emmental, Roquefort, Romano or any other cheeses for the Cheddar, Swiss and/or Parmesan.

Nutritional value per serving	
Calories	138
Fat, total	10 g
Fat, saturated	6 g
Cholesterol	30 mg
Sodium	142 mg
Carbohydrate	6 g
Fiber	0 g
Protein	6 g
Calcium	187 mg
Iron	1 mg

Red Onion Marmalade

Makes about 1½ cups (375 mL) (2 tbsp/25 mL per serving)

The sweet and tart flavors of Red Onion Marmalade make it a perfect accompaniment for pork dishes — a change from traditional applesauce.

Tips

Four red onions weigh about 2 lbs (1 kg).

Double the recipe and freeze it in smaller amounts to serve with your next pork roast.

2 tbsp	extra virgin olive oil	25 mL
4	red onions, finely sliced	4
¼ cup	balsamic vinegar	50 mL
2 tbsp	pure maple syrup	25 mL
1 tsp	salt	5 mL
½ tsp	freshly ground black pepper	2 mL

1. In a large saucepan, heat oil over medium-low heat. Add red onions and cook, stirring occasionally, for 45 to 60 minutes or until very soft and transparent.

2. Add vinegar, maple syrup, salt and pepper; cook, stirring often, for 20 to 25 minutes or until liquid has evaporated and onions are of marmalade consistency.

3. Store in an airtight container in the refrigerator for up to 1 week or in the freezer for up to 6 months.

Variation
Substitute Vidalia onions for the red.

Nutritional value per serving

Calories	38
Fat, total	2 g
Fat, saturated	0 g
Cholesterol	0 mg
Sodium	158 mg
Carbohydrate	5 g
Fiber	1 g
Protein	0 g
Calcium	9 mg
Iron	0 mg

Roasted Red Pepper Coulis

**Makes about 2 cups
(500 mL)
(2 tbsp/25 mL per
serving)**

*Choose one of the
many flavors that
follow to provide
variety. We like to
serve this with our
Chunky Crab Cakes
(page 134) and to
accompany asparagus
or any fresh vegetable.*

Tips

We recommend using only
red bell peppers, as the
skins of Sheppard peppers
are too difficult to remove
after roasting.

The main recipe and all
of the flavor variations
below can be stored in
an airtight container in
the refrigerator for up to
1 week.

• Preheat oven to 400°F (200°C)
• 13- by 9-inch (33 by 23 cm) square baking pan

| 6 | large red bell peppers | 6 |

1. Place peppers in baking pan and roast in preheated oven
   for 30 minutes. Turn and roast for 25 to 30 minutes
   longer or until skins are well charred and blistered and
   peppers are soft.

2. Remove from oven and place peppers in a plastic or
   paper bag. Close bag and let peppers steam for 10 to
   15 minutes or until skins loosen. Peel skin from peppers.
   Seed peppers and cut into strips.

3. Transfer peppers to a food processor and purée until
   smooth.

Oregano and Chive–Flavored

Egg-free / White sugar–free

1 cup	Roasted Red Pepper Coulis	250 mL
½ cup	snipped fresh oregano	125 mL
¼ cup	snipped fresh chives	50 mL
¼ cup	plain yogurt or GF sour cream	50 mL

1. In a food processor or blender, purée coulis, oregano,
   chives and yogurt until smooth.

2. Transfer to a bowl, cover and refrigerate overnight to
   let flavors develop and blend.

Oregano and Chive–Flavored • Nutritional value per serving			
Calories	17	Carbohydrate	4 g
Fat, total	0 g	Fiber	1 g
Fat, saturated	0 g	Protein	1 g
Cholesterol	0 mg	Calcium	18 mg
Sodium	3 mg	Iron	0 mg

Cilantro and Parsley–Flavored

Dairy-free / Lactose-free / Egg-free / White sugar–free

1 cup	Roasted Red Pepper Coulis	250 mL
2 tbsp	snipped fresh cilantro	25 mL
2 tbsp	snipped fresh parsley	25 mL
1 tbsp	extra virgin olive oil	15 mL

1. In a food processor or blender, purée coulis, cilantro, parsley and oil until smooth.
2. Transfer to a bowl, cover and refrigerate overnight to let flavors develop and blend.

Cilantro and Parsley–Flavored • Nutritional value per serving			
Calories	20	Carbohydrate	3 g
Fat, total	1 g	Fiber	1 g
Fat, saturated	0 g	Protein	0 g
Cholesterol	0 mg	Calcium	5 mg
Sodium	1 mg	Iron	0 mg

Horseradish-Flavored

Egg-free / White sugar–free

1 cup	Roasted Red Pepper Coulis	250 mL
1/4 cup	plain yogurt or GF sour cream	50 mL
1 tbsp	prepared horseradish	15 mL

1. In a food processor or blender, purée coulis, yogurt and horseradish until smooth.
2. Transfer to a bowl, cover and refrigerate overnight to let flavors develop and blend.

Horseradish–Flavored • Nutritional value per serving			
Calories	17	Carbohydrate	3 g
Fat, total	0 g	Fiber	1 g
Fat, saturated	0 g	Protein	1 g
Cholesterol	0 mg	Calcium	11 mg
Sodium	4 mg	Iron	0 mg

Hot Pepper–Flavored

Dairy-free / Lactose-free / White sugar–free

1 cup	Roasted Red Pepper Coulis	250 mL
2 tbsp	GF mayonnaise	25 mL
1 tbsp	extra virgin olive oil	15 mL
¼ tsp	cayenne pepper	1 mL
¼ tsp	hot pepper sauce	1 mL

1. In a food processor or blender, purée coulis, mayonnaise, oil, cayenne and hot pepper sauce until smooth.
2. Transfer to a bowl, cover and refrigerate overnight to let flavors develop and blend.

Hot Pepper–Flavored • Nutritional value per serving			
Calories	30	Carbohydrate	3 g
Fat, total	2 g	Fiber	1 g
Fat, saturated	0 g	Protein	0 g
Cholesterol	1 mg	Calcium	5 mg
Sodium	10 mg	Iron	0 mg

Chipotle-Flavored

Dairy-free/ Lactose-free / Egg-free / White sugar–free

1 cup	Roasted Red Pepper Coulis	250 mL
1	chipotle pepper in adobo sauce	1

1. In a food processor or blender, purée coulis and chipotle pepper in adobo sauce until smooth.
2. Transfer to a bowl, cover and refrigerate overnight to let flavors develop and blend.

Chipotle–Flavored • Nutritional value per serving			
Calories	13	Carbohydrate	3 g
Fat, total	0 g	Fiber	1 g
Fat, saturated	0 g	Protein	0 g
Cholesterol	0 mg	Calcium	4 mg
Sodium	4 mg	Iron	0 mg

Pineapple Mango Relish

**Makes about 2 cups
(500 mL)
(½ cup/125 mL per
serving)**

*Although Heather
grew up with the
California Ham Loaf
(page 142) topped
with canned pineapple
rings, she enjoys this
fresh relish in their
place.*

Tips

For information on fresh
mangos, see the Techniques
Glossary, page 397.

This recipe can be doubled.

Serve with luncheon ham
salad, entrée fish dishes or
a modern grilled cheese
sandwich.

1	mango, diced	1
1 cup	diced fresh pineapple	250 mL
¼ cup	diced green bell pepper	50 mL
2 tbsp	red onion, finely chopped	25 mL
1 tsp	snipped fresh cilantro	5 mL
¾ tsp	white (granulated) sugar	4 mL
¼ cup	freshly squeezed orange juice	50 mL
¾ tsp	red wine vinegar	4 mL
½ tsp	extra virgin olive oil	2 mL

1. In a large bowl, combine mango, pineapple, green
   pepper, red onion, cilantro, sugar, orange juice, vinegar
   and oil.

2. Cover and refrigerate for at least 2 hours to let flavors
   develop and blend. Store in an airtight container in the
   refrigerator for up to 2 weeks.

Variations

For a spicier relish, add ½ tsp (2 mL) finely chopped
seeded jalapeño pepper and 1 tsp (5 mL) snipped fresh
mint.

Substitute 1½ cups (375 mL) diced papaya or guava for
the mango.

Nutritional value per serving	
Calories	72
Fat, total	1 g
Fat, saturated	0 g
Cholesterol	0 mg
Sodium	2 mg
Carbohydrate	17 g
Fiber	2 g
Protein	1 g
Calcium	11 mg
Iron	0 mg

A Page from Deanna's Diary

GROWING UP ON a gluten-free diet can be challenging sometimes, because it feels like there is never enough variety to what you can eat. It only seems this way because there aren't as many convenient food choices available. The best strategy I've found to deal with this is to learn to cook and bake for yourself. You may or may not be the only one in your family on a gluten-free diet, but there are always more choices if you make the extra effort.

We have to use some extra initiative and creativity to learn to cook and bake at home. First, make sure all your ingredients are gluten-free, and that your utensils and work area are clean. When I was a young child, my mom and I started baking with prepared mixes we bought. These usually turned out quite well, and we started to experiment a bit. Later, we were able to find recipes to make our own mixes, which saved us lots of time. Typically, gluten-free baking recipes have about twice as many ingredients as wheat recipes, so plan ahead a bit and help make the grocery list.

As for cooking, you might be surprised by how many recipes you can easily make without changing them much at all. Cooking is all about trying new things and experimenting. I know from experience that things don't always work the way you want them to the first time.

In our kitchen, we have a container of gluten-free flour mix, which we substitute in a recipe if it calls for just a small amount of flour. But most of my favorite things to cook don't use any flour at all: rice pasta, hamburgers (on a gluten-free bun, of course), fried rice, French toast (again, gluten-free bread), taco salad and yogurt smoothies.

Start out by helping to make dinner a few times a week, and you'll learn so many new things. Your favorite recipes and a few good cookbooks will be your best resource as you learn to cook at home, with other family members, and then prepare to cope on your own. One day, you'll be able to make all these things without any help, and they'll taste even better because you made them yourself.

— *Deanna Jennett, Kingston, Ontario*

Authors' note: Deanna and her mother, Sue, have been celiac friends of ours since before we began developing gluten-free recipes in 2001. Deanna, now a teenager, shares her point of view in each of our gluten-free cookbooks to help other young celiacs.

Snacks, Starters, Salads and Soups

Lemon Pepper Thins

**Dairy-free
Lactose-free
Egg-free
White sugar–free**

**Makes about 32 crackers
(¹/₁₆ recipe per serving)**

Keep this thin, crisp cracker handy to serve with cheese, salsa or dip.

Tips

Spread batter to an even thickness, right to the edges of the pan; this ensures that the center is cooked before the edges become too dark.

Watch these carefully during baking — even as little as 1 minute too long can cause edges to burn.

Store in an airtight container at room temperature for up to 3 weeks.

If difficult to remove from the pan, place in a 300°F (150°C) oven for 2 to 3 minutes and remove immediately.

Nutritional value per serving

Calories	30
Fat, total	1 g
Fat, saturated	0 g
Cholesterol	0 mg
Sodium	76 mg
Carbohydrate	4 g
Fiber	1 g
Protein	1 g
Calcium	9 mg
Iron	1 mg

- Preheat oven to 300°F (150°C)
- 15- by 10-inch (40 by 25 cm) jelly roll pan, lightly greased

¹/₂ cup	water	125 mL
2 tbsp	grated lemon zest	25 mL
¹/₄ cup	freshly squeezed lemon juice	50 mL
1 tbsp	vegetable oil	15 mL
³/₄ cup	amaranth flour	175 mL
¹/₂ tsp	baking soda	2 mL
¹/₂ tsp	freshly cracked black pepper	2 mL
¹/₄ tsp	salt	1 mL

1. In a small bowl, whisk together water, lemon zest, lemon juice and oil. Set aside.

2. In a food processor, pulse amaranth flour, baking soda, pepper and salt until combined. With the motor running, through the feed tube, gradually add water mixture in a steady stream. Process for 30 seconds or until smooth and lump-free.

3. Drop dough by heaping spoonfuls onto prepared pan. Spread evenly right to the edges with a moist rubber spatula.

4. Bake on top rack of preheated oven for 15 to 20 minutes or until golden brown. (Watch carefully, as it browns and burns quickly.) Turn off oven and let cool in the oven for 1 hour. Remove from oven and break into pieces.

Variations

Add 2 tbsp (25 mL) chopped crumbled dried rosemary to the batter. Sprinkle with 2 tbsp (25 mL) freshly grated Parmesan cheese just before baking.

Substitute ¹/₄ tsp (1 mL) freshly ground black pepper for the cracked.

Sesame Crispbread

**Makes about 32 crackers
($\frac{1}{16}$ recipe per serving)**

Quick and easy to make, this crisp flatbread is similar to chapati in texture, appearance and use.

Tips

For information on toasting sesame seeds, see the Techniques Glossary, page 399. This is an important step for the flavor of the crispbread.

Spreading the dough is similar to patting out pizza dough; continue all the way to the edge, or it will be too thick.

During baking, the crispbread will crack and curl up.

Store in an airtight container at room temperature for up to 3 months.

- Preheat oven to 400°F (200°C)
- 15- by 10-inch (40 by 25 cm) jelly roll pan, lightly greased

$\frac{3}{4}$ cup	water	175 mL
1 tbsp	vegetable oil	15 mL
$\frac{3}{4}$ cup	brown rice flour	175 mL
$\frac{1}{3}$ cup	tapioca starch	75 mL
1 tsp	white (granulated) sugar	5 mL
$1\frac{1}{2}$ tsp	xanthan gum	7 mL
$\frac{1}{2}$ tsp	GF baking powder	2 mL
$\frac{1}{2}$ tsp	salt	2 mL
$\frac{1}{2}$ cup	sesame seeds, toasted	125 mL
1 to 2 tbsp	sweet rice flour	15 to 25 mL

1. In a small bowl, whisk together water and oil. Set aside.

2. In a food processor, pulse brown rice flour, tapioca starch, sugar, xanthan gum, baking powder, salt and sesame seeds until combined. With the motor running, through the feed tube, gradually add water mixture in a steady stream. Process for 15 seconds or until smooth and lump-free.

3. Drop dough by heaping spoonfuls onto prepared pan. Sprinkle with sweet rice flour. With floured fingers, gently and evenly pat out dough right to the edges of the pan, sprinkling with sweet rice flour as required.

4. Bake in preheated oven for 20 to 23 minutes or until lightly browned. Let cool in pan on a wire rack. Break into large pieces.

Variations

Add 1 to 2 tbsp (15 to 25 mL) dried herbs with the sesame seeds. Sprinkle the dough with 2 tbsp (25 mL) freshly grated Parmesan cheese just before baking.

For a stronger sesame flavor, substitute sesame oil for the vegetable oil.

Nutritional value per serving	
Calories	75
Fat, total	3 g
Fat, saturated	0 g
Cholesterol	0 mg
Sodium	74 mg
Carbohydrate	10 g
Fiber	1 g
Protein	1 g
Calcium	55 mg
Iron	1 mg

Sun-Dried Tomato Lavosh

Makes about 48 crackers ($\frac{1}{16}$ recipe per serving)

Keep this fat-free crisp on hand to serve as a snack, with fresh vegetables or with soup or salad. It's the perfect addition to a basket of fresh rolls.

- Preheat oven to 375°F (190°C)
- 15- by 10-inch (40 by 25 cm) jelly roll pan, lightly greased

$\frac{1}{2}$ cup	sorghum flour	125 mL
$\frac{1}{3}$ cup	whole bean flour	75 mL
$\frac{1}{4}$ cup	tapioca starch	50 mL
1 tsp	white (granulated) sugar	5 mL
$\frac{1}{2}$ tsp	xanthan gum	2 mL
$1\frac{1}{2}$ tsp	bread machine or instant yeast	7 mL
$\frac{1}{2}$ tsp	salt	2 mL
2 tbsp	dried basil	25 mL
$\frac{2}{3}$ cup	snipped sun-dried tomatoes (see tip, at right)	150 mL
$\frac{3}{4}$ cup	water	175 mL
1 tsp	cider vinegar	5 mL
2 tbsp	extra virgin olive oil	25 mL
$\frac{1}{2}$ cup	freshly grated Parmesan cheese, divided	125 mL

Bread Machine Method

1. In a large bowl or plastic bag, combine sorghum flour, whole bean flour, tapioca starch, sugar, xanthan gum, yeast, salt, basil and tomatoes. Mix well and set aside.

2. Pour water, vinegar and oil into the bread machine baking pan. Select the **Dough Cycle**. As the bread machine is mixing, gradually add the dry ingredients, scraping bottom and sides of pan with a rubber spatula. Try to incorporate all the dry ingredients within 1 to 2 minutes. Stop bread machine as soon as the kneading portion of the cycle is complete. Do not let bread machine finish the cycle.

Mixer Method

1. In a large bowl or plastic bag, combine sorghum flour, whole bean flour, tapioca starch, sugar, xanthan gum, yeast, salt, basil and tomatoes. Mix well and set aside.

2. In a separate bowl, using a heavy-duty electric mixer with paddle attachment, combine water, vinegar and oil until well blended. With the mixer on its lowest speed, slowly add the dry ingredients until combined. Stop the machine and scrape the bottom and sides of the bowl with a rubber spatula. With the mixer on medium speed, beat for 4 minutes.

Nutritional value per serving	
Calories	64
Fat, total	3 g
Fat, saturated	1 g
Cholesterol	2 mg
Sodium	178 mg
Carbohydrate	8 g
Fiber	1 g
Protein	3 g
Calcium	57 mg
Iron	1 mg

Tips

Purchase dry, not oil-packed, sun-dried tomatoes. Snip them with kitchen shears.

The thinner the dough is spread, the more authentic the cracker will be. To more easily spread the dough, moisten the rubber spatula as needed. Don't worry: you can't use too much water. If you create holes, that's fine — just leave them.

Store in an airtight container at room temperature for up to 3 months. If necessary, crisp the lavosh in a 300°F (150°C) oven for 5 minutes before serving.

For Both Methods

3. Sprinkle prepared pan with half the Parmesan. Remove dough to prepared pan. With a moistened rubber spatula, spread out the dough to fill the pan evenly, sprinkling with Parmesan if dough becomes too sticky to handle. Sprinkle with the remaining Parmesan and press lightly into dough.

4. Bake in preheated oven for 16 to 18 minutes or until golden brown. Turn off oven and let cool in the oven for 1 hour. Remove from oven and break into pieces.

Variations

Add 2 to 3 cloves of roasted garlic with the dry ingredients, or, for a stronger flavor, use minced fresh garlic.

Substitute Romano or Asiago cheese for the Parmesan.

Oatcakes

*A crunchy cracker
to serve with cheese!
Who can eat just one?*

Tips

Place one baking sheet
in the bottom third of
the oven and the other
in the top third. Rotate
the sheets and switch
their positions halfway
through the baking time.
Watch carefully during
baking — even a couple
of minutes extra can cause
the oatcakes to burn.

Store in an airtight
container at room
temperature for up to
3 days or in the freezer
for up to 1 month.

- 2-inch (5 cm) round cookie cutter
- 2 baking sheets, lined with parchment paper

2 cups	GF large-flake rolled oats	500 mL
1/2 cup	walnuts, coarsely chopped	125 mL
1/2 cup	amaranth flour	125 mL
1/4 cup	quinoa flour	50 mL
1/4 cup	potato starch	50 mL
2 tbsp	packed brown sugar	25 mL
1 1/2 tsp	GF baking powder	7 mL
1 1/2 tsp	xanthan gum	7 mL
1/2 tsp	salt	2 mL
1/2 cup	cold butter, cut into 1-inch (2.5 cm) cubes	125 mL
3/4 cup	buttermilk	175 mL

Food Processor Method

1. In a food processor, pulse oats, walnuts, amaranth
flour, quinoa flour, potato starch, brown sugar, baking
powder, xanthan gum and salt until combined. Add
butter and pulse for 5 to 7 seconds or until mixture
resembles coarse crumbs (about the size of small peas).
Add buttermilk all at once and process, stopping and
scraping the bottom and sides occasionally, until dough
begins to hold together.

Traditional Method

1. In a large bowl, combine oats, walnuts, amaranth
flour, quinoa flour, potato starch, brown sugar, baking
powder, xanthan gum and salt. Using a pastry blender
or two knives, cut in butter until mixture resembles
coarse crumbs (about the size of small peas). Add
buttermilk all at once, stirring with a fork to make a
thick dough.

Nutritional value per serving

Calories	45
Fat, total	3 g
Fat, saturated	1 g
Cholesterol	4 mg
Sodium	39 mg
Carbohydrate	5 g
Fiber	1 g
Protein	1 g
Calcium	15 mg
Iron	1 mg

Tip

If you don't have buttermilk on hand, add 1 tsp (5 mL) lemon juice to ¾ cup (175 mL) milk; let stand for 5 minutes, then use as a substitute.

For Both Methods

2. Divide dough in half and pat each half into a disc about ½ inch (1 cm) thick. Wrap in plastic wrap and refrigerate for at least 30 minutes, until chilled, or for up to 24 hours. Meanwhile, preheat oven to 325°F (160°C).

3. Remove from refrigerator and let stand for 5 minutes. Place each disc between 2 sheets of parchment paper and roll out to ⅛-inch (3 mm) thick. Using the cookie cutter, cut into rounds, rerolling scraps. Place 1 inch (2.5 cm) apart on prepared baking sheets.

4. Bake for 15 to 17 minutes or until edges are crisp and golden. Remove from pan and let cool completely on a wire rack.

Savory Onion Toastie

**Makes 8 wedges
(1 per serving)**

Instead of using this open-textured bread for a sandwich, we've put an onion topping on it.

Tip

Before measuring honey, coat the measuring spoon with vegetable spray — the honey will flow more easily and rapidly.

- 12-inch (30 cm) pizza pan, lightly greased and sprinkled with cornmeal

Onion Topping

2 tbsp	butter	25 mL
4	onions, finely chopped	4
2 tbsp	snipped fresh thyme	25 mL
2 tbsp	liquid honey	25 mL

Toastie

1½ cups	water	375 mL
¼ cup	vegetable oil	50 mL
2 tsp	cider vinegar	10 mL
1 cup	whole bean flour	250 mL
1 cup	sorghum flour	250 mL
⅓ cup	tapioca starch	75 mL
1 tsp	white (granulated) sugar	5 mL
1 tsp	xanthan gum	5 mL
1 tbsp	bread machine or instant yeast	15 mL
1 tsp	salt	5 mL
	Sweet rice flour	
½ cup	freshly grated Parmesan cheese	125 mL

1. *Topping:* In a skillet, melt butter over medium-low heat. Sauté onions for 20 minutes or until tender and light golden brown. Remove from heat and stir in thyme and honey. Let cool slightly.

2. *Toastie:* Meanwhile, in a small bowl, combine water, oil and vinegar. Set aside.

3. In a food processor, pulse whole bean flour, sorghum flour, tapioca starch, sugar, xanthan gum, yeast and salt until combined. With the motor running, through the feed tube, gradually add water mixture in a steady stream. Pulse until dough holds together.

4. Drop dough by large spoonfuls on prepared pan. Spread evenly with a water-moistened rubber spatula. Generously dust top with sweet rice flour. With well-floured fingers, make deep indents all over the dough, making sure to press all the way down to the pan. Let rise, uncovered, in a warm, draft-free place for 20 minutes.

Nutritional value per serving

Calories	260
Fat, total	12 g
Fat, saturated	4 g
Cholesterol	13 mg
Sodium	327 mg
Carbohydrate	32 g
Fiber	7 g
Protein	7 g
Calcium	116 mg
Iron	2 mg

5. Meanwhile, preheat oven to 400°F (200°C).

6. Sprinkle dough with Parmesan. Spread onion mixture over cheese.

7. Bake for 20 to 25 minutes or until top is golden. Remove from pan immediately, cut into 8 wedges and serve warm.

Variation
For a more tender crust, substitute GF beer for the water.

Crispy Calamari

Makes 4 servings

*Donna's nephew
and wife often enjoy
calamari (squid) as
an appetizer in their
favorite restaurant.
Serve with Yogurt Dill
Dip (page 76).*

Tips

The cayenne pepper helps
the batter to brown, but
if cayenne is too hot for
your taste, omit it and
add another $\frac{1}{2}$ tsp (2 mL)
paprika.

You can use cleaned fresh
squid rings instead of
frozen.

Use this coating to make
onion rings as well.

• Candy/deep-fry thermometer

$\frac{1}{4}$ cup	sweet rice flour	50 mL
2 tbsp	cornstarch	25 mL
$\frac{1}{2}$ tsp	paprika	2 mL
$\frac{1}{4}$ tsp	cayenne pepper	1 mL
1 lb	frozen calamari (squid) rings, thawed and patted dry	500 g
	Vegetable oil	
$\frac{1}{4}$ tsp	salt	1 mL
	Lemon wedges	

1. In a plastic bag, combine sweet rice flour, cornstarch, paprika and cayenne. Add calamari and shake to coat. Transfer to a sieve and shake off excess flour mixture.

2. In a wok or a deep saucepan, heat $1\frac{1}{2}$ to 2 inches (4 to 5 cm) of oil until it registers 375°F (190°C) on the thermometer. Working in batches, fry calamari for 2 to 3 minutes or until golden. Using a slotted spoon, transfer to a plate lined with paper towels. Sprinkle with salt just before serving. Serve with lemon wedges to squeeze over top.

Nutritional value per serving	
Calories	209
Fat, total	6 g
Fat, saturated	1 g
Cholesterol	320 mg
Sodium	248 mg
Carbohydrate	16 g
Fiber	0 g
Protein	22 g
Calcium	48 mg
Iron	1 mg

Mussels Provençal

Makes 8 servings as an appetizer or 4 servings as an entrée

Summer tomatoes, fresh basil and sweet tarragon make these mussels fit for any gourmet.

Tips

It's important to check to make sure mussels are alive before cooking them. If any are open, tap them with your finger; discard any that stay open. Then, using a paper towel, grab the beard and firmly tug to remove. Rinse mussels under cold running water, scrubbing the shells with a small firm brush to remove any sand.

Instead of fresh tomatoes, you can use a 28-oz (796 mL) can, drained.

6	cloves garlic, minced	6
¼ cup	snipped fresh tarragon	50 mL
1 cup	clam juice	250 mL
1 cup	dry white wine	250 mL
10	large tomatoes, coarsely chopped	10
½ cup	snipped fresh basil	125 mL
4 lbs	fresh mussels, scrubbed and debearded (see tip, at left)	2 kg
	Salt and freshly ground black pepper	

1. In a large saucepan, bring garlic, tarragon, clam juice and wine to a boil over medium heat. Boil for 6 to 8 minutes or until liquid is reduced by half. Stir in tomatoes, basil and mussels. Cover and boil for 6 to 8 minutes or until mussels have opened. Discard any mussels that have not opened. Season to taste with salt and pepper.

Nutritional value per serving	
Calories	254
Fat, total	6 g
Fat, saturated	1 g
Cholesterol	64 mg
Sodium	766 mg
Carbohydrate	17 g
Fiber	2 g
Protein	29 g
Calcium	87 mg
Iron	10 mg

Spinach Cheese Squares

**Makes 12 squares
(1 per serving)**

Serve warm or cold, as a starter or to accompany a salad.

Tips

For 4 cups (1 L) spinach, you'll need about 6 oz (175 g). All prepackaged greens should be washed under lots of cold running water just before use and drained well.

Refrigerate cheese squares in an airtight container for up to 3 days, or wrap airtight and freeze for up to 1 month.

- Preheat oven to 375°F (190°C)
- 9-inch (23 cm) square baking pan, lightly greased and lined with parchment paper

½ cup	low-fat soy flour	125 mL
¼ cup	brown rice flour	50 mL
¼ cup	tapioca starch	50 mL
1½ tsp	xanthan gum	7 mL
2 tsp	GF baking powder	10 mL
½ tsp	salt	2 mL
1 tsp	dry mustard	5 mL
3	eggs	3
1 cup	milk	250 mL
¼ cup	vegetable oil	50 mL
4 cups	packed spinach, trimmed and coarsely chopped	1 L
2 cups	shredded aged Cheddar cheese	500 mL

1. In a bowl or plastic bag, combine soy flour, brown rice flour, tapioca starch, xanthan gum, baking powder, salt and mustard. Mix well and set aside.

2. In a separate bowl, using an electric mixer, beat eggs, milk and oil until combined. Add dry ingredients and mix until smooth. With mixer on low speed, stir in spinach and cheese.

3. Spoon batter into prepared pan. Bake in preheated oven for 25 to 30 minutes or until golden brown and a tester inserted in the center comes out clean. Let cool in pan on a wire rack for 10 minutes.

Variations

Cook 5 slices of GF bacon until crisp. Crumble and fold into the batter with the spinach.

Add 1 to 2 tsp (5 to 10 mL) dried dillweed to the flour mixture in step 1.

Nutritional value per serving

Calories	181
Fat, total	12 g
Fat, saturated	5 g
Cholesterol	67 mg
Sodium	248 mg
Carbohydrate	9 g
Fiber	1 g
Protein	9 g
Calcium	224 mg
Iron	1 mg

Mediterranean Pasta Salad

**Makes 4 servings
(1 cup/250 mL per
serving)**

This easy make-ahead pasta salad bursts with savory Mediterranean flavor.

Tips

Chickpeas are also known as garbanzo beans.

We always wash packaged greens, even those labeled "prewashed."

Dressing

4	cloves garlic, minced	4
¼ cup	fresh oregano leaves, snipped	50 mL
½ cup	extra virgin olive oil	125 mL
3 tbsp	red wine vinegar	45 mL

Salad

4 cups	packed baby spinach	1 L
1½ cups	GF fusilli, rotini or small shell pasta, cooked and cooled	375 mL
1 cup	grape tomatoes	250 mL
1 cup	crumbled feta cheese	250 mL
½ cup	rinsed drained canned chickpeas	125 mL
½ cup	sliced kalamata olives	125 mL

1. *Dressing:* In a small bowl, whisk together garlic, oregano, oil and vinegar until well combined. Set aside.

2. *Salad:* In a large bowl, combine spinach, pasta, tomatoes, feta, chickpeas and olives. Pour in dressing and toss lightly to coat.

3. Cover and refrigerate for at least 2 hours, until chilled, or for up to 3 days.

Variation

Add sliced artichoke hearts and red onion rings to the salad.

Nutritional value per serving

Calories	512
Fat, total	40 g
Fat, saturated	10 g
Cholesterol	33 mg
Sodium	622 mg
Carbohydrate	30 g
Fiber	5 g
Protein	11 g
Calcium	292 mg
Iron	4 mg

Tuscan Black Bean Salad

Egg-free
White sugar–free

Makes 6 servings
(½ cup/125 mL per serving)

Here's a delicious way to add more legumes to your diet.

Tip

Purchase dry, not oil-packed, sun-dried tomatoes. Snip sun-dried tomatoes using kitchen shears.

3	cloves garlic, minced	3
¼ cup	extra virgin olive oil	50 mL
1 tbsp	grated lemon zest	15 mL
2 tbsp	freshly squeezed lemon juice	25 mL
¼ tsp	salt	1 mL
¼ tsp	freshly ground black pepper	1 mL
½ cup	thinly sliced sun-dried tomatoes	125 mL
1	can (14 to 19 oz/398 to 540 mL) black beans, drained and rinsed	1
½ cup	cubed Asiago cheese	125 mL

1. In a large bowl, whisk together garlic, oil, lemon zest, lemon juice, salt and pepper. Add tomatoes and beans; toss to coat.

2. Cover and refrigerate for at least 4 hours to let flavors develop and blend, or for up to 1 week. Add cheese right before serving.

Variation

Use a six-bean medley containing chickpeas (garbanzo beans), red kidney beans, black-eyed peas, white kidney beans, Romano beans and baby lima beans.

Nutritional value per serving

Calories	191
Fat, total	13 g
Fat, saturated	3 g
Cholesterol	10 mg
Sodium	588 mg
Carbohydrate	16 g
Fiber	4 g
Protein	7 g
Calcium	144 mg
Iron	2 mg

Lentil Squash Salad

Makes 12 servings (½ cup/125 mL per serving)

This is a good make-ahead dish for your next family get-together, and if you choose vegetable broth, it's vegetarian! It can be eaten cold or, if you prefer, heated in the microwave to serve hot.

Tips

A 3-lb (1.5 kg) butternut squash yields about 4 cups (1 L) diced.

For information on toasting seeds, see the Techniques Glossary, page 399.

Nutritional value per serving

Calories	129
Fat, total	4 g
Fat, saturated	1 g
Cholesterol	0 mg
Sodium	254 mg
Carbohydrate	19 g
Fiber	2 g
Protein	4 g
Calcium	36 mg
Iron	2 mg

• **Large microwave-safe casserole dish**

Dressing

1	clove garlic, minced	
2 tbsp	cider vinegar	25 mL
2 tbsp	liquid honey	25 mL
2 tbsp	vegetable oil	25 mL
2 tsp	Dijon mustard	10 mL

Salad

3 cups	GF vegetable or beef broth	750 mL
½ cup	dried red and/or green lentils	125 mL
½ cup	dried split peas	125 mL
1	butternut squash, diced	1
½ cup	dried cranberries	125 mL
½ cup	chopped green onions	125 mL
⅓ cup	green pumpkin seeds, toasted	75 mL
3 tbsp	snipped fresh tarragon	45 mL
	Salt and freshly ground black pepper	

1. *Dressing:* In a small bowl, whisk together garlic, vinegar, honey, oil and mustard. Set aside.

2. *Salad:* In a large saucepan, bring broth to a boil over high heat. Add lentils and split peas; return to a boil. Reduce heat to medium-low and simmer for 25 to 30 minutes or until tender. Drain and let cool.

3. In casserole dish, combine squash and 2 tbsp (25 mL) water. Cover and microwave on High for 10 to 12 minutes or until squash is fork-tender. Drain and set aside.

4. In a large bowl, combine lentils, split peas, squash, cranberries, green onions, pumpkin seeds and tarragon. Pour in dressing and toss to coat.

5. Cover and refrigerate for at least 8 hours, until chilled, or for up to 3 days. Season to taste with salt and pepper.

Variations

Substitute hubbard squash for the butternut, using about 4 cups (1 L) diced.

A 14- to 19-oz (398 to 540 mL) can of beans, drained and rinsed, can be substituted for the lentils and broth.

You can use all lentils or all split peas.

Substitute sunflower seeds for the pumpkin seeds.

...w with Lime ...Dressing

*We first tried Asian Slaw
as an accompaniment
to a delightful sandwich
at Milestones in
Kamloops, British
Columbia, on our way
home from speaking
at the Canadian Celiac
Association Conference
in Victoria.*

Tips

To maintain a crisp Asian
Slaw, do not let dressed
slaw stand for more than
1 hour before serving.

For a tangy slaw, decrease
the honey to 2 tbsp
(25 mL).

Dressing

2 tbsp	grated gingerroot	25 mL
2 tbsp	snipped fresh cilantro	25 mL
¼ cup	rice wine vinegar	50 mL
¼ cup	freshly squeezed lime juice	50 mL
¼ cup	liquid honey	50 mL
2 tbsp	sesame oil	25 mL
2 tbsp	extra virgin olive oil	25 mL

Slaw

1	bag (16 oz/454 g) coleslaw mix or shredded green and red cabbage	1
1	carrot, finely shredded	1
1	large stalk celery, thinly sliced	1
3	green onions, trimmed and thinly sliced	3
1	small red onion, thinly sliced	1
	Sesame seeds, toasted	

1. *Dressing:* In a small bowl, whisk together ginger, cilantro, vinegar, lime juice, honey, sesame oil and olive oil. Set aside for at least 1 hour or cover and refrigerate overnight to let flavors develop and blend. Store in an airtight container in the refrigerator for up to 3 weeks.

2. *Slaw:* In a large bowl, combine coleslaw, carrot, celery and green onions.

3. Thirty minutes before serving, whisk or shake dressing, pour over slaw and toss to coat. Garnish with red onion and sesame seeds.

Variation

Substitute 2 cups (500 mL) thinly sliced cucumber, parsnips and red or green bell pepper for the carrot and celery.

Nutritional value per serving

Calories	123
Fat, total	7 g
Fat, saturated	1 g
Cholesterol	0 mg
Sodium	23 mg
Carbohydrate	16 g
Fiber	2 g
Protein	1 g
Calcium	34 mg
Iron	1 mg

Springtime Salad with Maple Vinaigrette

Makes 4 servings

A CanolaInfo recipe

Light, refreshing, colorful — the perfect salad! Serve for a summer luncheon to accompany cold salmon.

Tips

The vinaigrette can be stored in an airtight container in the refrigerator for up to 3 weeks. Shake well before drizzling over salad.

We recommend that all prepackaged greens be washed under lots of cold running water before use, even if they are labeled "prewashed."

For information on toasting seeds, see the Techniques Glossary, page 399.

Vinaigrette		
3 tbsp	pure maple syrup	45 mL
2 tbsp	tarragon-flavored wine vinegar	25 mL
1 tsp	dried tarragon	5 mL
1/4 tsp	salt	1 mL
1/4 cup	vegetable oil	50 mL
Salad		
1	package (5 oz/142 g) mesclun (spring salad mix)	1
12	strawberries, sliced	12
1/4 cup	unsalted raw sunflower seeds, toasted	50 mL
1/4 cup	coarsely chopped pecans	50 mL

1. *Vinaigrette:* In a small bowl, whisk together maple syrup, vinegar, tarragon and salt. While whisking, slowly drizzle in oil. Set aside for at least 1 hour or cover and refrigerate overnight to let flavors develop and blend. Whisk well before drizzling over salad.

2. *Salad:* Divide mesclun evenly among four individual salad plates or bowls. Top with strawberries, sunflower seeds and pecans. Serve drizzled with vinaigrette.

Variations

To turn this into a dinner salad, top with julienne strips of roast beef.

Substitute mango cubes, mandarin orange sections or clementine sections for the strawberries.

Nutritional value per serving

Calories	285
Fat, total	24 g
Fat, saturated	2 g
Cholesterol	0 mg
Sodium	165 mg
Carbohydrate	16 g
Fiber	3 g
Protein	4 g
Calcium	50 mg
Iron	2 mg

Marilyn's Orange Salad with Orange Dressing

Dairy-free
Lactose-free
Egg-free
White sugar–free

Makes 4 servings

Donna's sister, Marilyn, served this salad for lunch topped with cooked roast beef when entertaining her celiac friend.

Tips

We recommend that all prepackaged greens be washed under lots of cold running water before use, even if they are labeled "prewashed."

If clementines are not in season, substitute a 10-oz (284 mL) can of mandarin oranges, drained.

1	package (10 oz/284 g) baby spinach	1
2	clementines, peeled and sectioned	2
½	red onion, sliced	½
½ cup	slivered almonds, toasted	125 mL
½ cup	Orange Dressing (see recipe, opposite)	125 mL

1. In a large salad bowl, combine spinach, clementines, red onion and almonds. Pour in dressing and toss to coat.

Variations

Substitute a 7-oz (198 g) package of baby romaine lettuce for the baby spinach.

Substitute 1 cup (250 mL) sliced strawberries for the clementines.

Nutritional value per serving	
Calories	493
Fat, total	36 g
Fat, saturated	3 g
Cholesterol	0 mg
Sodium	351 mg
Carbohydrate	40 g
Fiber	4 g
Protein	7 g
Calcium	131 mg
Iron	3 mg

**Makes 1¼ cups
(300 mL)
(2 tbsp/25 mL per
serving)**

Tip

To enhance the flavor of
the dressing, let it stand
at room temperature for
up to 30 minutes before
serving.

Orange Dressing

½	small red onion, chopped	½
½ cup	vegetable oil	125 mL
⅓ cup	liquid honey	75 mL
¼ cup	cider vinegar	50 mL
2 tbsp	frozen unsweetened orange juice concentrate, thawed	25 mL
1 tsp	dry mustard	5 mL
½ tsp	salt	2 mL
¼ tsp	freshly ground white pepper	1 mL

1. In a blender or food processor, combine onion, oil, honey, vinegar, orange juice concentrate, dry mustard, salt and pepper; process until smooth.

2. Set aside for at least 1 hour or cover and refrigerate overnight to let flavors develop and blend. Store in an airtight container in the refrigerator for up to 3 weeks.

Variation

Substitute balsamic or red wine vinegar for the cider vinegar.

Nutritional value per serving	
Calories	117
Fat, total	9 g
Fat, saturated	1 g
Cholesterol	0 mg
Sodium	97 mg
Carbohydrate	10 g
Fiber	0 g
Protein	0 g
Calcium	3 mg
Iron	0 mg

Caprese Salad

Egg-free
White sugar–free

Makes 4 servings

This simple salad from the Italian region of Campania displays the colors of the Italian flag with sliced fresh mozzarella, tomatoes and basil. We've added extra flavor with our Sun-Dried Tomato Pesto.

Tips

For the mozzarella, use 1½-inch (4 cm) bocconcini or ¾-inch (2 cm) ciliegini.

Tomatoes and cheese both have the best flavor at room temperature.

If you can't find heirloom tomatoes, use regular plum (Roma) tomatoes instead.

¼ cup	Sun-Dried Tomato Pesto (page 74)	50 mL
¼ cup	extra virgin olive oil	50 mL
7 oz	baby arugula	210 g
1 lb	mixed heirloom tomatoes, cored and cut into ¼-inch (0.5 cm) thick slices	500 g
8 oz	fresh mozzarella cheese (see tip, at left), cut into ¼-inch (5 mm) thick slices	250 g
⅔ cup	pitted black olives	150 mL
12	fresh basil leaves, thinly sliced	12
	Salt and freshly ground black pepper	

1. In a small bowl, whisk together pesto and oil until combined.

2. Arrange arugula on a large platter. Top with tomatoes, mozzarella and olives. Sprinkle with basil and pesto mixture. Season to taste with salt and pepper.

Variations

You can use any commercial GF basil pesto in place of the Sun-Dried Tomato Pesto.

Substitute baby spinach or baby romaine lettuce for the arugula.

Nutritional value per serving

Calories	388
Fat, total	30 g
Fat, saturated	9 g
Cholesterol	33 mg
Sodium	652 mg
Carbohydrate	12 g
Fiber	2 g
Protein	20 g
Calcium	560 mg
Iron	2 mg

Sedona Salad

Makes 6 servings

On November 21, 2007, on our way home from the Grand Canyon, we lunched in Sedona, Arizona. We enjoyed our lunch so much, we modified this salad just for you.

Tips

We recommend that all prepackaged greens be washed under lots of cold running water before use, even if they are labeled "prewashed." When preparing leafy greens in advance, wash and dry them, then refrigerate, covered with a damp, lint-free tea towel.

Small, delicate baby spinach leaves are milder than the mature ones.

For information on toasting nuts, see the Techniques Glossary, page 398.

Nutritional value per serving	
Calories	442
Fat, total	27 g
Fat, saturated	7 g
Cholesterol	100 mg
Sodium	443 mg
Carbohydrate	11 g
Fiber	3 g
Protein	38 g
Calcium	215 mg
Iron	4 mg

8 cups	packed baby spinach, trimmed	2 L
2	boneless skinless chicken breasts, cooked and sliced	2
2	Granny Smith apples, cut into wedges	2
1 cup	crumbled feta cheese	250 mL
½ cup	pecan halves, toasted	125 mL
⅓ cup	raspberry-flavored dried cranberries	75 mL
	Raspberry Vinaigrette (page 77)	

1. Divide spinach evenly among four individual luncheon plates. Top with chicken, apples, feta, pecans and cranberries. Serve drizzled with vinaigrette.

Variations

Substitute hazelnuts or almonds for the pecans.

Substitute GF blue cheese or Emmental for the feta. For the best flavor, serve at room temperature.

Honey Pecan Salmon Salad

We first tried this salad when we visited Texas and spoke to the Dallas–Fort Worth GIG Support Group. We selected this from Johnny Carino's Italian Grill gluten-free lunch menu and have adapted it for you.

Tips

We recommend that all prepackaged greens be washed under lots of cold running water before use, even if they are labeled "prewashed."

Don't use the same utensils for the raw and cooked salmon.

Fold the thin part of the salmon under to make the fillets an even thickness.

Nutritional value per serving	
Calories	596
Fat, total	38 g
Fat, saturated	5 g
Cholesterol	78 mg
Sodium	531 mg
Carbohydrate	37 g
Fiber	4 g
Protein	33 g
Calcium	70 mg
Iron	3 mg

- Rimmed baking sheet, lined with foil

Honey Pecan Salmon

¼ cup	freshly squeezed lemon juice	50 mL
¼ cup	liquid honey, divided	50 mL
2 tbsp	extra virgin olive oil	25 mL
4	salmon fillets (each 5 oz/150 g)	4
½ cup	pecan halves, coarsely chopped	125 mL

Salad

½	head romaine lettuce, torn	½
4	plum (Roma) tomatoes, cut into wedges	4
½	red onion, cut into rings	½
½ cup	sun-dried tomatoes, thinly sliced	125 mL
¼ cup	drained capers	50 mL
½ cup	Lemon Vinaigrette (see recipe, opposite)	125 mL

1. *Salmon:* In a large shallow dish or sealable plastic bag, whisk together lemon juice, 2 tbsp (25 mL) of the honey and oil. Add fillets and turn to coat. Cover or seal and refrigerate for at least 20 minutes or for up to 1 hour.

2. Place oven rack in top third of oven and preheat oven to 450°F (230°C).

3. Remove salmon from marinade, discarding marinade. Place salmon, skin side down, on prepared baking sheet. Bake for 10 to 12 minutes per inch (2.5 cm) of thickness or until salmon is opaque and flakes easily with a fork. During the last 4 minutes, brush the top of the salmon with the remaining honey and top with pecans.

4. *Salad:* Divide romaine evenly among four individual salad plates. Top with plum tomatoes, red onion, sun-dried tomatoes and capers.

5. Top each salad with a salmon fillet. Serve drizzled with vinaigrette.

Variations

Soak an untreated cedar plank in cold water for 2 hours. Place the plank on the barbecue over high heat and preheat for 5 to 10 minutes or until the wood begins to smoke. Place the salmon on the plank and cook, without turning, for 10 to 12 minutes per inch (2.5 cm) of thickness or until salmon is opaque and flakes easily with a fork.

If you want to serve the salmon cold, let it cool, cover and refrigerate for at least 2 hours or for up to 2 days.

Lemon Vinaigrette

2 tbsp	grated lemon zest	25 mL
½ cup	freshly squeezed lemon juice	125 mL
¼ cup	water	50 mL
3 tbsp	extra virgin olive oil	45 mL
1 tbsp	liquid honey	15 mL

1. In a small bowl, whisk together lemon zest, lemon juice, water, oil and honey. Cover and refrigerate for at least 1 hour to let flavors develop and blend, or for up to 3 weeks.

**Nutritional value
per serving**

Calories	86
Fat, total	7 g
Fat, saturated	1 g
Cholesterol	0 mg
Sodium	1 mg
Carbohydrate	7 g
Fiber	0 g
Protein	0 g
Calcium	3 mg
Iron	0 mg

Scallop Salad with Asian Dressing

Makes 4 servings

Perfect for a special-occasion summer luncheon, this warm salad is as pleasing to the eye as it is to the palate.

Tips

A pound (500 g) of sea scallops contains 20 to 30 scallops, depending on size.

Sixteen ounces (454 g) of mesclun yields about 10 cups (2.5 L). Mesclun is a mixture of baby greens, often including endive and radicchio.

We recommend that all prepackaged greens be washed under lots of cold running water before use, even if they are labeled "prewashed."

Nutritional value per serving	
Calories	477
Fat, total	28 g
Fat, saturated	4 g
Cholesterol	37 mg
Sodium	281 mg
Carbohydrate	35 g
Fiber	5 g
Protein	23 g
Calcium	117 mg
Iron	3 mg

¼ cup	dry white wine	50 mL
1 lb	sea scallops, trimmed of hard side muscles	500 g
8 cups	packed mesclun (spring salad mix)	2 L
1½ cups	mixed chopped kiwifruit, mango and papaya	375 mL
½ cup	Asian Dressing (see recipe, opposite)	125 mL
¼ cup	sesame seeds, toasted	50 mL

1. In a large skillet, heat wine over medium-low heat. Add scallops, cover and cook for 5 minutes or until firm and opaque.

2. Divide mesclun evenly among four individual luncheon plates. Top with scallops and fruit. Serve drizzled with dressing and sprinkled with sesame seeds.

Variations

Substitute grapes, pineapple chunks, strawberries, melon balls or any fresh fruit you like for the tropical fruit.

Substitute water or GF chicken broth for the wine.

**Makes about 1 cup
(250 mL)
(2 tbsp/25 mL per
serving)**

Tip

To extend the shelf life of specialty oils such as walnut or sesame, store in the refrigerator.

Asian Dressing

⅓ cup	extra virgin olive oil	75 mL
¼ cup	liquid honey	50 mL
¼ cup	rice wine vinegar	50 mL
2 tbsp	freshly squeezed lime juice	25 mL
1 tbsp	sesame oil	15 mL
2 tsp	Dijon mustard	10 mL
1 tsp	ground ginger	5 mL
¼ tsp	hot pepper flakes	1 mL

1. In a small bowl, whisk together olive oil, honey, vinegar, lime juice, sesame oil, mustard, ginger and hot pepper flakes. Use immediately or cover and refrigerate for up to 3 weeks.

Variation
Substitute 1 tbsp (15 mL) grated gingerroot for the ground ginger.

Nutritional value per serving	
Calories	108
Fat, total	9 g
Fat, saturated	1 g
Cholesterol	0 mg
Sodium	26 mg
Carbohydrate	8 g
Fiber	0 g
Protein	0 g
Calcium	2 mg
Iron	0 mg

Caesar Salad with Pork Tenderloin Strips

Egg-free

Makes 4 servings

Pork tenderloin is convenient to have on hand, as it can be used in so many ways — and it's economical, as there is no waste.

Tip

Wash the romaine under lots of cold running water before use.

- **Preheat oven to 400°F (200°C)**
- **13- by 9-inch (33 by 23 cm) baking pan**

1	pork tenderloin (12 to 16 oz/375 to 500 g)	1
1	head romaine lettuce, torn into bite-size pieces	1
½ cup	Roasted Garlic Caesar Dressing (page 80)	125 mL
24	Whole-Grain Croutons (page 81)	24
½ cup	freshly shaved Parmesan cheese	125 mL
	Freshly ground black pepper	

1. Place tenderloin in baking pan, tucking thin end underneath. Roast in preheated oven for 20 minutes or until a meat thermometer inserted in the thickest part registers 155°F (68°C). Transfer to a cutting board, tent with foil and let rest for 10 minutes.

2. Cut tenderloin in half lengthwise, then cut across the grain into thin slices. Set aside.

3. In a large serving bowl, combine romaine and dressing, tossing to coat.

4. Divide salad evenly among individual salad plates. Top with pork, croutons and Parmesan. Season to taste with pepper.

Variations

To serve the pork tenderloin cold, let it cool, then cover and refrigerate for up to 24 hours before slicing.

Barbecue the pork tenderloin, using medium-high indirect heat, for 10 to 15 minutes, turning once, until a meat thermometer inserted in the thickest part registers 155°F (68°C).

Nutritional value per serving	
Calories	445
Fat, total	26 g
Fat, saturated	7 g
Cholesterol	98 mg
Sodium	213 mg
Carbohydrate	15 g
Fiber	3 g
Protein	37 g
Calcium	234 mg
Iron	4 mg

Pork Quinoa Salad with Indian Dressing

Makes 4 servings

We love this make-ahead salad when we're entertaining houseguests for the weekend — no need to worry about their arrival time!

Tips

The dressing can be stored in an airtight container in the refrigerator for up to 1 week.

Leave the peel on the cucumber for great color and added fiber.

Cardamom Dressing

⅔ cup	plain yogurt	150 mL
1 tsp	ground coriander	5 mL
1 tsp	ground cardamom	5 mL
1 tsp	ground cumin	5 mL

Salad

⅓ cup	quinoa, rinsed	75 mL
1 cup	GF chicken broth	250 mL
8 oz	cooked pork tenderloin, thinly sliced	250 g
16	strawberry or grape tomatoes	16
½	seedless cucumber, cubed	½
½ cup	dried currants	125 mL
2 tbsp	snipped fresh cilantro	25 mL

1. *Dressing:* In a small bowl, whisk together yogurt, coriander, cardamom and cumin. Set aside for at least 1 hour or cover and refrigerate overnight to let flavors develop and blend.

2. *Salad:* In a saucepan, bring quinoa and broth to a boil over high heat. Reduce heat to low, cover and simmer for 18 to 20 minutes or until quinoa is transparent and the tiny, spiral-like germ is separated. Remove from heat and let stand, covered, for 5 to 10 minutes or until stock is absorbed.

3. In a large bowl, combine quinoa, pork, tomatoes, cucumber, currants and cilantro. Pour in dressing and toss well to coat.

4. Cover and refrigerate for at least 4 hours to let flavors develop and blend, or overnight.

Variations

Substitute an equal amount of brown rice or wild rice for the quinoa. See "Cooking Rice," page 23, for information on cooking brown rice and wild rice.

Substitute raisins or peanuts for the currants.

Nutritional value per serving

Calories	211
Fat, total	4 g
Fat, saturated	1 g
Cholesterol	41 mg
Sodium	235 mg
Carbohydrate	21 g
Fiber	3 g
Protein	23 g
Calcium	121 mg
Iron	3 mg

Taco Salad

Makes 2 servings

Quick, easy, nutritious — and a meal with hardly any cleanup!

Tips

We used a mild GF barbecue sauce, but you could certainly choose a hotter one. Just be sure it is gluten-free. Make your own, if you prefer.

If you purchase a sirloin steak, cut it across the grain into thin strips for a tender result.

2	Tortilla Bowls (see recipe, opposite)	2
4 cups	shredded lettuce	1 L
2	tomatoes, diced	2
1/4	orange bell pepper, finely chopped	1/4
1/4	yellow bell pepper, finely chopped	1/4
1/4 cup	GF barbecue sauce	50 mL
3/4 tsp	chili powder	4 mL
Pinch	ground hot pepper	Pinch
1 tsp	extra virgin olive oil	5 mL
6 oz	beef sirloin stir-fry strips	175 g

1. Place tortilla bowls on individual plates. Divide the lettuce evenly among the tortilla bowls. Top each with tomatoes, orange pepper and yellow pepper. Set aside.

2. In a small bowl, combine barbecue sauce, chili powder and hot pepper. Set aside.

3. In a skillet, heat oil over medium-high heat. Brown beef strips, turning occasionally, for 2 to 3 minutes or until just slightly pink in the center. Pour in the barbecue sauce mixture and heat just until steaming.

4. Top each tortilla bowl with half the beef mixture.

Variations

Top the salad with shredded cheese, sour cream, guacamole or salsa.

Marinate the beef strips in the sauce for 30 minutes before cooking them. Drain beef and discard marinade before browning.

Nutritional value per serving

Calories	344
Fat, total	8 g
Fat, saturated	2 g
Cholesterol	40 mg
Sodium	548 mg
Carbohydrate	45 g
Fiber	8 g
Protein	24 g
Calcium	159 mg
Iron	4 mg

Makes 2 servings

Make these neat containers to hold anything from salads to entrées. Children and adults alike will love to eat from them.

Tip

Warm the tortillas in the oven slightly before molding them into the bowl, for easier handling.

Tortilla Bowls

- Preheat oven to 350°F (180°C)
- 5½-inch (14 cm) ovenproof bowl, at least 3½ inches (9 cm) deep

| 2 | 8-inch (20 cm) GF tortillas | 2 |

1. Gently place a tortilla in the bowl, easing it in to fit the bottom and up the sides. Bake in preheated oven for 15 minutes or until crisp. Let cool in bowl for 5 minutes. Carefully remove from bowl and repeat for remaining tortilla. Let cool completely before filling.

Nutritional value per serving	
Calories	120
Fat, total	2 g
Fat, saturated	0 g
Cholesterol	0 mg
Sodium	10 mg
Carbohydrate	23 g
Fiber	3 g
Protein	3 g
Calcium	72 mg
Iron	1 mg

Classic French Onion Soup

**Makes 8 servings
(1 cup/250 mL per
serving)**

*This classic, traditional
soup is a family
favorite.*

Tips

This soup can be made
ahead through step 2. Let
cool, transfer to an airtight
container and refrigerate
for up to 2 days. Reheat
over medium heat until
steaming, then continue
with step 3.

Don't try to rush when
browning the onions.
The longer and slower
they are cooked, the richer
and deeper the flavor of
the soup.

Nutritional value per serving

Calories	225
Fat, total	9 g
Fat, saturated	5 g
Cholesterol	25 mg
Sodium	888 mg
Carbohydrate	27 g
Fiber	3 g
Protein	9 g
Calcium	203 mg
Iron	1 mg

• Eight 1½-cup (375 mL) ovenproof bowls

3 tbsp	butter	45 mL
6 cups	thinly sliced onions	1.5 L
1 tsp	white (granulated) sugar	5 mL
2 tbsp	amaranth flour	25 mL
8 cups	GF beef broth	2 L
8	thick slices GF bread	8
1 cup	shredded Swiss cheese	250 mL
2 tbsp	freshly shaved Parmesan cheese	25 mL

1. In a large saucepan, melt butter over medium heat.
   Cook onions, stirring occasionally, for about 15 minutes
   or until soft and transparent. Reduce heat to low, stir in
   sugar and cook, stirring frequently, for 30 to 40 minutes
   or until onions are deep golden brown. Stir in amaranth
   flour and cook, stirring constantly, for 3 minutes.

2. Gradually stir in broth and bring to a boil. Reduce heat
   to medium-low and simmer, stirring occasionally, for
   30 minutes.

3. Meanwhile, preheat broiler. Place ovenproof bowls on a
   baking sheet. Divide soup among bowls, top each bowl
   with a slice of bread and sprinkle evenly with Swiss
   cheese and Parmesan.

4. Broil until cheeses are bubbly and lightly browned.

Variations

Substitute an equal amount of sorghum flour for the
amaranth flour.

Stir in ½ cup (125 mL) Madeira, dry white wine or dry
sherry just before ladling the soup into the bowls.

For ease of eating, cube rather than slice leftover bread.

Some folks like to use aged Cheddar, Emmental and/or
Gruyère cheese in place of the Swiss.

Minestrone

**Makes 10 servings
(1 cup/250 mL per
serving)**

*A steaming bowl
of minestrone is as
comforting as it gets!*

Tips

Soup can be divided into
2-cup (500 mL) portions
and frozen for up to
1 month. Reheat in the
microwave on High for
5 to 7 minutes or until
steaming.

Use the shape of pasta
you prefer, from small
shells to small elbows.
Follow package directions
to be sure pasta is not
overcooked. Rinse the
cooked pasta with cold
water to stop the cooking
process and remove excess
starch.

2 tsp	extra virgin olive oil	10 mL
2	carrots, chopped	2
1	stalk celery, chopped	1
1	clove garlic, minced	1
1	small onion, chopped	1
1	small zucchini, diced	1
1	can (28 oz/796 mL) diced tomatoes, with juice	1
1	can (14 to 19 oz/398 to 540 mL) kidney beans, drained and rinsed	1
1 cup	diced cooked GF ham	250 mL
1 cup	GF chicken or vegetable broth	250 mL
2 tbsp	tomato paste	25 mL
1 cup	packed spinach, trimmed and coarsely chopped	250 mL
1 cup	cooked small GF pasta	250 mL
¼ cup	snipped fresh basil	50 mL
	Salt and freshly ground black pepper	

1. In a large saucepan, heat oil over medium-low heat. Add carrots, celery, garlic and onion; cover and cook, stirring occasionally, for about 20 minutes or until tender but not brown.

2. Add zucchini, tomatoes with juice, beans, ham, broth and tomato paste; bring to a boil over medium-high heat. Reduce heat to low and simmer for 10 minutes or until soup is hot. Stir in spinach, pasta and basil; heat until spinach is wilted. Season to taste with salt and pepper.

Variations

Substitute an equal amount of shredded cabbage or cooked green beans for the spinach.

Substitute 6 slices GF bacon, chopped and cooked crisp, or 1 cup (250 mL) diced cooked chicken, beef or turkey for the ham.

For a spicier soup, substitute GF pepperoni for the ham.

Sprinkle with freshly grated Parmesan cheese.

Nutritional value per serving

Calories	138
Fat, total	3 g
Fat, saturated	1 g
Cholesterol	13 mg
Sodium	439 mg
Carbohydrate	21 g
Fiber	3 g
Protein	9 g
Calcium	45 mg
Iron	2 mg

Autumn Squash Soup

**Makes 8 servings
(1 cup/250 mL
per serving)**

*We always look
forward to autumn,
when we make this
thick, rich, nutritious
soup.*

- Preheat oven to 425°F (220°C)
- 2 large roasting pans, brushed with oil

2	large carrots, halved lengthwise	2
1	small butternut squash, quartered and seeds removed	1
1	large sweet potato, quartered	1
1 tbsp	extra virgin olive oil	15 mL
2	large leeks, white and light green parts only, halved lengthwise	2
4 cups	GF chicken or vegetable broth	1 L
1½ tsp	ground cumin	7 mL
	Salt and freshly ground white pepper	

1. Spread carrots, squash and sweet potato, cut side down, in a single layer in prepared pans, dividing evenly. Brush with oil. Roast in preheated oven for 30 minutes. Turn vegetables, add leeks and brush leeks with oil. Roast for 30 to 45 minutes or until vegetables are tender. Let cool in pan on a wire rack for 10 minutes.

2. Meanwhile, in a large saucepan, heat broth and cumin over medium heat.

3. Scoop out squash and sweet potato flesh and discard the skins.

4. Working in small batches, transfer vegetables to a food processor or blender. Add enough broth to allow you to purée until smooth (you'll use about 1 cup/250 mL broth total, among all the batches).

5. Add puréed vegetables to the broth remaining in saucepan and heat over medium-low heat just until steaming. Season to taste with salt and pepper.

Nutritional value per serving

Calories	95
Fat, total	2 g
Fat, saturated	0 g
Cholesterol	0 mg
Sodium	451 mg
Carbohydrate	18 g
Fiber	3 g
Protein	2 g
Calcium	69 mg
Iron	1 mg

Tips

If you're using a dark-colored roasting pan, turn vegetables frequently during the last half of roasting.

We always double this recipe, as it's just as quick to make more and freeze the extra. Soup can be divided into 2-cup (500 mL) portions and frozen for up to 1 month. Reheat in the microwave on High for 5 to 7 minutes or until steaming.

Variations

Use other kinds of squash, such as pepper, hubbard, turban or pumpkin, in place of the butternut. Use about 2 lbs (1 kg) of any variety.

Substitute 3 onions for the leeks and add 1 bulb of garlic with the leeks.

Substitute 1 to 2 tbsp (15 to 25 mL) GF mild or hot curry paste for the cumin.

For a thinner soup, add extra GF broth or milk in step 5.

Add 1 tbsp (15 mL) dried rosemary with the cumin.

Beef and Quinoa Soup

**Makes 14 servings
(1 cup/250 mL per
serving)**

*This hearty, rich soup
is a meal in a bowl.*

Tips

Soup can be divided into
2-cup (500 mL) portions
and frozen for up to
1 month. Reheat in the
microwave on High for
5 to 7 minutes or until
steaming.

Browning the beef in small
batches before adding the
broth results in a richer
beef flavor.

This recipe can be halved
or quartered.

2 tbsp	extra virgin olive oil (approx.)	25 mL
1½ lbs	stewing beef, cut into ¾-inch (2 cm) cubes	750 g
1	large onion, coarsely chopped	1
4 cups	GF beef broth	1 L
3	carrots, coarsely chopped	3
2	stalks celery, coarsely chopped	2
¼ cup	quinoa, rinsed	50 mL
1	can (28 oz/796 mL) diced tomatoes, with juice	1
1 tbsp	snipped fresh thyme	15 mL
	Salt and freshly ground black pepper	

1. In a large saucepan, heat 1 tbsp (15 mL) of the oil over medium heat. Working in small batches, sauté beef and onion for 20 minutes or until beef is browned on all sides, adding oil as needed between batches. Transfer each batch to a plate lined with paper towels as completed. Drain off fat.

2. Add broth and scrape up any brown bits from bottom of pan. Return the beef mixture to the pan. Reduce heat to low and simmer for 35 minutes or until beef is tender.

3. Add carrots, celery and quinoa; simmer for 30 minutes or until vegetables are tender and quinoa is transparent and the tiny, spiral-like germ is separated.

4. Add tomatoes with juice and thyme, increase heat to medium-high and heat until steaming. Season to taste with salt and pepper.

Variation

After step 1, transfer beef mixture to the stoneware of a large (minimum 5-quart) slow cooker. Add broth, carrots, celery, tomatoes and thyme. Cover and cook on Low for 8 to 10 hours. Meanwhile, cook quinoa as per the instructions in the Techniques Glossary, page 398. Fifteen minutes before you're ready to serve, add the quinoa to the slow cooker.

Nutritional value per serving

Calories	228
Fat, total	17 g
Fat, saturated	7 g
Cholesterol	39 mg
Sodium	358 mg
Carbohydrate	8 g
Fiber	2 g
Protein	10 g
Calcium	32 mg
Iron	2 mg

Ham and Bean Soup

**Makes 12 servings
(1 cup/250 mL per
serving)**

*A wintertime staple
of years gone by! We
like the deep, rich
flavor that develops
when you store this
soup overnight in the
refrigerator, but it's
also delicious served
right away.*

Tips

Soup can be divided into
2-cup (500 mL) portions
and frozen for up to
1 month. Reheat in the
microwave on High for
5 to 7 minutes or until
steaming.

To reduce the gas-
producing properties of
beans, always discard the
soaking water and cook
the beans in fresh liquid.

Nutritional value per serving

Calories	202
Fat, total	3 g
Fat, saturated	1 g
Cholesterol	22 mg
Sodium	559 mg
Carbohydrate	27 g
Fiber	4 g
Protein	17 g
Calcium	59 mg
Iron	2 mg

- **Large microwave-safe casserole dish**

¾ cup	dried navy beans	175 mL
¾ cup	dried green split peas	175 mL
¾ cup	dried yellow split peas	175 mL
10 oz	cooked GF ham, diced	300 g
1	large onion, chopped	1
1	bay leaf	1
1 tbsp	dried savory	15 mL
8 cups	GF chicken, beef or vegetable broth	2 L
2	stalks celery, diced	2
1	large carrot, diced	1
	Salt and freshly ground black pepper	

1. Sort and rinse the beans, green peas and yellow peas. Place beans and peas in casserole dish and cover with 6 cups (1.5 L) water. Cover and microwave on High for 10 to 15 minutes, or until boiling. Let stand for 1 hour. Drain and discard liquid. Rinse beans and peas well with cold water.

2. In a large saucepan, combine beans and peas, ham, onion, bay leaf, savory and broth; bring to a boil over high heat. Reduce heat to medium-low, cover and simmer for 1½ hours.

3. Add celery and carrot; cover and simmer for 30 minutes or until beans, peas and vegetables are tender. Season to taste with salt and pepper.

Variations

Use any variety of dried pea or bean. Or, for a quicker method, use rinsed drained canned dried peas and beans and add to the soup with the carrot.

For a deeper ham flavor, add a ham bone and remove it just before serving the soup.

Salmon Corn Chowder

**Makes 6 servings
(1 cup/250 mL per
serving)**

*The perfect soup to
serve when company
drops in for lunch!*

Tips

If you can't find a 14½-oz
(418 g) can of salmon, use
two 7-oz (210 g) cans.

Check to be sure cream-
style corn is gluten-free.

1	can (14½ oz/418 g) salmon, drained	1
2 tsp	vegetable oil	10 mL
1	carrot, diced	1
1	stalk celery, diced	1
½	small onion, finely chopped	½
1	large potato, chopped	1
1 cup	GF chicken or vegetable broth	250 mL
1	can (14 oz/398 mL) GF cream-style corn	1
1 cup	milk	250 mL
	Salt and freshly ground white pepper	

1. Remove skin from salmon and mash bones. Break
   salmon into large chunks; set aside.

2. In a large saucepan, heat oil over medium heat. Sauté
   carrot, celery and onion for 5 to 7 minutes or until
   tender. Add potato and broth; bring to a boil over high
   heat. Reduce heat to medium-low and simmer for
   6 to 10 minutes or until potato is tender. Add salmon,
   corn and milk; reduce heat to low and heat, stirring
   occasionally, just until steaming. Do not let boil, or
   chowder may curdle. Season to taste with salt and
   pepper.

Variations

Add 2 tsp (10 mL) snipped fresh dill or tarragon with the
salt and pepper.

For a chunkier chowder, add a 14-oz (398 mL) can of corn
kernels with the cream-style corn.

Nutritional value per serving	
Calories	214
Fat, total	7 g
Fat, saturated	2 g
Cholesterol	32 mg
Sodium	815 mg
Carbohydrate	20 g
Fiber	2 g
Protein	18 g
Calcium	233 mg
Iron	1 mg

Main Dishes

Cheese Soufflé

This savory French dish can be made for any occasion with common ingredients always on hand in your refrigerator and pantry.

Tips

The soufflé can be prepared through step 3, covered and refrigerated for up to 4 hours before baking.

See the Equipment Glossary, page 388, for information on soufflé dishes.

Be sure not to open the oven door during baking, or the soufflé will deflate.

Nutritional value per serving

Calories	432
Fat, total	34 g
Fat, saturated	20 g
Cholesterol	275 mg
Sodium	680 mg
Carbohydrate	9 g
Fiber	1 g
Protein	23 g
Calcium	519 mg
Iron	3 mg

- Preheat oven to 300°F (150°C)
- 10-cup (2.5 L) soufflé dish, at least 3 inches (7.5 cm) deep, buttered

¼ cup	butter	50 mL
¼ cup	amaranth flour	50 mL
1 cup	milk	250 mL
2 cups	shredded extra sharp (extra old) Cheddar cheese	500 mL
¼ tsp	salt	1 mL
¼ tsp	paprika	1 mL
Pinch	cayenne pepper	Pinch
4	eggs, separated	4
¼ tsp	cream of tartar	1 mL

1. In a microwave-safe bowl, microwave butter on High for 1 to 2 minutes or until melted. Stir in amaranth flour and microwave on High for 1 to 2 minutes or until mixture is the consistency of dry sand. Stir in milk and microwave on High for 3 to 5 minutes, stopping to stir occasionally, until mixture comes to a boil and has thickened. Stir in cheese, salt, paprika and cayenne. Set aside.

2. In a small bowl, using an electric mixer, beat egg yolks for 5 minutes or until thick and lemon-colored. Fold in cheese mixture.

3. In a large bowl, using an electric mixer with clean wire whisk attachment, beat egg whites and cream of tartar until stiff but not dry. Fold in cheese mixture. Spoon into prepared soufflé dish.

4. Bake in preheated oven for 60 to 75 minutes or until puffed and golden brown. Serve immediately, before it deflates.

Variations

Try substituting Asiago, Gruyère or a commercial blend of cheeses for the Cheddar.

Add ½ tsp (2 mL) Dijon or dry mustard with the cheese.

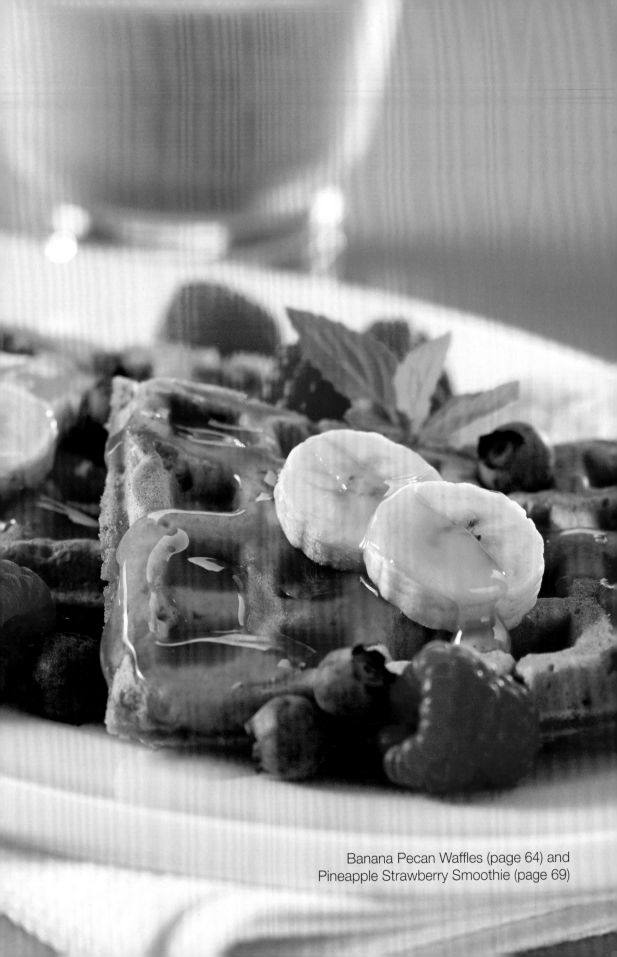

Banana Pecan Waffles (page 64) and
Pineapple Strawberry Smoothie (page 69)

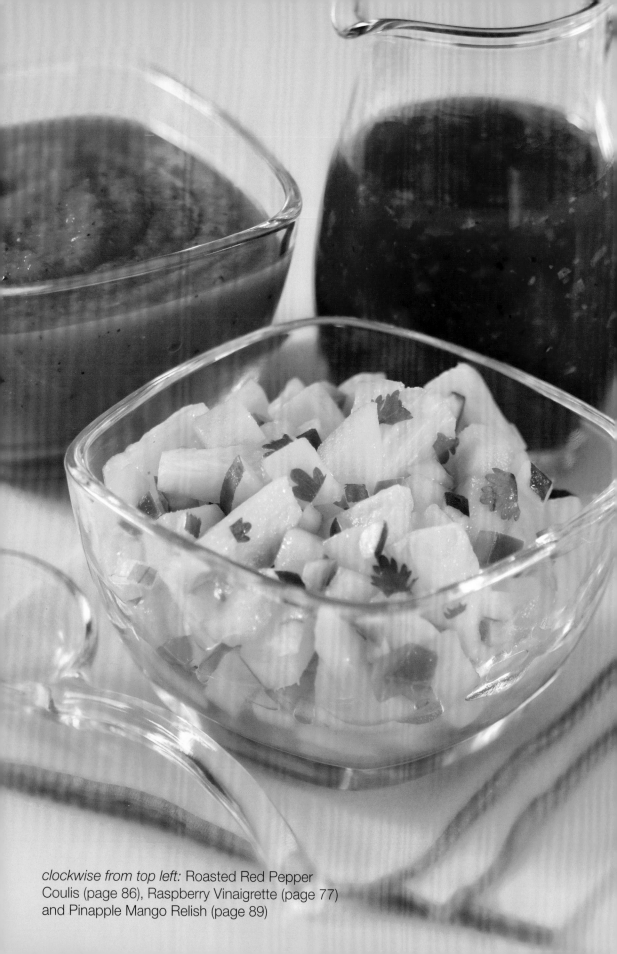

clockwise from top left: Roasted Red Pepper
Coulis (page 86), Raspberry Vinaigrette (page 77)
and Pinapple Mango Relish (page 89)

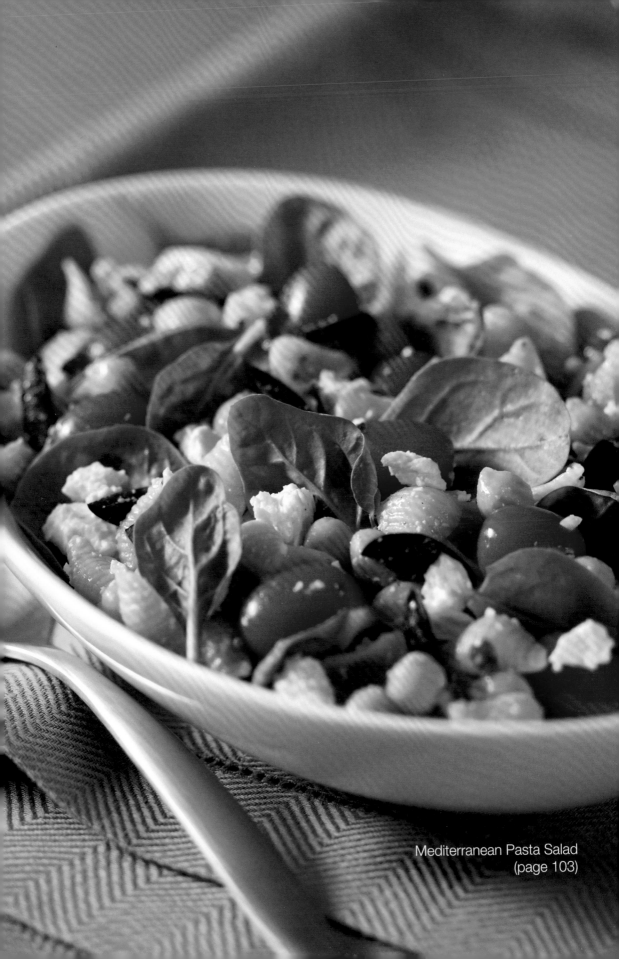

Mediterranean Pasta Salad
(page 103)

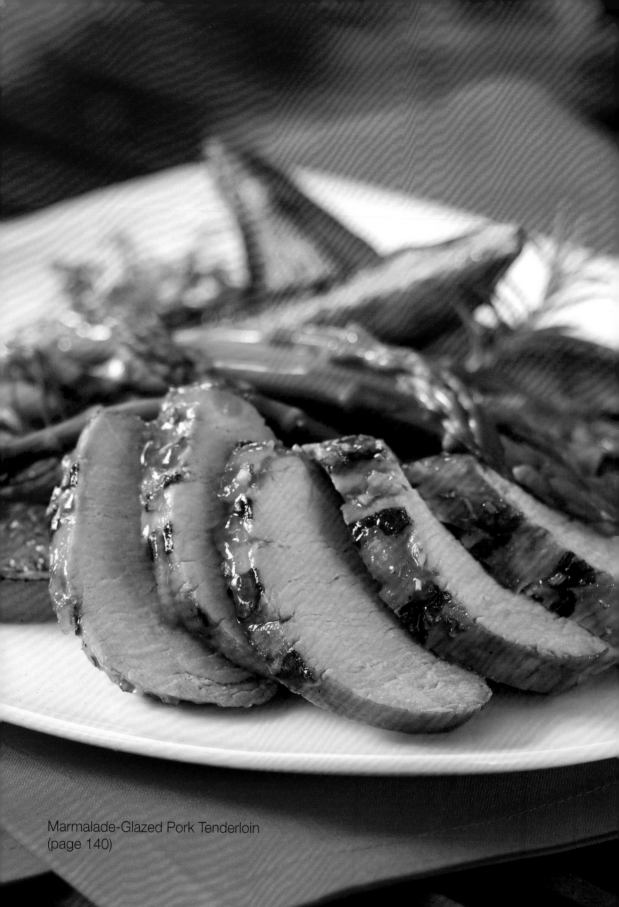

Marmalade-Glazed Pork Tenderloin
(page 140)

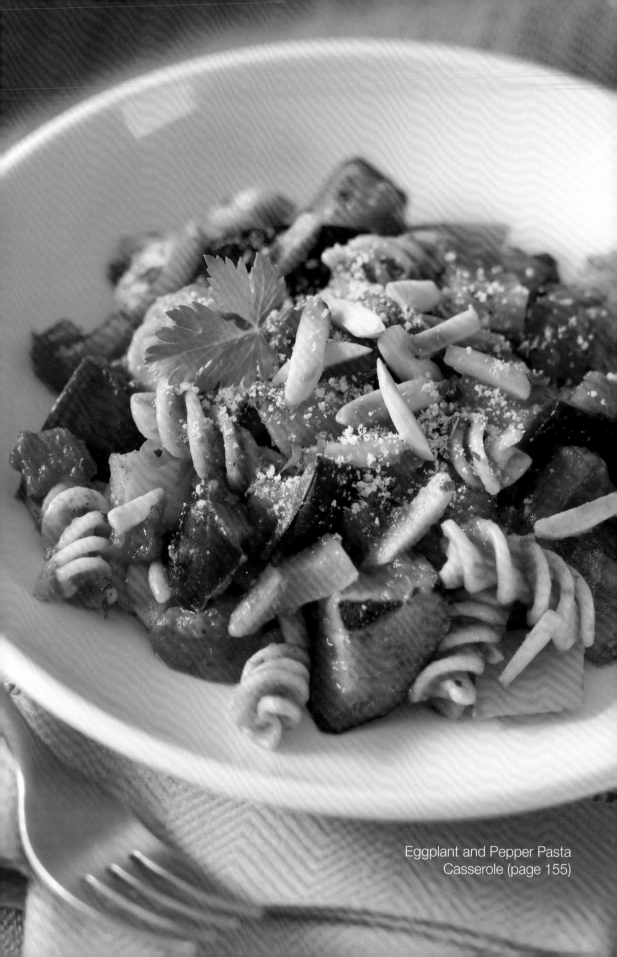

Eggplant and Pepper Pasta
Casserole (page 155)

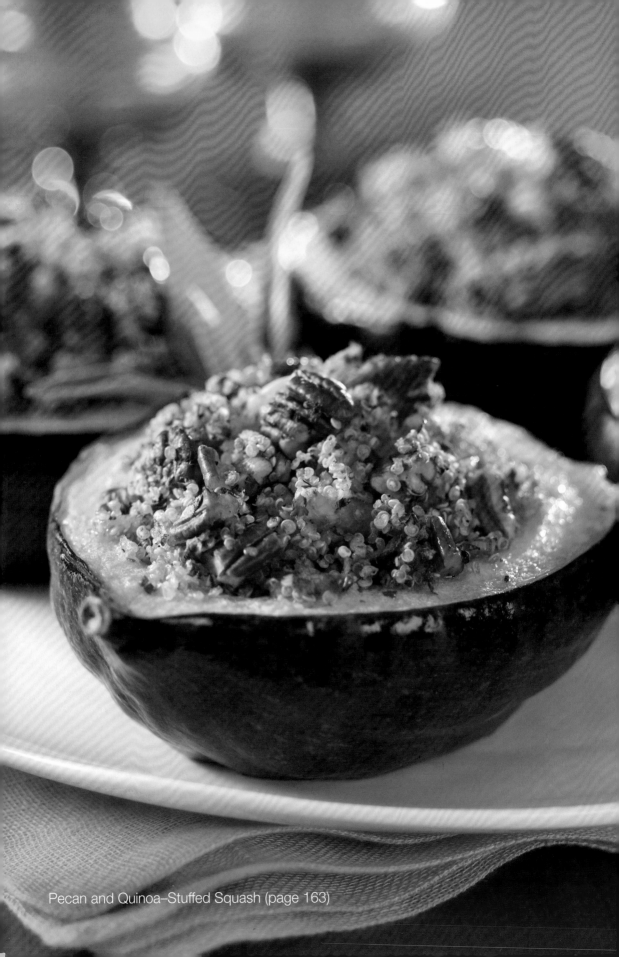

Pecan and Quinoa–Stuffed Squash (page 163)

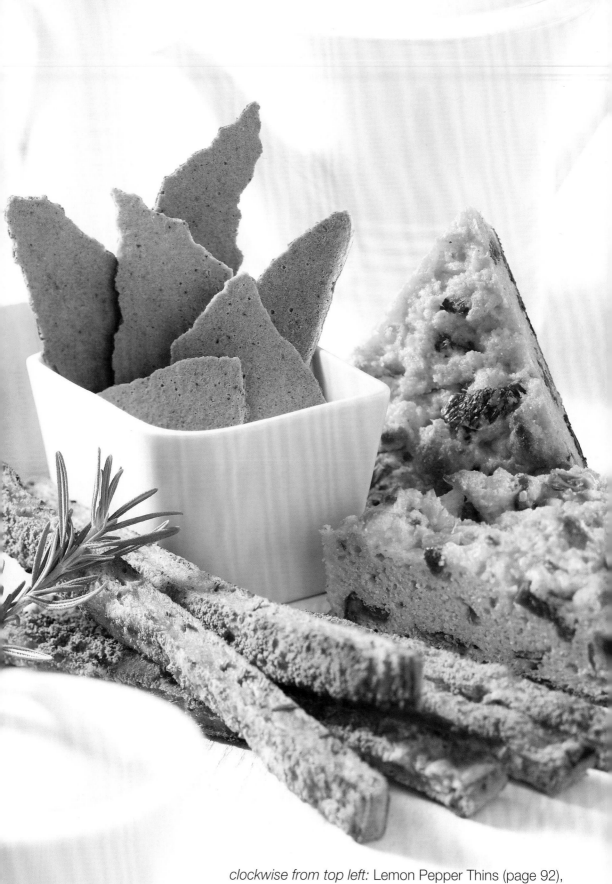

clockwise from top left: Lemon Pepper Thins (page 92),
Sun-Dried Tomato Green Onion Cornbread (page 239)
and Rosemary Breadsticks (pages 187 and 219)

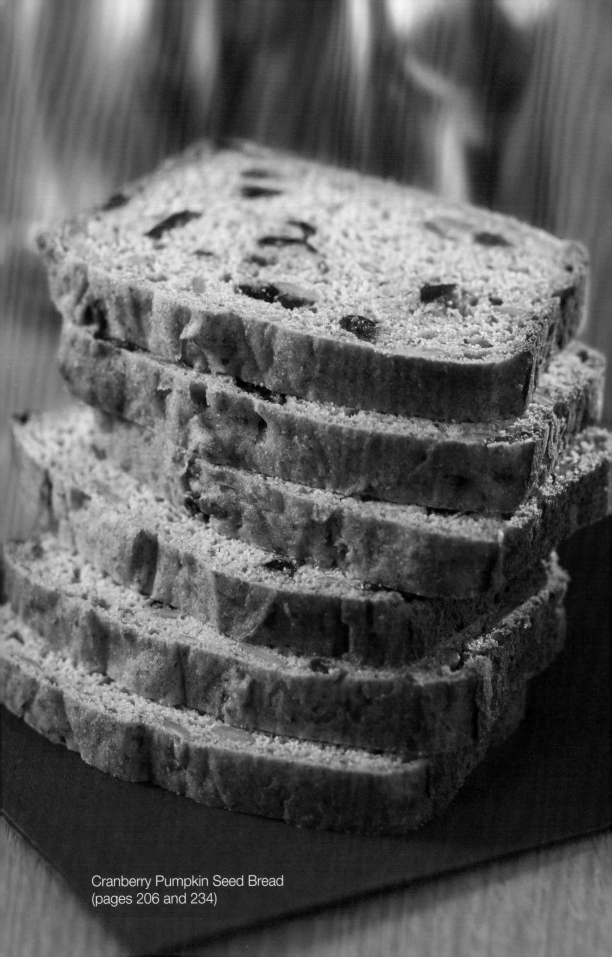

Cranberry Pumpkin Seed Bread
(pages 206 and 234)

Poached Tilapia
with Peppers

Makes 4 servings

Fish is the ideal dish to serve when time is short.

Tips

Fold thinner pieces of fish in half to ensure even thickness when cooking.

To prevent fish from breaking or becoming tough, be sure the wine is just simmering, not boiling rapidly.

1 tbsp	extra virgin olive oil	15 mL
1	red bell pepper, cut into 8 slices	1
1	yellow bell pepper, cut into 8 slices	1
1	orange bell pepper, cut into 8 slices	1
1	onion, cut into wedges	1
2 tbsp	snipped fresh tarragon	25 mL
	Salt and freshly ground white pepper	
½ cup	dry white wine	125 mL
4	skinless tilapia fillets (each 6 oz/175 g), about 1 inch (2.5 cm) thick	4

1. In a large skillet, heat oil over medium heat. Sauté red, yellow and orange peppers and onion for 8 to 10 minutes or until softened. Stir in tarragon, salt and pepper. Reduce heat to low, cover and cook, stirring occasionally, for 20 to 25 minutes or until peppers are very tender.
2. Meanwhile, in a skillet, bring wine to a boil over medium-low heat. Reduce heat to low and add tilapia. Cover and simmer gently for 7 minutes or until fish is opaque and flakes easily with a fork.
3. Serve tilapia topped with pepper mixture.

Variations

Cook fish in GF·vegetable broth instead of wine.

The pepper mixture is also delicious over chicken, scallops or shrimp.

Nutritional value per serving

Calories	285
Fat, total	7 g
Fat, saturated	2 g
Cholesterol	23 mg
Sodium	96 mg
Carbohydrate	19 g
Fiber	3 g
Protein	39 g
Calcium	86 mg
Iron	3 mg

Sole Florentine

Makes 4 servings

Fish is always nutritious and quick to prepare. Select your favorite for this recipe.

- Preheat oven to 400°F (200°C)
- 10-cup (2.5 L) casserole dish, lightly greased

1	package (10 oz/300 g) baby spinach	1
1½ lbs	skinless sole fillets	750 g
1	red onion, chopped	1
1	small bay leaf	1
3	whole black peppercorns	3
¼ tsp	salt	1 mL
¾ cup	dry white wine	175 mL
2 tbsp	freshly squeezed lemon juice	25 mL
¼ cup	amaranth flour	50 mL
2 tbsp	butter, melted	25 mL
¼ cup	milk	50 mL
¼ cup	freshly grated Parmesan cheese	50 mL

1. Using a salad spinner, wash and spin-dry the spinach. Place spinach in prepared casserole and set aside.

2. Divide sole fillets into four equal portions. Loosely roll each portion around your finger (see tip, at right). Set aside.

3. In a medium saucepan, combine onion, bay leaf, peppercorns, salt, wine and lemon juice. Bring to a boil over medium-low heat. Reduce heat to low and add fillet rolls. Cover and simmer for 5 minutes. Place fillet rolls on top of the spinach.

4. Strain the simmering liquid, reserving 1 cup (250 mL) liquid and discarding solids.

5. In a microwave-safe bowl, combine flour and butter. Microwave on High for 1 minute or until mixture is the consistency of dry sand. Stir in milk and reserved liquid. Microwave on High for 3 minutes, stopping to stir occasionally, or until mixture comes to a boil and has thickened. Pour over fish. Sprinkle with cheese.

Nutritional value per serving

Calories	328
Fat, total	11 g
Fat, saturated	5 g
Cholesterol	102 mg
Sodium	412 mg
Carbohydrate	12 g
Fiber	3 g
Protein	39 g
Calcium	234 mg
Iron	5 mg

Tips

If you've purchased frozen sole fillets, thaw overnight in the refrigerator. Packages of frozen sole may be slightly smaller than 1½ lbs (750 g); this will be fine for this recipe.

If fish fillets are small, you may need to roll several together to form four rolls.

6. Bake in preheated oven for 10 to 12 minutes or until fish is opaque, flakes easily with a fork and reaches an internal temperature of 155°F (68°C).

Variations

Use any other white fish, such as tilapia, halibut, cod or haddock.

For a real change, substitute 20 large scallops for the sole. Skip step 2 and proceed with the recipe.

Salmon en Papillote

Makes 4 servings

These packets are impressive, yet easy, and you can assemble them ahead of time. Relax and enjoy your guests, and just pop the parcels into the oven at a convenient time. Be sure not to eat the parchment paper!

Tips

In early spring, when only thin asparagus spears are available, use 16 spears and leave them whole.

Julienned vegetables are about the size of matchsticks and cook quickly.

You can use foil in place of the parchment.

Nutritional value per serving

Calories	183
Fat, total	5 g
Fat, saturated	1 g
Cholesterol	21 mg
Sodium	259 mg
Carbohydrate	23 g
Fiber	6 g
Protein	12 g
Calcium	104 mg
Iron	3 mg

- Preheat oven to 400°F (200°C)
- Parchment paper

1 cup	GF vegetable broth	250 mL
1/4 cup	quinoa, rinsed	50 mL
16	fresh spinach leaves, trimmed	16
4	skinless salmon fillets (each 5 oz/150 g)	4
1/2 cup	dry white wine	125 mL
8	asparagus spears, trimmed and halved lengthwise	8
6	shallots, quartered	6
1	yellow bell pepper, julienned	1
1	carrot, julienned	1
2	lemons, thinly sliced	2

1. In a saucepan, bring broth and quinoa to a boil over high heat. Reduce heat to low, cover and simmer for 18 to 20 minutes or until tender. Remove from heat. Let stand, covered, for 5 to 10 minutes or until quinoa has turned from white to transparent and the tiny, spiral-like germ is separated. Drain, if necessary.

2. Cut four 15-inch (38 cm) squares of parchment paper. Fold each square in half and cut out the shape of half of a heart, with the center fold as the center of the heart, covering as much of the paper as possible. When you open up the paper, you'll have a heart-shaped piece.

3. On each open piece of parchment paper, spread 1/4 cup (50 mL) quinoa a little off-center on one side of the heart. Top with one-quarter of the spinach. Center a salmon fillet on top of the spinach, then add 2 tbsp (25 mL) white wine and one-quarter of the vegetables. Top with one-quarter of the lemon slices. Fold one edge of the parchment paper over to meet the other edge, enclosing the filling. Seal the packet by making small folds, starting at the top, all around the outer edge of the paper, twisting the paper at the end. Place on a baking sheet. Repeat with the remaining paper hearts and ingredients.

Tips

Packets can be prepared through the end of step 3 and refrigerated for up to 4 hours. Increase the baking time to 25 to 30 minutes.

If the packets are not completely sealed, overwrap with another layer of parchment paper to prevent leaking.

Open packets carefully, as steam will escape. To avoid being burned, do not unseal along the outer edge; instead, cut an X in the center.

4. Bake in preheated oven for 20 to 25 minutes or until parchment puffs up with steam and a meat thermometer inserted into a salmon fillet registers 155°F (68°C).

Variations

Substitute GF vegetable broth for the white wine.

Substitute julienned green beans for the asparagus.

Substitute ½ fennel bulb, 1 cup (250 mL) broccoli florets or 12 snow peas for any of the vegetables.

Make packets using the full square instead of cutting hearts. Place ingredients in the center, then seal packets by making a drugstore fold (see the Techniques Glossary, page 396).

Chunky Crab Cakes

**Makes 8 crab cakes
(2 per serving)**

*For the last several
years, we've spent
a month in Georgia,
going from restaurant
to restaurant to
evaluate crab cakes.
Hope you like our
modified favorite.*

Tip

You can purchase roasted
red peppers or make your
own (see box, opposite).

- Preheat oven to 450°F (230°C)
- 2 baking sheets, one lined with parchment paper,
  the other brushed with olive oil

Crab Cakes

1	green onion, finely chopped	1
1/2 cup	chopped roasted red bell peppers	125 mL
2 tbsp	snipped fresh parsley or dill	25 mL
1 tbsp	grated lemon zest	15 mL
2	eggs	2
1/4 cup	GF mayonnaise	50 mL
1 tsp	Dijon mustard	5 mL
1/2 cup	fine dry GF bread crumbs	125 mL
1 lb	shelled cooked crabmeat, cut into large chunks	500 g

Coating

2	eggs	2
2 cups	fine dry GF bread crumbs	500 mL

Roasted Red Pepper Coulis
(page 86)

1. *Crab cakes:* In a bowl, combine green onion, roasted
   peppers, parsley, lemon zest, eggs, mayonnaise and
   mustard. Gently stir in bread crumbs and crabmeat.
   Form into 8 patties about 3/4 inch (2 cm) thick.

2. *Coating:* In a pie plate or shallow dish, beat eggs.
   Place the bread crumbs in another pie plate or shallow
   dish. Coat both sides of each patty with egg, then with
   bread crumbs (use two spatulas to turn them, as they
   are very crumbly and soft). Discard any excess egg
   and bread crumbs. Place crab cakes on paper-lined
   baking sheet.

Nutritional value per serving	
Calories	646
Fat, total	24 g
Fat, saturated	4 g
Cholesterol	278 mg
Sodium	1,164 mg
Carbohydrate	68 g
Fiber	8 g
Protein	40 g
Calcium	284 mg
Iron	6 mg

Tips

Either purchase GF bread crumbs or make your own. Use at least 2-day-old thin slices of bread and dry them in a 250°F (120°C) oven until crisp but not too dark, let cool to room temperature then pulse in food processor until fine.

You can use fresh cooked, canned or frozen crabmeat. If using canned, drain it. If using frozen, thaw it, place in a sieve and press firmly to remove any excess liquid.

For portion control, use an ice cream scoop to transfer crabmeat mixture to the egg, then flatten slightly.

3. Place oiled baking sheet in preheated oven for 5 minutes or until very hot. Gently transfer crab cakes to hot baking sheet. Bake for 10 minutes or until top is golden. Turn and bake for 5 minutes or until top is golden.

4. Serve crab cakes with Roasted Red Pepper Coulis.

Roasting Red Bell Peppers

To roast red bell peppers, place whole peppers on a baking sheet, piercing each near the stem with a knife. Bake at 425°F (220°C) for 18 minutes. Turn and bake for 15 minutes or until the skins blister. (Or roast on the barbecue, turning frequently, until skin is completely charred.) Place in a paper or plastic bag. Seal and let cool for 10 minutes or until skin is loose. Peel and discard seeds.

Seafood Mushroom Risotto

Makes 4 to 6 servings

Just add a salad and dessert to this quick, easy risotto for a complete meal.

Tip

Mushrooms can be stored in a paper bag in the refrigerator for up to 4 days.

1 tbsp	extra virgin olive oil	15 mL
2	cloves garlic, minced	2
1	onion, chopped	1
½	red bell pepper, cut into 1-inch (2.5 cm) pieces	½
½	yellow bell pepper, cut into 1-inch (2.5 cm) pieces	½
2 cups	chopped mushrooms	500 mL
1 cup	Arborio rice	250 mL
2½ cups	GF chicken broth	625 mL
½ cup	dry white wine	125 mL
24	mussels, scrubbed and debearded (see tip, page 101)	24
12	jumbo or colossal shrimp (about 1 lb/500 g), peeled and deveined	12
	Salt and freshly ground white pepper	
½ cup	freshly grated Parmesan cheese	125 mL

1. In a large pot, heat olive oil over medium heat. Add garlic, onion, red and yellow peppers, mushrooms and rice; sauté for 5 to 7 minutes or until vegetables are soft.

2. Stir in broth and wine; bring to a boil. Reduce heat to medium-low, cover and simmer for 15 minutes. Add mussels and shrimp, cover and simmer for 10 minutes or until mussels have opened, shrimp is pink and opaque, rice is tender and liquid is absorbed. Discard any mussels that have not opened. Season to taste with salt and pepper. Sprinkle with Parmesan. Serve immediately.

Variations

Use a variety of mushrooms. Plan to include shiitake, cremini (firmer and with a stronger flavor than a regular white button) and portobellini, as well as portobello (mature cremini with a strong, concentrated flavor).

Substitute any short-grain rice for the Arborio rice.

If you prefer not to use white wine, increase the GF broth to 3 cups (750 mL).

For a creamier, more traditional risotto, increase the amount of liquid to up to 5 cups (1.25 L). Cook, uncovered, adding 1 cup (250 mL) broth at a time, stirring frequently and allowing all the broth to be absorbed before adding more.

Nutritional value per serving

Calories	355
Fat, total	7 g
Fat, saturated	2 g
Cholesterol	22 mg
Sodium	765 mg
Carbohydrate	39 g
Fiber	2 g
Protein	27 g
Calcium	191 mg
Iron	5 mg

Speedy Chicken Florentine

Makes 4 servings

Who says you can't improve on a classic? This quick and easy dish will become a favorite.

Tip

Today it is recommend that all prepackaged greens be washed under lots of cold running water, even if they are labeled "prewashed."

- Preheat broiler
- 9-inch (23 cm) square baking pan, lightly greased

2 tbsp	snipped fresh rosemary	25 mL
2 tbsp	extra virgin olive oil	25 mL
1 tbsp	white balsamic vinegar	15 mL
4	small boneless skinless chicken breasts	4
1	package (10 oz/300 g) baby spinach	1
1 tbsp	freshly squeezed lemon juice	15 mL
2	thin slices GF ham, cut in half	2
1⅓ cups	shredded Swiss cheese	325 mL

1. In a large skillet, over medium heat, combine rosemary, oil and vinegar. Add chicken and cook for 5 to 7 minutes per side or until no longer pink inside and an instant-read thermometer inserted in the thickest part registers 165°F (74°C).

2. Meanwhile, using a salad spinner, wash and spin-dry the spinach. In a large saucepan, over medium-high heat, combine spinach and lemon juice; cover and cook for 1 to 2 minutes or until spinach is wilted.

3. Transfer spinach to prepared baking pan. Top with chicken. Top each chicken breast with ham and cheese.

4. Broil for 4 to 5 minutes or until cheese is melted.

Variation

Substitute boneless pork chops for the chicken and, in step 1, cook for 5 to 10 minutes per side (depending on thickness) or until just a hint of pink remains inside.

Nutritional value per serving

Calories	504
Fat, total	22 g
Fat, saturated	9 g
Cholesterol	178 mg
Sodium	491 mg
Carbohydrate	5 g
Fiber	2 g
Protein	69 g
Calcium	447 mg
Iron	4 mg

Sun-Dried Tomato Pesto Chicken

**Egg-free
White sugar–free**

Makes 4 servings

Everybody we talk to enjoys our recipes containing sun-dried tomatoes. We know you'll want to serve chicken this way. You can serve this dish hot or cold.

Tip

Choose chicken breasts of equal size to ensure all will be cooked at the same time.

- Preheat oven to 350°F (180°C)
- 9-inch (23 cm) square glass baking dish, lightly greased

| 4 | bone-in skin-on chicken breasts | 4 |
| 1 cup | Sun-Dried Tomato Pesto (page 74) | 250 mL |

1. Using a knife or spatula, gently lift skin of chicken breast. Stuff pesto under skin, spreading to coat chicken completely. Press down on skin to smooth and spread pesto mixture. Place chicken in prepared baking dish.

2. Roast in preheated oven for 30 to 40 minutes or until chicken is no longer pink inside and an instant-read thermometer inserted in the thickest part registers 165°F (74°C).

Variation

Use a whole roasting chicken (3 to 4 lbs/1$\frac{1}{2}$ to 2 kg) instead of the chicken breasts. Increase the roasting time to 1$\frac{1}{2}$ to 1$\frac{3}{4}$ hours or until a meat thermometer inserted in the thickest part of the thigh registers 165°F (74°C).

Nutritional value per serving

Calories	423
Fat, total	16 g
Fat, saturated	4 g
Cholesterol	145 mg
Sodium	398 mg
Carbohydrate	6 g
Fiber	2 g
Protein	60 g
Calcium	178 mg
Iron	3 mg

Chicken Quesadillas

**Makes 3 servings
(6 wedges per serving)**

Donna's grandson, Martin, thinks of this as Mexican grilled cheese.

Tips

Serve with guacamole, GF salsa and/or sour cream.

A pizza wheel makes cutting the quesadillas into wedges easier.

• 9- to 10-inch (23 to 25 cm) nonstick skillet, or griddle

6	8-inch (20 cm) GF tortillas	6
3/4 cup	GF salsa	175 mL
2 cups	diced cooked chicken breasts	500 mL
1 1/2 cups	shredded GF Tex-Mex blend cheese	375 mL

1. Spread half of each tortilla evenly with 2 tbsp (25 mL) salsa. Top with 1/3 cup (75 mL) chicken and 1/4 cup (50 mL) cheese. Fold remaining half of tortilla over filling.

2. Heat skillet over medium heat. Cook quesadillas for 4 to 5 minutes per side or until both sides are golden brown and cheese is melted. Cut each quesadilla into 3 wedges.

Variation

Add 2 tbsp (25 mL) refried beans to each quesadilla before cooking.

Nutritional value per serving	
Calories	636
Fat, total	26 g
Fat, saturated	12 g
Cholesterol	138 mg
Sodium	608 mg
Carbohydrate	50 g
Fiber	8 g
Protein	50 g
Calcium	596 mg
Iron	4 mg

Marmalade-Glazed Pork Tenderloin

Makes 4 servings

A CanolaInfo recipe

Try this for a weeknight supper — buy the tenderloin on the way home from work one night, marinate it overnight and bake or grill it the next.

Tips

To prevent the thin tip of pork tenderloin from drying out, turn it under before baking.

Tenderloin can be frozen in the marinade for up to 2 months, thawed in the refrigerator overnight and then baked or grilled (see variation, below).

Nutritional value per serving

Calories	371
Fat, total	8 g
Fat, saturated	2 g
Cholesterol	84 mg
Sodium	294 mg
Carbohydrate	42 g
Fiber	0 g
Protein	35 g
Calcium	56 mg
Iron	3 mg

- 13- by 9-inch (33 by 23 cm) baking pan, lightly greased

Marinade

¾ cup	orange marmalade	175 mL
2 tbsp	Dijon mustard	25 mL
1 tbsp	vegetable oil	15 mL
3	cloves garlic, minced	3
2 tbsp	finely snipped fresh rosemary	25 mL
2	pork tenderloins (each about 10 oz/300 g)	2

1. *Marinade:* In a small microwave-safe bowl, combine marmalade, mustard and oil. Microwave on Medium (50%) for 1 to 2 minutes or until marmalade is melted. Stir in garlic and rosemary. Let cool.

2. Pour marinade into a large sealable plastic bag set in a bowl. Add pork, seal and turn to coat. Refrigerate for at least 4 hours or for up to 2 days, turning occasionally.

3. Preheat oven to 400°F (200°C).

4. Remove pork from marinade, discarding marinade. Place pork tenderloins in prepared baking pan, making sure they are not touching.

5. Bake in preheated oven for 20 to 25 minutes or until just a hint of pink remains inside and a meat thermometer inserted in the thickest part registers 155°F (68°C). Transfer to a cutting board, tent loosely with foil and let rest for 5 minutes. Slice across the grain.

Variations

If you're short on time, cut tenderloin into 1-inch (2.5 cm) thick slices and grill over high heat for 3 to 4 minutes per side or until just a hint of pink remains inside. Avoid overcooking. (The cooking time will be much shorter if you're using an indoor contact grill. Check the manufacturer's instructions for timing.)

For a sweet ginger flavor, add 1 tbsp (15 mL) grated gingerroot with the garlic.

Pesto Pork

Egg-free
White sugar–free

Makes 4 servings

Pork tenderloin is just the right size for four — share it with good friends!

Tips

Remove any fat, along with the membrane, from the outside of the tenderloin before butterflying it (step 1).

Secure the filling with toothpicks instead of string. Count them to be sure you remove them all at the end.

- Preheat oven to 400°F (200°C)
- 13- by 9-inch (33 by 23 cm) baking pan, lightly greased
- Kitchen string

1	pork tenderloin (about 1 lb/500 g)	1
⅓ cup	Greek Pesto (page 73)	75 mL
½ cup	shredded Asiago cheese	125 mL

1. Cut tenderloin in half lengthwise, almost but not all the way through. Open and lie flat. Spread pesto down both sides and top with cheese. Fold the two sides together, like closing a book. Tie tightly with kitchen string and place in prepared baking pan.

2. Roast in preheated oven for 25 to 30 minutes or until just a hint of pink remains inside and a meat thermometer inserted in the thickest part registers 155°F (68°C). Transfer to a cutting board, tent with foil and let rest for 10 minutes. Remove string and slice across the grain.

Variations

Substitute Sun-Dried Tomato Pesto (page 74) for the Greek Pesto.

Nutritional value per serving	
Calories	290
Fat, total	16 g
Fat, saturated	6 g
Cholesterol	88 mg
Sodium	234 mg
Carbohydrate	2 g
Fiber	1 g
Protein	33 g
Calcium	204 mg
Iron	2 mg

California Ham Loaf

Makes 4 servings

Heather grew up with this easy-to-make ham loaf. Today, we would serve Pineapple Mango Relish (page 89) to complement it.

Tip
If you can't find ground ham, finely diced ham works well.

- Preheat oven to 350°F (180°C)
- 8-inch (20 cm) square baking pan

8 oz	GF ground ham	250 g
4 oz	lean ground beef or veal	125 g
4 oz	lean ground pork	125 g
1 cup	GF corn flakes cereal	250 mL
1 cup	milk	250 mL
1	egg	1
½	large green bell pepper, coarsely chopped	½

1. In a large bowl, combine ham, beef, pork, corn flakes, milk, egg and green pepper. Spoon into baking pan.

2. Bake in preheated oven for 1 hour or until a meat thermometer inserted in the center registers 160°F (71°C). Drain off accumulated liquid and cut into squares or slices.

Variations
Add ⅓ cup (75 mL) each chopped onion and mushrooms.
Use two 9- by 5-inch (23 by 12.5 cm) loaf pans.

Nutritional value per serving	
Calories	410
Fat, total	23 g
Fat, saturated	8 g
Cholesterol	127 mg
Sodium	336 mg
Carbohydrate	24 g
Fiber	1 g
Protein	25 g
Calcium	91 mg
Iron	5 mg

Second-Day Beef Quinoa Salad

Makes 2 servings

This delightful dinner salad for a hot summer's evening can be put together quickly with leftovers from the night before.

Tip

The asparagus should be cooked just until tender-crisp and then well chilled.

½ cup	Onion Purée (page 147)	125 mL
1 tbsp	cider vinegar	15 mL
1 tbsp	vegetable oil	15 mL
¼ tsp	salt	1 mL
¼ tsp	freshly ground black pepper	1 mL
2	green onions, thinly sliced	2
¼	large red bell pepper, cut into ¼-inch (0.5 cm) pieces	¼
2 cups	Quinoa Pilaf (page 173)	500 mL
1 cup	cooked asparagus pieces (2-inch/ 5 cm pieces)	250 mL
1 cup	shaved or thinly sliced cooked Rubbed Roast Beef (page 146)	250 mL
⅓ cup	shredded Havarti or smoked Gouda cheese	75 mL

1. In a large salad bowl, combine Onion Purée, vinegar, oil, salt and pepper. Add green onions, red pepper, Quinoa Pilaf, asparagus, beef and cheese; toss to combine.

2. Cover and refrigerate for at least 2 hours to let flavors develop and blend, or for up to 3 days.

Variation

Other vegetables that could be substituted or added include cooked broccoli florets, green or yellow beans or snow peas.

Nutritional value per serving

Calories	177
Fat, total	14 g
Fat, saturated	5 g
Cholesterol	21 mg
Sodium	419 mg
Carbohydrate	7 g
Fiber	2 g
Protein	8 g
Calcium	177 mg
Iron	1 mg

Slow Cooker Beef Stew with Winter Vegetables and Biscuit Topping

Makes 4 to 6 servings

A CanolaInfo recipe

Winter stews have always been considered true comfort food. We've included lots of root vegetables in ours, as they are readily available and economical all winter long.

Tips

Use less or more meat, according to the meat-to-vegetable ratio you like in your stew.

For a deeper color and a richer gravy, take the time to brown the beef in 2 tbsp (25 mL) vegetable oil over medium heat, in batches if necessary, before adding it to the slow cooker.

Nutritional value per serving

Calories	503
Fat, total	13 g
Fat, saturated	3 g
Cholesterol	90 mg
Sodium	480 mg
Carbohydrate	51 g
Fiber	8 g
Protein	47 g
Calcium	149 mg
Iron	8 mg

- Cheesecloth
- 5- to 7-quart slow cooker

Beef Stew

2	bay leaves	2
2 tsp	whole black peppercorns	10 mL
1 tsp	whole cloves	5 mL
1/2 tsp	whole allspice berries	2 mL
4	parsnips, cut into 2-inch (5 cm) pieces	4
4	potatoes, cut into 2-inch (5 cm) pieces	4
3	cloves garlic	3
2	small white turnips, peeled and thinly sliced	2
2	onions, cut into wedges	2
1	package (12 oz/340 g) baby carrots	1
1/4	winter squash, peeled and cut into 2-inch (5 cm) pieces (about 1 cup/250 mL)	1/4
1	can (28 oz/796 mL) diced tomatoes, with juice	1
1/2 cup	GF beef broth	125 mL
1/4 cup	tomato paste	50 mL
2 to 3 lbs	stewing beef	1 to 1.5 kg
	Salt and freshly ground black pepper	
1/4 cup	amaranth flour	50 mL
2 tbsp	vegetable oil	25 mL

Biscuit Topping

2/3 cup	amaranth flour	150 mL
2/3 cup	whole bean flour	150 mL
1/4 cup	potato starch	50 mL
2 tbsp	white (granulated) sugar	25 mL
1 tsp	xanthan gum	5 mL
1 tbsp	GF baking powder	15 mL
1/2 tsp	baking soda	2 mL
1/4 tsp	salt	1 mL
3 tbsp	vegetable oil	45 mL
1 cup	buttermilk	250 mL

Tip

The stew must be bubbling hot to ensure that the bottom of the biscuits bake.

Stovetop Method

In a large Dutch oven, heat 1 tbsp (15 mL) vegetable oil over medium heat. Brown beef, in batches, adding oil as needed between batches. Drain off fat and return all beef to the pan. Add all other stew ingredients, except for the flour and oil, and bring to a boil over medium-high heat. Reduce heat to low and simmer gently, stirring occasionally, for 1 to 1½ hours or until beef is tender. Discard the spice bag and preheat oven as in step 3. Combine amaranth flour and oil, stir into stew, increase heat to medium and simmer for about 15 minutes or until thickened. Transfer Dutch oven to oven and continue with recipe from step 5 on.

1. *Beef stew:* Tie bay leaves, peppercorns, cloves and allspice in a 6-inch (15 cm) square of cheesecloth.

2. In slow cooker stoneware, combine parsnips, potatoes, garlic, turnips, onions, carrots and squash. Top with tomatoes with juice, broth, tomato paste and stewing beef. Add spice bag. Cover and cook on Low for 8 hours or until meat and vegetables are tender. Remove and discard spice bag. Season to taste with salt and pepper.

3. Preheat oven to 425°F (220°C).

4. In a bowl, combine amaranth flour and oil; stir into liquid in slow cooker. Cover and cook on High for about 15 minutes or until thickened.

5. Transfer slow cooker stoneware to oven and bake for 15 minutes or until stew is hot and bubbly.

6. *Biscuit topping:* Meanwhile, in a food processor, pulse amaranth flour, whole bean flour, potato starch, sugar, xanthan gum, baking powder, baking soda and salt until combined. Whisk together oil and buttermilk. With the motor running, through the feed tube, gradually add oil mixture in a steady stream. Process for 5 to 10 seconds or until dough just holds together. Do not overprocess.

7. Drop biscuit topping by heaping spoonfuls onto hot stew. Bake for 15 to 20 minutes or until tops are golden. Serve immediately.

Variations

Substitute ¼ rutabaga for the turnips.

Substitute 3 to 4 lbs (1.5 to 2 kg) beef short ribs for the stewing beef.

To make a vegetarian stew, substitute 2 cans (14 to 19 oz/ 398 to 540 mL) kidney beans or black beans, drained and rinsed, for the stewing beef.

Add 2 tsp (10 mL) dried summer savory to the dry ingredients in the biscuit topping.

For a quick and easy biscuit to serve with any meal, drop biscuit topping by heaping spoonfuls onto a lightly greased baking sheet. Bake in a 425°F (220°C) oven for 10 to 13 minutes or until tops are golden. Immediately transfer biscuits to a wire rack. Serve hot.

Rubbed Roast Beef with Onion Purée and Quinoa Pilaf

Makes 8 to 10 servings

This idea is right for today's busy lifestyle. Due to time restraints and smaller families, we no longer have time to cook for just one meal. Planned leftovers are "in" and save time and energy.

Tips

Choose any beef oven roast, such as sirloin tip, eye of round or any other tender cut.

Prepare the Quinoa Pilaf while the roast is in the oven, and prepare the Onion Purée while the roast is resting.

Roast Beef • Nutritional value per serving

Calories	240
Fat, total	8 g
Fat, saturated	2 g
Cholesterol	86 mg
Sodium	381 mg
Carbohydrate	2 g
Fiber	0 g
Protein	39 g
Calcium	49 mg
Iron	5 mg

- **Preheat oven to 450°F (230°C)**
- **Roasting pan**

4	cloves garlic, minced	4
1/4 cup	Dijon mustard	50 mL
1 tbsp	dried thyme	15 mL
1 tsp	freshly ground black pepper	5 mL
1/2 tsp	salt	2 mL
4 to 5 lb	beef oven roast	2 to 2.5 kg
	Onion Purée (see recipe, opposite)	
	Quinoa Pilaf (page 173)	

1. In a small bowl, combine garlic, mustard, thyme, pepper and salt. Spread rub on roast, coating all over. Place roast, fat side up, in roasting pan. Insert a meat thermometer in center of roast, avoiding fat.

2. Bake in preheated oven for 10 minutes. Reduce heat to 275°F (140°C) and bake for 2¼ to 2¾ hours, until thermometer registers 150°F (65°C) for medium, or until desired doneness. Transfer to a cutting board, tent with foil and let rest for 15 minutes.

3. Carve roast across the grain into thin slices. Serve with Onion Purée and Quinoa Pilaf.

Variation

Substitute green peppercorn Dijon mustard for the regular.

Makes about 4 cups (1 L)
(¼ cup/50 mL per
serving)

Onion Purée has a rich tangy flavor — your guests will want seconds! Serve with Rubbed Roast Beef and use to make Second-Day Beef Quinoa Salad (page 143).

Tips

If your roasting pan isn't safe for stovetop use, transfer the pan drippings to a saucepan before proceeding with the recipe.

If your pan drippings don't quite equal ¼ cup (50 mL), add olive oil to make up the difference.

Nutritional value per serving

Calories	32
Fat, total	0 g
Fat, saturated	0 g
Cholesterol	5 mg
Sodium	187 mg
Carbohydrate	4 g
Fiber	1 g
Protein	3 g
Calcium	20 mg
Iron	0 mg

Onion Purée

	Pan drippings from roast beef	
4	large onions, cut into wedges	4
1 tsp	freshly ground black pepper	5 mL
3 cups	GF beef broth	750 mL
2 tbsp	prepared horseradish	25 mL
2 tbsp	Dijon mustard	25 mL

1. Drain all but ¼ cup (50 mL) drippings from roasting pan and place over medium-high heat. Sauté onions and pepper for 5 to 10 minutes or until onions are softened. Add broth, horseradish and mustard; bring to a boil. Reduce heat to medium-low and simmer for about 5 minutes or until slightly thickened.

2. Working in batches as necessary, transfer to a food processor or blender and process until the consistency of applesauce.

Variation

Use ¼ cup (50 mL) of either mustard or horseradish instead of 2 tbsp (25 mL) of each.

Kerry's Shepherd's Pie

Makes 4 servings

Donna's daughter-in-law makes and freezes shepherd's pie to have ready for a quick yet hearty dinner for her husband and two hungry growing boys.

- Preheat oven to 350°F (180°C)
- Four 1½-cup (375 mL) baking dishes, lightly greased

4	boiling potatoes, peeled and quartered	4
⅓ cup	milk	75 mL
1 tbsp	butter	15 mL
2 lbs	lean ground beef	1 kg
2	cloves garlic, minced	2
1	small onion, chopped	1
1	carrot, diced	1
½	green bell pepper, chopped	½
¾ cup	sliced mushrooms	175 mL
1	can (14 oz/398 mL) GF cream-style corn	1
1 cup	tomato sauce	250 mL
	Salt and freshly ground black pepper	

1. In a saucepan, bring 1 inch (2.5 cm) of water to a rapid boil over high heat. Add potatoes, reduce heat to low, cover and simmer for 15 to 20 minutes or until tender. Drain well.

2. In a large bowl, using an electric mixer, beat potatoes, milk and butter until light and fluffy. Set aside.

3. Meanwhile, in a large skillet, over medium-high heat, cook beef, garlic and onion, breaking beef up with a fork, for 3 to 5 minutes or until beef is browned. Add carrot, green pepper and mushrooms; sauté for 5 to 10 minutes or until vegetables are softened. Add corn and tomato sauce; bring to a simmer. Reduce heat to medium-low, cover and simmer for 10 minutes or until carrot is tender. Season to taste with salt and pepper.

Nutritional value per serving

Calories	796
Fat, total	38 g
Fat, saturated	16 g
Cholesterol	136 mg
Sodium	942 mg
Carbohydrate	66 g
Fiber	6 g
Protein	50 g
Calcium	98 mg
Iron	6 mg

4. Spoon beef mixture into prepared baking dishes, dividing evenly, and spread mashed potatoes over top.

5. Bake in preheated oven for 25 to 30 minutes or until potatoes are slightly browned and meat mixture bubbles around the edges.

Variations

Make 1 large shepherd's pie in a 10-cup (2.5 L) casserole and bake for 25 to 30 minutes or until potatoes are slightly browned and meat mixture bubbles around the edges.

Add 1 to 2 tbsp (15 to 25 mL) caraway seeds or dried thyme or marjoram or $\frac{1}{4}$ to $\frac{1}{2}$ cup (50 to 125 mL) chopped fresh thyme or marjoram with the ground beef.

Sprinkle the top with 2 cups (500 mL) shredded Cheddar cheese for the last 10 minutes of baking.

Substitute 3 cups (750 mL) mashed cooked winter squash or sweet potatoes for the potato topping.

Lasagna

White sugar–free

Makes 8 to 9 servings

Here's another example of a dish adopted by North Americans that has become a staple of our diet.

Tips

Either make your own pasta sauce or purchase a gluten-free one.

To save time, purchase 7 oz (210 g) shredded mozzarella cheese.

- Preheat oven to 350°F (180°C)
- 13- by 9-inch (33 by 23 cm) baking pan

1½ lbs	lean ground beef	750 g
1	onion, diced	1
4 cups	GF pasta sauce	1 L
1½ cups	water	375 mL
1 cup	cottage cheese	250 mL
2	eggs, lightly beaten	2
12	GF oven-ready brown rice lasagna noodles	12
2 cups	shredded mozzarella cheese	500 mL
½ cup	freshly grated Parmesan cheese	125 mL

1. In a large skillet, over medium heat, cook beef and onion, breaking beef up with a fork, for 5 minutes or until beef is browned and onion is tender. Drain off fat. Add pasta sauce and water; bring to a boil. Reduce heat and simmer for 10 minutes. Set aside.

2. In a small bowl, combine cottage cheese and eggs. Set aside.

3. Spread a thin layer of beef mixture in baking pan. Top with 4 lasagna noodles, making sure they don't overlap. Cover with one-third of the remaining beef mixture and half the cottage cheese mixture. Sprinkle with half the mozzarella. Cover with 4 lasagna noodles and layer with half the remaining beef mixture and the remaining cottage cheese mixture and mozzarella. Cover with the remaining lasagna noodles, beef mixture and Parmesan cheese. Cover with foil.

Nutritional value per serving	
Calories	486
Fat, total	22 g
Fat, saturated	9 g
Cholesterol	103 mg
Sodium	953 mg
Carbohydrate	38 g
Fiber	4 g
Protein	32 g
Calcium	290 mg
Iron	3 mg

Tips

We found that, for each layer, 3 noodles lengthwise and 1 crosswise fit nicely in the pan without overlapping.

Be sure the noodles in each layer are completely covered with beef mixture.

Freeze leftover lasagna in individual portions for up to 1 month. Thaw and reheat in the microwave.

4. Bake in preheated oven for 1 hour. Remove foil and bake for 15 minutes or until bubbly, noodles are cooked and cheese is golden brown. Let stand for 10 to 15 minutes before serving.

Variations

Add 6 oz (175 g) baby spinach, washed and dried, layering it between the beef mixture and the cottage cheese mixture.

Substitute tomato juice or garden vegetable juice for the water.

Taco Bake

White sugar–free

Makes 6 to 8 servings

This is like a Mexican shepherd's pie.

Tips

Be sure the milk is no more than 130°F (55°C), or the yeast will be killed.

Yes, we really mean to start it in a cold oven. No need to preheat.

Let cooked Taco Bake cool, wrap tightly and freeze for up to 1 month. Thaw in the refrigerator overnight and reheat in the microwave until steaming.

• 9-inch (23 cm) glass baking dish, lightly greased

Filling

1 lb	extra-lean ground beef	500 g
2 tbsp	Taco Seasoning (see recipe, opposite)	25 mL

Base

½ cup	pea flour	125 mL
¼ cup	cornstarch	50 mL
½ tsp	xanthan gum	2 mL
½ cup	cornmeal	125 mL
4½ tsp	bread machine or instant yeast	22 mL
1 tbsp	white (granulated) sugar	15 mL
½ tsp	salt	2 mL
¾ cup	milk, warmed to 120°F to 130°F (50°C to 55°C)	175 mL
3 tbsp	vegetable oil	45 mL
1	egg	1

Topping

1¼ cups	GF salsa	300 mL
1½ cups	shredded GF Tex-Mex blend cheese	375 mL
1 cup	partially crushed GF tortilla chips	250 mL

1. *Filling:* In a skillet, over medium heat, cook beef, breaking it up with a fork, for 5 minutes or until browned. Drain off fat. Add taco seasoning and mix well. Set aside.

2. *Base:* In a small bowl or plastic bag, combine pea flour, cornstarch, xanthan gum, cornmeal, yeast, sugar and salt. Set aside.

3. In a large bowl, using an electric mixer, combine milk, oil and egg. Add dry ingredients and mix until smooth. Spoon batter into prepared baking dish. Top with filling.

4. *Topping:* Pour salsa evenly over meat. Sprinkle with cheese and tortilla chips.

5. Place in a cold oven. Set temperature to 350°F (180°C) and bake for 35 to 40 minutes or until cheese is bubbly, chips are crisp and an instant-read thermometer inserted in the center of the base registers 200°F (100°C).

Variations

Substitute ground chicken or turkey for the beef.

Substitute GF corn chips or wraps for the tortilla chips. Two 10-inch (25 cm) wraps, cut with a pizza wheel into 1-inch (2.5 cm) pieces, yield about 1 cup (250 mL).

Nutritional value per serving

Calories	350
Fat, total	20 g
Fat, saturated	8 g
Cholesterol	68 mg
Sodium	477 mg
Carbohydrate	21 g
Fiber	2 g
Protein	21 g
Calcium	218 mg
Iron	2 mg

Makes ½ cup (125 mL) (2 tbsp/25 mL per serving)

Unable to find a gluten-free, salt-free taco seasoning? Here's the answer.

Tip

Check to be sure all the seasonings are fresh and gluten-free.

Taco Seasoning

¼ cup	dried minced onion	50 mL
2 tbsp	chili powder	25 mL
2 tsp	cornstarch	10 mL
2 tsp	garlic powder	10 mL
2 tsp	ground cumin	10 mL
1 tsp	dried oregano	5 mL
¼ tsp	cayenne pepper	1 mL

1. In a small bowl, combine onion, chili powder, cornstarch, garlic powder, cumin, oregano and cayenne. Mix well.

2. Store in an airtight container in a cool, dry place for up to 1 year.

Variations

To make this corn-free, substitute potato starch (not potato flour) for the cornstarch.

Increase or decrease the chili powder and cayenne pepper according to the amount of heat you prefer.

To increase the heat, add hot pepper flakes to taste.

Nutritional value per serving	
Calories	35
Fat, total	1 g
Fat, saturated	0 g
Cholesterol	0 mg
Sodium	33 mg
Carbohydrate	6 g
Fiber	1 g
Protein	1 g
Calcium	30 mg
Iron	1 mg

Layered Enchilada Bake

Egg-free
White sugar–free

Makes 8 servings

No need to roll the wraps individually — just layer and bake.

Tip

We found that a pizza wheel cut this dish into individual servings without disturbing the layers.

- Preheat oven to 400°F (200°C)
- 10-inch (25 cm) springform pan, lightly greased

1 lb	lean ground beef	500 g
1	onion, chopped	1
1	can (14 to 19 oz/398 to 540 mL) black beans, drained and rinsed	1
2 cups	GF salsa	500 mL
2 tbsp	Taco Seasoning (page 153)	25 mL
4	10-inch (25 cm) GF tortillas	4
1 cup	sour cream	250 mL
2 cups	shredded GF Tex-Mex blend cheese	500 mL
2 to 4	tomatoes, diced	2 to 4
1 cup	shredded lettuce	250 mL

1. In a skillet, over medium heat, cook beef and onion, breaking beef up with a fork, for 5 minutes or until beef is browned. Drain off fat. Stir in beans, salsa and taco seasoning; cook, stirring occasionally, for 5 minutes.

2. Center prepared pan on a large square of heavy-duty foil and press foil up sides of pan. Layer 2 tortillas in bottom of pan. Cover with half the meat mixture. Top with half the sour cream and half the cheese. Repeat the layers. Cover with foil.

3. Bake in preheated oven for 30 minutes. Remove the foil and bake for 10 to 15 minutes or until casserole is heated through and cheese starts to brown. Let stand for 5 minutes. Remove springform ring and cut into wedges. Serve tomatoes and lettuce as an accompaniment.

Variations

Substitute drained yogurt for the sour cream. See the Techniques Glossary, page 399, for information on draining yogurt.

Add 1/2 cup (125 mL) drained canned corn with the beans.

Nutritional value per serving

Calories	367
Fat, total	21 g
Fat, saturated	11 g
Cholesterol	71 mg
Sodium	680 mg
Carbohydrate	23 g
Fiber	2 g
Protein	24 g
Calcium	313 mg
Iron	3 mg

Eggplant and Pepper Pasta Casserole

Makes 4 servings

Looking for something different to serve for dinner this weekend? Try this vegetarian casserole.

Tips

Select an eggplant that is heavy for its size and firm to the touch. The skin should be deep, glossy purple to black. The thin skin is edible, so there's no need to peel. Store eggplant in the refrigerator, unwrapped, for 1 to 2 days.

In the past, it was the practice to sprinkle eggplant slices with salt and let stand for 15 minutes to remove some moisture and bitterness. There's no need to do this with the varieties we purchase today.

Nutritional value per serving	
Calories	299
Fat, total	17 g
Fat, saturated	2 g
Cholesterol	0 mg
Sodium	260 mg
Carbohydrate	33 g
Fiber	5 g
Protein	8 g
Calcium	107 mg
Iron	3 mg

2 tbsp	extra virgin olive oil	25 mL
2	orange bell peppers, cut into 1/2-inch (1 cm) pieces	2
2	cloves garlic, minced	2
1	eggplant, cut into 1-inch (2.5 cm) cubes	1
1/2 cup	slivered almonds	125 mL
1 1/2 cups	canned diced tomatoes, with juice	375 mL
2 tbsp	tomato paste	25 mL
1/2 tsp	ground cumin	2 mL
1/4 tsp	ground cinnamon	1 mL
2 oz	GF pasta (rotini, elbow or small tubes)	60 g
1/4 cup	snipped fresh parsley	50 mL
	Freshly grated Parmesan cheese	

1. In a large skillet, heat oil over medium heat. Sauté orange peppers for 5 minutes. Add garlic, eggplant and almonds; sauté for 3 to 5 minutes or until peppers are tender. Add tomatoes with juice, tomato paste, cumin and cinnamon; bring to a boil. Reduce heat to low and simmer for 5 minutes or until heated through.

2. Meanwhile, in a large saucepan of boiling water, cook pasta according to package directions until just tender. Rinse under cold running water and drain well.

3. Add pasta and parsley to the skillet and bring to a boil over medium heat. Reduce heat to low and simmer for 5 to 10 minutes or until heated through. Serve sprinkled with Parmesan.

Variations

For more heat, add 1/4 tsp (1 mL) hot pepper flakes with the spices.

Use 1 1/2 cups (375 mL) GF pasta sauce (any flavor) in place of the tomatoes and tomato paste.

Black Beans and Squash with Pasta

Egg-free
White sugar–free

Makes 6 servings

This colorful autumn main dish is quick and easy for family or company.

Tips

If the GF broth tastes salty, omit the salt in the recipe.

If your skillet doesn't have a lid, use foil to cover it.

1 tbsp	vegetable oil	15 mL
2	cloves garlic, minced	2
1	onion, chopped	1
1	red bell pepper, chopped	1
1/4 cup	snipped fresh sage	50 mL
1/4 tsp	salt	1 mL
1/4 tsp	freshly ground black pepper	1 mL
4 cups	cubed peeled butternut squash (1-inch/2.5 cm cubes)	1 L
1/2 cup	GF vegetable broth	125 mL
1 cup	rinsed drained canned black beans	250 mL
2 oz	GF pasta (rotini, elbow or small tubes)	60 g
1 cup	cubed cooked GF ham (1/2-inch/1 cm cubes)	250 mL
1/3 cup	freshly grated Parmesan cheese	75 mL
1/4 cup	snipped fresh cilantro	50 mL

1. In a large skillet, heat oil over medium heat. Sauté garlic, onion, red pepper, sage, salt and pepper for 5 minutes or until onion is soft. Add squash and broth; bring to a boil. Reduce heat to low, cover and simmer for 12 to 15 minutes or until squash is tender.

2. Add beans and simmer for about 5 minutes or until heated through.

3. Meanwhile, in a large saucepan of boiling water, cook pasta according to package directions until just tender. Rinse under cold running water and drain well.

4. Return pasta to the saucepan. Add squash mixture, ham, Parmesan and cilantro; bring to a boil over medium heat. Reduce heat to low and simmer, stirring occasionally, for 5 to 10 minutes or until heated through.

Variations

Use any other variety of beans in place of the black beans.

Substitute 2 cups (500 mL) cooked quinoa or brown rice for the cooked pasta.

Nutritional value per serving

Calories	168
Fat, total	5 g
Fat, saturated	2 g
Cholesterol	17 mg
Sodium	780 mg
Carbohydrate	21 g
Fiber	6 g
Protein	11 g
Calcium	160 mg
Iron	2 mg

Pasta, Spinach and Clams

Makes 3 to 4 servings

You'll enjoy this refreshing mixture of tomatoes, basil and clams.

Tips

When you are purchasing clams, remember that they are alive. They should feel heavy for the size. When you bring them home from the store, place them in a bowl, cover with wet paper towels and refrigerate. Use the same day. If any clams are open, tap them; if they don't snap shut, discard them. Also discard any that don't open after cooking. If you feel it's simpler, you can substitute a drained 10-oz (284 mL) can of clams.

If you prefer, you can use fresh tomatoes; you'll need about 6 large to get the same amount.

You can use 2 to 3 tbsp (25 to 45 mL) dried basil instead of the fresh.

Nutritional value per serving	
Calories	444
Fat, total	10 g
Fat, saturated	3 g
Cholesterol	87 mg
Sodium	591 mg
Carbohydrate	43 g
Fiber	7 g
Protein	41 g
Calcium	440 mg
Iron	35 mg

3 oz	GF wild rice penne or linguine pasta	90 g
1 tbsp	extra virgin olive oil	15 mL
3 to 4	cloves garlic, minced	3 to 4
1	large onion, coarsely chopped	1
1	can (28 oz/796 mL) diced tomatoes, drained	1
½ cup	snipped fresh basil	125 mL
1 cup	GF tomato basil pasta sauce	250 mL
½ cup	dry white wine	125 mL
2 lbs	clams, scrubbed	1 kg
1	package (10 oz/300 g) baby spinach	1
½ cup	freshly grated Parmesan cheese	125 mL

1. In a large saucepan of boiling water, cook pasta according to package directions until just tender. Rinse under cold running water and drain well.

2. Meanwhile, in a large saucepan, heat oil over medium heat. Sauté garlic and onion for 3 to 5 minutes or until onion begins to soften. Add tomatoes, basil, pasta sauce and wine; bring to a boil over medium-high heat and boil for 5 minutes. Add clams, reduce heat to medium, cover and simmer for 7 to 10 minutes or until clams open. Discard any clams that do not open. Top with spinach, cover and simmer for 1 minute or until wilted. Stir in pasta and simmer until heated through. Serve sprinkled with Parmesan.

Variations

Substitute clam juice for the white wine.

Use 10 oz (300 g) sea scallops instead of clams and cook for 3 to 5 minutes (depending on size) or until firm and opaque.

Use oregano-based GF pasta sauce and substitute fresh oregano for the basil.

Beefy Mac 'n' Cheese

Makes 6 servings

*Here is yet another
version of mac and
cheese.*

- **Preheat oven to 350°F (180°C)**
- **10-cup (2.5 L) casserole dish, lightly greased**

1 lb	lean ground beef	500 g
1	can (28 oz/796 mL) diced tomatoes, with juice	1
1/2 cup	snipped fresh oregano	125 mL
2 cups	GF wild rice elbow pasta	500 mL
1 tbsp	butter	15 mL
1 tbsp	amaranth flour	15 mL
1/2 tsp	dry mustard	2 mL
1/2 tsp	salt	2 mL
1/4 tsp	freshly ground white pepper	1 mL
Pinch	cayenne pepper	Pinch
1 1/2 cups	milk	375 mL
1/4 tsp	GF Worcestershire sauce	1 mL
1 cup	shredded aged Cheddar cheese	250 mL
1/2 cup	shredded Swiss cheese	125 mL

1. In a large skillet, over medium heat, cook beef, breaking it up with a fork, for 5 minutes or until browned. Drain off fat, if necessary. Add tomatoes and oregano; bring to a boil. Reduce heat to medium-low and simmer for 10 minutes.

2. Meanwhile, in a large saucepan of boiling water, cook pasta according to package directions until just tender. Rinse under cold running water and drain well. Set aside.

3. In a microwave-safe bowl, microwave butter on High for 30 to 60 seconds or until melted. Stir in amaranth flour, mustard, salt, white pepper and cayenne. Microwave on High for 1 to 3 minutes or until mixture is the consistency of dry sand. Stir in milk and Worcestershire sauce. Microwave on High for 3 to 5 minutes, stopping to stir occasionally, until mixture comes to a boil and has thickened. Stir in Cheddar and Swiss cheese.

**Nutritional value
per serving**

Calories	420
Fat, total	23 g
Fat, saturated	12 g
Cholesterol	78 mg
Sodium	612 mg
Carbohydrate	26 g
Fiber	3 g
Protein	26 g
Calcium	352 mg
Iron	3 mg

Tips

Rinsing the cooked pasta well prevents the macaroni and cheese from becoming too thick.

Be sure to use orange-colored Cheddar cheese for a more attractive dish.

4. In prepared casserole, combine pasta, cheese sauce and beef mixture.

5. Bake in preheated oven for 10 minutes or until heated through.

Variations

Add 1 onion, diced, with the ground beef.

Substitute ground chicken or turkey for the beef.

Just before baking, top with extra shredded cheese.

Broccoli Chicken Pasta

Makes 4 to 6 servings

Supper on the table in 20 minutes or less! Most of the preparation is done ahead of time.

Tips

Cook broccoli just until tender-crisp in a steamer or microwave. Plunge into a bowl or sink of ice water to stop the cooking. Drain well.

Slice the chicken breasts across the grain for a tender bite.

You can purchase roasted red peppers or roast your own. If you buy them, drain well before slicing. See the Techniques Glossary, page 398, for information on roasting peppers.

2 cups	GF brown rice fusilli pasta	500 mL
4	roasted red bell peppers, halved then sliced	4
2	cloves garlic, minced	2
4 cups	GF tomato basil pasta sauce	1 L
4	cooked chicken breasts, thickly sliced	4
4 cups	broccoli florets, cooked tender-crisp	1 L

1. In a large saucepan of boiling water, cook pasta according to package directions until just tender. Rinse under cold running water and drain well. Set aside.

2. In a saucepan, combine roasted peppers, garlic and pasta sauce; bring to a boil over medium heat. Reduce heat to low and simmer for 5 to 10 minutes or until heated through. Stir in chicken, broccoli and pasta; simmer until heated through.

Variations

Try vegetable brown rice pasta, brown rice and navy bean pasta or corn rotini. Or choose a shape that extra sauce clings to, such as elbows and shells.

Substitute 2 cups (500 mL) diced tomatoes for half the pasta sauce.

Nutritional value per serving

Calories	362
Fat, total	5 g
Fat, saturated	1 g
Cholesterol	97 mg
Sodium	348 mg
Carbohydrate	37 g
Fiber	6 g
Protein	43 g
Calcium	197 mg
Iron	3 mg

Side Dishes

Asparagus with Mock Hollandaise Sauce

Makes 4 servings

Enjoy fresh asparagus in the spring, with a light, easy-to-make, tangy sauce.

Tips

You'll need 15 to 20 asparagus spears for 1 lb (500 g).

To avoid overcooking the tender tips of the asparagus, cut spears in half crosswise and cook the thicker stalks for 5 minutes before adding the tips.

Be sure to use low heat so the hollandaise does *not* come to a boil.

The mock hollandaise can be stored in an airtight container in the refrigerator for up to 1 day and served chilled.

1 lb	thin asparagus spears, trimmed	500 g
½ cup	GF mayonnaise	125 mL
½ cup	low-fat plain yogurt	125 mL
1 tsp	freshly squeezed lemon juice	5 mL
¼ tsp	dry mustard	1 mL

1. In a steamer, cook asparagus for 5 to 7 minutes or until tender-crisp. (Or microwave on High in a microwave-safe bowl for 5 to 7 minutes or until tender-crisp.)

2. Meanwhile, in a small saucepan, over low heat, combine mayonnaise, yogurt, lemon juice and mustard. Cook, stirring constantly, for 5 minutes or until heated through. (Or microwave on High in a microwave-safe bowl for 3 to 4 minutes, stopping to stir occasionally, until heated through. Do not let boil.)

3. Serve asparagus drizzled with mock hollandaise.

Variations

Serve mock hollandaise over green beans, broccoli or snow peas.

Chilled mock hollandaise can be used as a dip or salad dressing. Season with 2 tbsp (25 mL) snipped fresh dill or cilantro.

Asparagus

Select firm, plump spears with tightly closed tips. The full length of the spear should be a bright green color. Store asparagus upright in the refrigerator in ½ inch (1 cm) of water or with the ends wrapped in a moist paper towel. It should not be washed until just before use. Don't cut asparagus spears while cleaning — simply bend the spear and snap off the woody end at the natural breaking point.

Nutritional value per serving

Calories	251
Fat, total	23 g
Fat, saturated	4 g
Cholesterol	22 mg
Sodium	172 mg
Carbohydrate	7 g
Fiber	2 g
Protein	4 g
Calcium	81 mg
Iron	1 mg

Pecan and Quinoa–Stuffed Squash

Makes 4 servings

Make this in the fall, when squash are plentiful, for an excellent accompaniment to Thanksgiving turkey.

Tips

Fresh herbs keep longer if wrapped in a slightly dampened paper towel and placed in a sealed plastic bag in your refrigerator.

For information on cooking quinoa, see the Techniques Glossary, page 398.

Prepare through step 3, cover and refrigerate. An hour before serving time, preheat oven. Bake for 45 minutes or until tops are golden.

Double the filling recipe and serve the extra as a pilaf. (Cook once and serve twice.)

Nutritional value per serving

Calories	347
Fat, total	15 g
Fat, saturated	2 g
Cholesterol	0 mg
Sodium	188 mg
Carbohydrate	50 g
Fiber	9 g
Protein	8 g
Calcium	132 mg
Iron	6 mg

- Preheat oven to 375°F (190°C)
- 9-inch (23 cm) square baking pan, lightly greased

2	small acorn squash	2
2 tsp	olive oil	10 mL
2	stalks celery, diced	2
½ cup	chopped onion	125 mL
1 tbsp	snipped fresh sage	15 mL
½ cup	snipped fresh parsley	125 mL
¾ tsp	dried marjoram	4 mL
¼ tsp	salt	1 mL
¼ tsp	freshly ground pepper	1 mL
Pinch	ground nutmeg	Pinch
1 cup	cooked quinoa	250 mL
½ cup	coarsely chopped pecans	125 mL

1. With a small knife, pierce each squash through to the center in four places. Place one squash on a paper towel in the microwave. Microwave on High for 6 to 8 minutes, turning once, until tender when pierced with a knife. Remove from microwave and let stand for 5 minutes. Repeat with the other squash.

2. Cut squash in half crosswise and remove seeds. Trim a thin slice off the bottom of each to allow them to lie flat. Place hollow side up in prepared baking pan and set aside.

3. In a large skillet, heat olive oil over medium heat. Sauté celery, onion and sage for 6 to 8 minutes or until just softened. Remove from heat and stir in parsley, marjoram, salt, pepper and nutmeg. Stir in quinoa and pecans. Spoon the mixture evenly into the squash halves.

4. Bake in preheated oven for 15 to 20 minutes or until tops are golden.

Variation

Substitute wild rice for the quinoa.

Roasted Turnips and Carrots

Makes 4 servings

With the arrival of fall, our thoughts go once again to enjoying root vegetables.

Tips

This recipe can be prepared up to 2 days ahead, stored in a covered container in the refrigerator and reheated in the microwave on Medium-High (70%) for 4 to 6 minutes, stirring once.

We like to double this recipe and freeze it in single-serving airtight containers for up to 1 month. Reheat in the microwave on Medium-High (70%) for 3 to 5 minutes.

Nutritional value per serving	
Calories	101
Fat, total	4 g
Fat, saturated	1 g
Cholesterol	0 mg
Sodium	281 mg
Carbohydrate	16 g
Fiber	4 g
Protein	2 g
Calcium	54 mg
Iron	1 mg

- **Preheat oven to 400°F (200°C)**
- **Roasting pan**

6	carrots, cut into 2-inch (5 cm) pieces	6
1	large turnip, peeled and cut into 2-inch (5 cm) cubes	1
2 tbsp	snipped fresh rosemary	25 mL
1 tbsp	extra virgin olive oil	15 mL
¾ cup	GF chicken broth	175 mL
	Salt and freshly ground black pepper	

1. In roasting pan, combine carrots and turnip. Sprinkle with rosemary and drizzle with oil, stirring to coat vegetables. Spread out in a single layer. Roast in preheated oven, stirring occasionally, for 75 minutes or until well browned and fork-tender.

2. Transfer to a food processor and add broth. Process for 2 to 3 minutes, scraping the sides occasionally, until smooth. Serve hot.

Variations

Thin with cream, milk or extra GF chicken broth for a quick and easy soup.

For a milder turnip flavor, add ½ cup (125 mL) unsweetened applesauce with the broth.

Roast 3 leeks, white and light green parts only, cut into 2-inch (5 cm) pieces, along with the carrots and turnip. Watch carefully, as leeks roast more quickly than other vegetables.

Tex-Mex Potato Fries

Makes 6 to 8 servings

Because these thick-cut fries are baked, you don't have to worry about cross-contamination in the deep fryer. They're lower in fat — and healthier too!

Tips

Use any variety of baking potatoes, such as russet, white or Idaho. Two large potatoes weigh about 1 pound (500 g).

For safety's sake, always cut vegetables with a flat side down, and cut away from yourself with a sharp knife.

- Preheat oven to 450°F (230°C)
- 2 baking sheets

2	large baking potatoes, cut into ½-inch (1 cm) sticks	2
2	large sweet potatoes, cut into ½-inch (1 cm) sticks	2
¼ cup	chili powder	50 mL
1 tbsp	dried thyme	15 mL
1 tbsp	dried oregano	15 mL
1 tsp	salt	5 mL
1 tsp	freshly ground black pepper	5 mL
¼ cup	extra virgin olive oil	50 mL

1. Place baking sheets in preheated oven for 5 minutes.

2. Meanwhile, in a large bowl, toss together potatoes, sweet potatoes, chili powder, thyme, oregano, salt, pepper and oil. Spread out in a single layer on hot baking sheets.

3. Bake for 10 to 15 minutes, turning once, until potatoes are browned and tender.

Variation

Add thickly sliced onion rings with the potatoes.

Nutritional value per serving

Calories	164
Fat, total	8 g
Fat, saturated	1 g
Cholesterol	0 mg
Sodium	337 mg
Carbohydrate	22 g
Fiber	4 g
Protein	2 g
Calcium	38 mg
Iron	2 mg

Zucchini Latkes

**Makes 10 latkes
(1 per serving)**

Serve as an appetizer or as a side to accompany a main course.

Tips

Choose small to medium zucchini, heavy for their size, with deep green skin.

Select a high-starch potato variety, such as Yukon gold or russet.

To grate zucchini and potatoes, use the grating disc of a food processor or the coarse side of a box grater.

Nutritional value per serving	
Calories	71
Fat, total	1 g
Fat, saturated	0 g
Cholesterol	37 mg
Sodium	178 mg
Carbohydrate	13 g
Fiber	1 g
Protein	3 g
Calcium	15 mg
Iron	1 mg

- Preheat oven to 250°F (120°C)
- Baking sheet, lined with paper towels

2 cups	grated zucchini	500 mL
1 cup	grated potatoes (unpeeled)	250 mL
1/4 cup	finely chopped onion	50 mL
1	clove garlic, minced	1
2	eggs, beaten	2
1 cup	cooked long- or short-grain brown rice	250 mL
1/4 cup	brown rice flour	50 mL
1/2 tsp	salt	2 mL
	Vegetable oil	

1. In a sieve set over the sink or a bowl, combine zucchini, potatoes, onion and garlic. Using your hands, firmly squeeze to remove as much liquid as possible. Transfer to a large bowl and add eggs, rice, brown rice flour and salt. Mix well.

2. In a large, wide skillet, over medium-high heat, heat just enough oil to cover the bottom of the pan in a thin layer. In batches, using 2 tbsp (25 mL) of the batter per latke, drop latkes about 1 inch (2.5 cm) apart in pan. Flatten to 1/4-inch (0.5 cm) thickness with the back of a spoon. Fry for 3 to 5 minutes per side, using two spatulas to turn latkes once, until crisp and golden. Drain on prepared baking sheet and keep warm in preheated oven. Repeat with the remaining batter, adding oil and reheating pan between batches as needed. Serve hot.

Tips

Remove any small cooked bits from the skillet between batches, if necessary.

If you find that a lot of liquid accumulates in the batter, drain well before frying.

To make ahead, fry latkes and place on prepared baking sheet to cool. Stack between layers of waxed paper in an airtight container. Refrigerate for up to 3 days or freeze for up to 1 month. Thaw overnight in the refrigerator. Bake in a single layer in the center of a 400°F (200°C) oven for 5 minutes. Using two spatulas, turn latkes over. Bake for 5 to 8 minutes or until crisp. Serve immediately.

Variation

Substitute 1 cup (250 mL) grated carrot for 1 cup (250 mL) of the grated zucchini.

Great Latkes

- To ensure crisp latkes, be sure to squeeze excess water from potatoes before mixing. The drier they are, the less likely they are to break during frying.
- For a fluffy latke, don't grate the onion, just thinly slice.
- Use only small amounts of latke batter; larger amounts tend to absorb more oil during frying.
- Test the temperature of the oil by adding a small amount of latke batter; it should turn golden in 1 to 2 minutes.

Two-Potato Latkes

**Makes 10 latkes
(1 per serving)**

A CanolaInfo recipe

We've added sweet potato to a traditional Jewish pancake. Serve as an appetizer or as a side to a main course.

Tips

Select a high-starch potato variety, such as Yukon gold or russet.

To grate potatoes, use the grating disc of a food processor or the coarse side of a box grater.

- Preheat oven to 250°F (120°C)
- Baking sheet, lined with paper towels

2 cups	grated potatoes (unpeeled)	500 mL
½ cup	grated peeled sweet potato	125 mL
½ cup	finely chopped onion	125 mL
2	eggs, beaten	2
½ cup	cooked long- or short-grain brown rice	125 mL
3 tbsp	brown rice flour	45 mL
½ tsp	GF baking powder	2 mL
½ tsp	salt	2 mL
	Vegetable oil	

1. In a sieve set over the sink or a bowl, combine potatoes, sweet potato and onion. Using your hands, firmly squeeze to remove as much liquid as possible. Transfer to a large bowl and add eggs, rice, brown rice flour, baking powder and salt. Mix well.

2. In a large, wide skillet, over medium-high heat, heat just enough oil to cover the bottom of the pan in a thin layer. In batches, using 2 tbsp (25 mL) of the batter per latke, drop latkes about 1 inch (2.5 cm) apart in pan. Flatten to ¼-inch (0.5 cm) thickness with the back of a spoon. Fry for 3 to 5 minutes per side, using two spatulas to turn latkes once, until crisp and golden. Drain on prepared baking sheet and keep warm in preheated oven. Repeat with the remaining batter, adding oil and reheating pan between batches as needed. Serve hot.

Nutritional value per serving	
Calories	71
Fat, total	1 g
Fat, saturated	0 g
Cholesterol	37 mg
Sodium	132 mg
Carbohydrate	13 g
Fiber	1 g
Protein	2 g
Calcium	21 mg
Iron	1 mg

Tips

To check that vegetable oil is the correct temperature, drop a small amount of the mixture into the hot vegetable oil. After 1 to 2 minutes, it should be golden in color.

Remove any small cooked bits from the skillet between batches, if necessary.

To make ahead, fry latkes and place on prepared baking sheet to cool. Stack between layers of waxed paper in an airtight container. Refrigerate for up to 3 days or freeze for up to 1 month. Thaw overnight in the refrigerator. Bake in a single layer in the center of a 400°F (200°C) oven for 5 minutes. Using two spatulas, turn latkes over. Bake for 5 to 8 minutes or until crisp. Serve immediately

Cooking Brown Rice

To get 3 to 4 cups (750 mL to 1 L) cooked brown rice, combine 1 cup (250 mL) rice and 2 to 2½ cups (500 to 625 mL) water or GF stock in a saucepan and bring to a boil. Reduce heat, cover and simmer for 45 to 50 minutes. After rice begins to simmer, do not remove the cover and peek. Peeking allows the steam to escape and the rice to become too dry. If rice is not quite tender or liquid is not absorbed after the specified cooking time, replace the lid and cook for 2 to 4 minutes longer. Remove from heat and let stand, covered, for 5 to 10 minutes or until all liquid is absorbed. Fluff with a fork. Use ½ cup (125 mL) cooked rice in this recipe and save the remainder for another use.

Potatoes and Carrots au Gratin

Makes 8 servings

This dish is similar to scalloped potatoes, only much more flavorful because of the sun-dried tomato pesto. You'll want to take it to your next potluck.

Tip

To easily slice the potatoes and carrots, use a food processor fitted with a slicing plate.

- Preheat oven to 400°F (200°C)
- 10-cup (2.5 L) casserole dish, lightly greased

4 cups	thinly sliced baking potatoes	1 L
2 cups	thinly sliced carrots	500 mL
½ cup	water	125 mL
1	recipe Sun-Dried Tomato Pesto (page 74)	1
1 cup	shredded aged Cheddar cheese	250 mL
½ cup	freshly grated Parmesan cheese	125 mL
1 cup	hot GF chicken broth	250 mL

1. In a large microwave-safe bowl, combine potatoes, carrots and water. Cover and microwave on High for 10 minutes or until vegetables are tender-crisp. Drain well.

2. Layer half the vegetable mixture in prepared casserole. Top with half the pesto, Cheddar and Parmesan. Repeat layers. Pour in hot broth.

3. Cover and bake in preheated oven for 30 minutes. Uncover and bake for about 15 minutes or until cheese is bubbling and starting to brown.

Variation

Omit the carrots and increase the potatoes to 6 cups (1.5 L).

Nutritional value per serving

Calories	365
Fat, total	24 g
Fat, saturated	8 g
Cholesterol	30 mg
Sodium	616 mg
Carbohydrate	25 g
Fiber	4 g
Protein	16 g
Calcium	396 mg
Iron	2 mg

Minted Lentils with Vegetables

Makes 4 servings

Lentils are high in fiber and are easier to prepare than dried beans, as they don't require soaking.

Tips

If you prefer vegetables in smaller, more uniform pieces, dice rather than chop.

Depending on the sodium content of the GF broth, you may need to add a little salt.

1 tbsp	vegetable oil	15 mL
2	cloves garlic, minced	2
2	stalks celery, chopped	2
1	carrot, diced	1
1	onion, chopped	1
1	red bell pepper, chopped	1
1 tsp	ground cumin	5 mL
1 cup	dried green lentils, rinsed	250 mL
2 cups	GF chicken broth	500 mL
¼ cup	snipped fresh mint	50 mL

1. In a saucepan, heat oil over medium heat. Sauté garlic, celery, carrot, onion, red pepper and cumin for 5 minutes or until onion is softened.

2. Stir in lentils and broth; bring to a boil. Reduce heat and simmer gently for 30 to 40 minutes or until lentils are tender. Drain, if necessary. Stir in mint.

Variation

Add leftover diced cooked chicken, GF ham or beef for a quick and easy entrée.

Nutritional value per serving	
Calories	237
Fat, total	4 g
Fat, saturated	0 g
Cholesterol	0 mg
Sodium	412 mg
Carbohydrate	39 g
Fiber	10 g
Protein	13 g
Calcium	101 mg
Iron	4 mg

Mushroom Leek Pilaf

Dairy-free
Lactose-free
Egg-free
White sugar–free

Makes 4 to 6 servings

A CanolaInfo recipe

Want to incorporate more whole grains into your diet? Try this nutritious side dish.

Tips

We used a mixture of cremini, shiitake, portobello and oyster mushrooms.

Dice carrots, rather than leaving them in larger pieces, so they cook in the same time as the leek and mushrooms.

See the Techniques Glossary, page 398, for information on toasting quinoa.

1 tbsp	vegetable oil	15 mL
2	cloves garlic, minced	2
1	leek, white and light green parts only, chopped	1
2 cups	sliced assorted mushrooms	500 mL
1 cup	diced carrots	250 mL
3 tbsp	snipped fresh rosemary	45 mL
½ cup	wild rice	125 mL
1½ cups	GF chicken broth	375 mL
¼ cup	quinoa, rinsed and toasted	50 mL
	Salt and freshly ground black pepper	

1. In a large saucepan, heat oil over medium-low heat. Sauté garlic, leek, mushrooms, carrots and rosemary for 6 to 8 minutes or until tender.

2. Add wild rice and broth; increase heat to medium-high and bring to a boil. Reduce heat to low, cover and simmer gently for 40 minutes.

3. Add quinoa, cover and simmer for 15 minutes or until quinoa is transparent and the tiny, spiral-like germ is separated, and rice is tender. Remove from heat and let stand for 5 to 10 minutes or until liquid is absorbed. Season to taste with salt and pepper.

Variation

Substitute GF vegetable or beef broth for the chicken broth.

Nutritional value per serving

Calories	130
Fat, total	3 g
Fat, saturated	0 g
Cholesterol	0 mg
Sodium	244 mg
Carbohydrate	22 g
Fiber	3 g
Protein	4 g
Calcium	38 mg
Iron	2 mg

Quinoa Pilaf

Makes 12 servings

A pleasant change from mashed potatoes! Serve with Rubbed Roast Beef (page 146) and use to make Second-Day Beef Quinoa Salad (page 143).

Tip

See the Techniques Glossary, page 398, for information on toasting nuts.

1 tbsp	extra virgin olive oil	15 mL
2	cloves garlic, minced	2
1	large onion, finely chopped	1
1 cup	diced carrots	250 mL
¾ cup	sliced portobello mushroom caps	175 mL
½ cup	diced celery	125 mL
½ cup	wild rice	125 mL
½ tsp	freshly ground black pepper	2 mL
3½ cups	GF beef broth	875 mL
½ cup	quinoa, rinsed	125 mL
1½ cups	chopped walnuts, toasted	375 mL
½ cup	chopped red bell pepper	125 mL
2 tbsp	minced fresh parsley	25 mL

1. In a large saucepan, heat oil over medium heat. Sauté garlic, onion, carrots, mushrooms and celery for about 5 minutes or until tender.

2. Add wild rice, pepper and broth; bring to a boil. Reduce heat to low, cover and simmer gently for 40 minutes.

3. Add quinoa, cover and simmer for 20 minutes or until quinoa is transparent and the tiny, spiral-like germ is separated, rice is tender and liquid is absorbed. Remove from heat and stir in walnuts, red pepper and parsley.

Variation

Substitute brown or white rice for either the wild rice or the quinoa and adjust the amount of liquid and the simmering time according to package directions. Be sure to choose long-grain rice if substituting for the quinoa.

Nutritional value per serving

Calories	175
Fat, total	11 g
Fat, saturated	1 g
Cholesterol	0 mg
Sodium	251 mg
Carbohydrate	16 g
Fiber	3 g
Protein	6 g
Calcium	33 mg
Iron	1 mg

Oat Groat Pilaf

Egg-free
White sugar–free

Makes 8 servings

Beth Armour of Cream Hill Estates developed this recipe and has given us permission to include it in our cookbook for you. You can serve this hot as a side or cold as a salad.

Tips

Store in an airtight container in the refrigerator for up to 3 days or in the freezer for up to 3 weeks.

While you're taking the time to cook oat groats anyway, cook extra and freeze for up to 1 month for another use, such as a salad or stir-fry.

If you're planning to serve this as a cold salad, use the olive oil instead of the butter.

7 cups	water	1.75 L
2½ cups	GF whole oat groats	625 mL
¼ cup	butter or extra virgin olive oil	50 mL
½ cup	minced onion	125 mL
¼ cup	slivered almonds	50 mL
2	tomatoes, chopped	2
2 cups	cooked green peas	500 mL
2 tbsp	snipped fresh rosemary	25 mL
1 tsp	freshly ground black pepper	5 mL
½ tsp	salt	2 mL

1. In a saucepan, bring water to a boil over high heat. Add oat groats and return to a boil. Remove from heat, cover and let stand for 30 minutes.

2. Return saucepan to medium-low heat and bring to a simmer. Simmer for 35 to 45 minutes or until groats are tender. Remove from heat, drain and set aside.

3. In a skillet, melt butter over medium heat. Sauté onion and almonds for 5 minutes or until onion is tender and almonds are golden. Stir in cooked oat groats, tomatoes, peas, rosemary, pepper and salt.

4. Serve hot or let cool, transfer to an airtight container, cover and refrigerate until chilled.

Nutritional value per serving	
Calories	238
Fat, total	10 g
Fat, saturated	4 g
Cholesterol	13 mg
Sodium	238 mg
Carbohydrate	30 g
Fiber	6 g
Protein	8 g
Calcium	45 mg
Iron	4 mg

Polenta

Makes 10 servings (1/2 cup/125 mL per serving)

Polenta is a staple in northern Italy. It can be served warm or cold, and is often cut into rounds or squares and fried or grilled.

Tip

Divide cooked polenta in half. Serve half plain and turn the other half into Maple Pumpkin Polenta (page 176).

5 cups	GF chicken broth	1.25 L
1 tbsp	extra virgin olive oil	15 mL
1¼ cups	cornmeal	300 mL
	Salt and freshly ground black pepper	

1. In a saucepan, bring broth to a boil over high heat. Add oil, reduce heat to medium and gradually whisk in cornmeal. Cook, stirring frequently, for 12 to 15 minutes or until cornmeal is tender and pulls away from the sides of the pan. Season to taste with salt and pepper.

2. Serve warm or form into two 2-inch (5 cm) diameter rolls. Wrap in plastic wrap and store in the refrigerator for up to 3 days.

Variation

For grilled or fried polenta squares, line a 9-inch (23 cm) glass baking dish with parchment paper and grease the parchment. Spread warm polenta about 2 inches (5 cm) thick in prepared dish. Let stand at room temperature until firm. Cover and refrigerate for up to 3 days. To serve, cut into squares, then grill or fry in a nonstick pan over medium-high heat.

Nutritional value per serving

Calories	86
Fat, total	2 g
Fat, saturated	0 g
Cholesterol	0 mg
Sodium	390 mg
Carbohydrate	15 g
Fiber	1 g
Protein	2 g
Calcium	14 mg
Iron	0 mg

Maple Pumpkin Polenta

Makes 6 servings
(½ cup/125 mL per serving)

We're sure you'll enjoy this delicious version of polenta, replete with the flavors of autumn.

Tip

For grilled or fried polenta squares, line a 9-inch (23 cm) glass baking dish with parchment paper and grease the parchment. Spread warm polenta about 2 inches (5 cm) thick in prepared dish. Let stand at room temperature until firm. Cover and refrigerate for up to 3 days. To serve, cut into squares, then grill or fry in a nonstick pan over medium-high heat.

2½ cups	GF chicken broth	625 mL
1½ tsp	extra virgin olive oil	7 mL
⅔ cup	cornmeal	150 mL
1½ cups	canned pumpkin purée (not pie filling)	375 mL
2 tbsp	pure maple syrup	25 mL
⅛ tsp	cayenne pepper	0.5 mL
¼ cup	freshly grated Parmesan cheese	50 mL
1½ tsp	butter	7 mL
	Salt and freshly ground black pepper	

1. In a saucepan, bring broth to a boil over high heat. Add oil, reduce heat to medium and gradually whisk in cornmeal. Cook, stirring frequently, for 12 to 15 minutes or until cornmeal is tender and pulls away from the sides of the saucepan.

2. Stir in pumpkin purée, maple syrup and cayenne. Cook for 1 to 2 minutes or until heated through. Stir in Parmesan and butter. Season to taste with salt and pepper.

3. Serve warm or form into two 2-inch (5 cm) diameter rolls. Wrap in plastic wrap and store in the refrigerator for up to 3 days.

Variation

Substitute mashed sweet potato for the pumpkin purée and ½ tsp (2 mL) ground cumin for the cayenne.

Nutritional value per serving

Calories	142
Fat, total	4 g
Fat, saturated	2 g
Cholesterol	6 mg
Sodium	441 mg
Carbohydrate	23 g
Fiber	2 g
Protein	4 g
Calcium	90 mg
Iron	1 mg

Bread Machine Yeast Breads

Using Your Bread Machine

WE ARE FREQUENTLY asked to speak at international celiac conferences and support groups. Our favorite topic is bread machine baking, using the more nutritious flours, of course. We have worked with many different brands and models of bread machines over the years and enjoy the challenges. Each is so individual. Don't wait for your bread machine to bake an unacceptable loaf. The bread machine manual will help you become familiar with your make and model. Happy baking depends on it.

There is a great deal of variation among bread machines on the market today. Some models have a more vigorous and longer knead than others, resulting in slightly different loaves from the same recipe. We baked eight loaves in eight different bread machines using the White Bread Mix, and they were all slightly different.

The recipes in this cookbook are developed for either 1½-lb (750 g) or 2-lb (1 kg) bread machines. The 2½- to 3-lb (1.25 to 1.5 kg) bread machines with two kneading blades are too large to properly knead the amount of dough in the recipes.

When purchasing a new bread machine, make sure it has at least one of the following choices: both a Dough Cycle and a Bake Cycle; a Programmable mode or a dedicated Gluten-Free Cycle. Neither the 58-minute nor the 70-minute Rapid Cycles are long enough to rise and bake loaves successfully. The old 2-Hour Rapid Cycle works well. If your bread machine doesn't have any of these four selections, try baking the loaves using a Basic, White or Sweet Cycle.

To Use the Dough Cycle, Then the Bake Cycle

Select the Dough Cycle first. Remove the kneading blade at the end of the long knead, then allow the cycle to finish. Immediately select the Bake Cycle, setting it to 350°F or 360°F (180°C or 185°C) for 60 minutes. Allow the Bake Cycle to finish. It is important to get to know your own bread machine. For instance, we have one that is a lot hotter than the rest, and we find that we have to lower the baking temperature. However, with other machines of the same make and model, the loaf bakes with a thin, tender crust. In most machines, the default temperature is 350°F (180°C). Check your bread machine manual to learn how to change time and temperature. Take the internal temperature of the loaf. It should reach 200°F (100°C).

To Use the Dedicated Gluten-Free Cycle

If an information box appears below the recipe, read it first. We found that, for many loaves, we had to increase the liquid in the recipes. In addition, some ingredients, including liquids and eggs, needed to be warmed, not used directly from the refrigerator. (See the Techniques Glossary, page 396, for info on safely warming eggs). Select the Gluten-Free Cycle, removing the kneading blade when the machine signals or at the end of the long knead.

To Use the Programmable Cycle

Set the Programmable Cycle to a short knead of 2 minutes (the machine stirs slowly, allowing for the addition of dry ingredients). Then set a knead of 20 minutes, then a rise of 70 minutes and a 60-minute Bake Cycle at 350°F (180°C). When prompted, set all other cycles to 0, eliminating the extra cycles. No need to remove the paddle.

Tips for Bread Machine Baking

- If your bread machine has a Preheat Cycle, keep the top down until mixing starts, so the heat does not escape. As soon as the liquids begin to mix, add the dry ingredients, scraping the corners, sides and bottom of the baking pan and the kneading blade while adding. Watch that the rubber spatula does not get caught under the rotating blade. Continue scraping until no dry ingredients remain and dough is well mixed. Some machines require more "help" mixing than others.

- The consistency of the dough is closer to a cake batter than the traditional yeast dough ball. You should see the motion of the kneading blade turning. The mixing mark of the kneading blade remains on top of the dough. Some doughs are thicker than others, but do not adjust by adding more liquid or dry ingredients.

- The kneading blade needs to be removed at the end of the long knead to prevent the collapse of the final loaf. However, some bread machines knead intermittently rather than continuously, so the first few times you use a new machine, listen carefully for the sounds of the different cycles. Make notes of the times the cycles change. Then set an auxiliary timer for the time the kneading finishes and the rising starts. This will alert you to when to remove the kneading blade. The dough is sticky, so rinse the rubber spatula and your hand with cold water before removing the blade. Smooth the top of the loaf quickly.

- When we developed recipes for our first two gluten-free cookbooks, we found we needed close to 1 tbsp (15 mL) of yeast for a quality loaf; however, with the new bread machine models on the market today, many of the original loaves now rise and collapse slightly during baking and cooling. If this happens, decrease the yeast by almost half.

- Some bread machines and some recipes bake darker-colored crusts than others. If you find certain loaves are too dark, next time set the Bake Cycle temperature lower. When baking on a Gluten-Free Cycle, a Basic Cycle or a 2-Hour Rapid Cycle, select a lighter crust setting, if possible.

- At the end of the baking cycle, before turning the machine off, take the temperature of the loaf using an instant-read thermometer. It should read 200°F (100°C). If it has not reached the recommended temperature, leave the loaf in the machine for 15 to 20 minutes on the Keep Warm Cycle.

- Refer to How to Calibrate Your Thermometer (page 46).

- Slice the cooled baked loaf with an electric knife or bread knife with a serrated blade. Place one or two slices in individual plastic bags, then place bags in a larger resealable bag. Freeze for up to 3 weeks. Remove a slice or two at a time.

Single-Loaf White Bread Mix for Bread Machine

Makes about 3½ cups (875 mL), enough for 1 loaf

You asked us for a white bread mix you could use to make a variety of nutritious loaves and rolls. We've done you one better and given you the recipe in three different batch sizes. Here's a single-loaf mix you can try before making the larger batches on pages 182 and 183. You can use this mix to make Sandwich Bread (page 184), Dinner Rolls (page 186), Rosemary Breadsticks (page 187) or Orange Chocolate Chip Loaf (page 188).

1¼ cups	brown rice flour	300 mL
½ cup	almond flour	125 mL
½ cup	amaranth flour	125 mL
½ cup	quinoa flour	125 mL
⅓ cup	potato starch	75 mL
¼ cup	tapioca starch	50 mL
1 tbsp	xanthan gum	15 mL
1¼ tsp	bread machine or instant yeast	6 mL
1¼ tsp	salt	6 mL

1. In a large bowl or plastic bag, combine brown rice flour, almond flour, amaranth flour, quinoa flour, potato starch, tapioca starch, xanthan gum, yeast and salt. Mix well.

2. Use right away or seal tightly in a plastic bag, removing as much air as possible. Store at room temperature for up to 3 days or in the freezer for up to 6 months.

Working with Bread Mix

Label and date the package if not using bread mix immediately. We add the page number of the recipe to the label as a quick reference.

Let bread mix warm to room temperature, and mix well before using.

Nutritional value per serving (¹⁄₁₅ recipe)

Calories	105
Fat, total	3 g
Fat, saturated	0 g
Cholesterol	0 mg
Sodium	198 mg
Carbohydrate	18 g
Fiber	2 g
Protein	3 g
Calcium	14 mg
Iron	1 mg

Four-Loaf White Bread Mix for Bread Machine

**Makes about 14 cups
(3.5 L), enough for
4 loaves**

*Here's the four-loaf
version of our bread
machine white bread
mix. Use it to make
Sandwich Bread (page
184), Dinner Rolls
(page 186), Rosemary
Breadsticks (page 187)
and Orange Chocolate
Chip Loaf (page 188).*

Tip

For accuracy, use a 1-cup
(250 mL) dry measure
several times to measure
each type of flour and
starch. If you use a 4-cup
(1 L) liquid measure, it's
difficult to get an accurate
volume and you'll end up
with extra flour in the mix.

5 cups	brown rice flour	1.25 L
2 cups	almond flour	500 mL
2 cups	amaranth flour	500 mL
2 cups	quinoa flour	500 mL
1⅓ cups	potato starch	325 mL
1 cup	tapioca starch	250 mL
¼ cup	xanthan gum	50 mL
2 tbsp	bread machine or instant yeast	25 mL
2 tbsp	salt	25 mL

1. In a very large container or roasting pan, combine brown rice flour, almond flour, amaranth flour, quinoa flour, potato starch, tapioca starch, xanthan gum, yeast and salt. Mix well.

2. Divide into four equal portions of about 3½ cups (875 mL) each. Seal tightly in plastic bags, removing as much air as possible. Store at room temperature for up to 3 days or in the freezer for up to 6 weeks.

Working with Bread Mix

In step 2, stir the mix before spooning it very lightly into the dry measures. Do not pack.

Be sure to divide the mix into equal portions. Depending on how much air you incorporate into the mix, and the texture of the individual gluten-free flours, the total volume of the mix can vary slightly. The important thing is to make the number of portions specified in the recipe.

Label and date the packages before storing. We add the page number of the recipe to the labels as a quick reference.

Let bread mix warm to room temperature, and mix well before using.

Nutritional value per serving (¹⁄₆₀ recipe)	
Calories	120
Fat, total	3 g
Fat, saturated	0 g
Cholesterol	0 mg
Sodium	236 mg
Carbohydrate	21 g
Fiber	2 g
Protein	3 g
Calcium	18 mg
Iron	2 mg

Six-Loaf White Bread Mix for Bread Machine

Makes about 21 cups (5.25 L), enough for 6 loaves

When you want to make a really big batch of white bread mix, this is the recipe for you. Use it to make Sandwich Bread (page 184), Dinner Rolls (page 186), Rosemary Breadsticks (page 187) and Orange Chocolate Chip Loaf (page 188).

Tip

For accuracy, use a 1-cup (250 mL) dry measure several times to measure each type of flour and starch. If you use a 4-cup (1 L) liquid measure, it's difficult to get an accurate volume and you'll end up with extra flour in the mix.

Nutritional value per serving (¹⁄₉₀ recipe)	
Calories	119
Fat, total	3 g
Fat, saturated	0 g
Cholesterol	0 mg
Sodium	237 mg
Carbohydrate	21 g
Fiber	2 g
Protein	3 g
Calcium	18 mg
Iron	2 mg

7½ cups	brown rice flour	1.875 L
3 cups	almond flour	750 mL
3 cups	amaranth flour	750 mL
3 cups	quinoa flour	750 mL
2 cups	potato starch	500 mL
1½ cups	tapioca starch	375 mL
⅓ cup	xanthan gum	75 mL
2½ tbsp	bread machine or instant yeast	32 mL
3 tbsp	salt	45 mL

1. In a very large container or roasting pan, combine brown rice flour, almond flour, amaranth flour, quinoa flour, potato starch, tapioca starch, xanthan gum, yeast and salt. Mix well. (When working with this large volume of ingredients, it is especially important to mix them very well before portioning.)

2. Divide into six equal portions of about 3½ cups (875 mL) each. Seal tightly in plastic bags, removing as much air as possible. Store at room temperature for up to 3 days or freeze for up to 6 weeks.

Working with Bread Mix

In step 2, stir the mix before spooning it very lightly into the dry measures. Do not pack.

Be sure to divide the mix into equal portions. Depending on how much air you incorporate into the mix, and the texture of the individual gluten-free flours, the total volume of the mix can vary slightly. The important thing is to make the number of portions specified in the recipe.

Label and date the packages before storing. We add the page number of the recipe to the labels as a quick reference.

Let bread mix warm to room temperature, and mix well before using.

Sandwich Bread

**Makes 15 slices
(1 per serving)**

This is sure to become your favorite nutritious white sandwich bread. It won't crumble in your packed lunch.

1¼ cups	water	300 mL
2 tbsp	vegetable oil	25 mL
2 tbsp	liquid honey	25 mL
1 tsp	cider vinegar	5 mL
2	eggs, lightly beaten	2
2	egg whites, lightly beaten	2
3½ cups	White Bread Mix for Bread Machine (pages 181–183)	875 mL

1. Pour water, oil, honey and vinegar into the bread machine baking pan. Add eggs and egg whites.

2. Select the **Dough Cycle**. As the bread machine is mixing, gradually add the bread mix, scraping bottom and sides of pan with a rubber spatula. Try to incorporate all the bread mix within 1 to 2 minutes. When the mixing and kneading are complete, remove the kneading blade, leaving the bread pan in the bread machine. Quickly smooth the top of the loaf. Allow the cycle to finish. Turn off the bread machine.

3. Select the **Bake Cycle**. Set time to 60 minutes and temperature to 350°F (180°C). Allow the cycle to finish. Do not turn machine off before taking the internal temperature of the loaf with an instant-read thermometer. It should be 200°F (100°C). If it's between 180°F (85°C) and 200°F (100°C), leave machine on the **Keep Warm Cycle** until baked. If it's below 180°F (85°C), turn on the **Bake Cycle** and check the internal temperature every 10 minutes. (Some bread machines are automatically set for 60 minutes; others need to be set by 10-minute intervals.)

4. Once the loaf has reached 200°F (100°C), remove it from the pan immediately and let cool completely on a rack.

Nutritional value per serving

Calories	141
Fat, total	5 g
Fat, saturated	1 g
Cholesterol	25 mg
Sodium	213 mg
Carbohydrate	21 g
Fiber	2 g
Protein	4 g
Calcium	18 mg
Iron	1 mg

Variation

To turn this into a raisin loaf, add ½ cup (125 mL) raisins and 1 tsp (5 mL) ground cinnamon with the bread mix.

Tip

To ensure success, see page 178 for extra information on using your bread machine and page 179 for general tips on bread machine baking.

Gluten-Free Cycle

If your bread machine has a Gluten-Free Cycle, you will need to make these adjustments:

1. Increase the water in the recipe to 1½ cups (375 mL).

2. Warm the water to between 110°F and 115°F (43°C and 46°C).

3. Warm the eggs and egg whites (see the Techniques Glossary, page 396).

4. Follow the recipe instructions, but select the **Gluten-Free Cycle** rather than the Dough Cycle and Bake Cycle.

5. At the end of the Gluten-Free Cycle, take the temperature of the loaf using an instant-read thermometer. It is baked at 200°F (100°C). If it's between 180°F (85°C) and 200°F (100°C), leave machine on the **Keep Warm Cycle** until baked. If it's below 180°F (85°C), turn on the **Bake Cycle** and check the internal temperature every 10 minutes. (Some bread machines are automatically set for 60 minutes; others need to be set by 10-minute intervals.)

Dinner Rolls

Makes 12 rolls
(1 per serving)

Everyone loves a golden brown dinner roll, and they're so easy to make from our mix.

Tips

To ensure success, see page 178 for extra information on using your bread machine and page 179 for general tips on bread machine baking.

For a softer crust, brush with melted butter as soon as you remove the rolls from the oven.

You can use ½ cup (125 mL) liquid whole eggs and 2 tbsp (25 mL) liquid egg white, if you prefer.

• **12-cup muffin tin, lightly greased**

1¼ cups	water	300 mL
2 tbsp	vegetable oil	25 mL
¼ cup	liquid honey	50 mL
1 tsp	cider vinegar	5 mL
2	eggs, lightly beaten	2
1	egg white, lightly beaten	1
3½ cups	White Bread Mix for Bread Machine (pages 181–183)	875 mL

1. Pour water, oil, honey and vinegar into the bread machine baking pan. Add eggs and egg white.

2. Select the **Dough Cycle**. As the bread machine is mixing, gradually add the bread mix, scraping bottom and sides of pan with a rubber spatula. Try to incorporate all the bread mix within 1 to 2 minutes. Stop bread machine as soon as the kneading portion of the cycle is complete. Do not let bread machine finish the cycle.

3. Using a ¼-cup (50 mL) scoop, drop dough into prepared muffin cups. Let rise, uncovered, in a warm, draft-free place for 60 to 75 minutes or until dough has risen to the top of the cups. Meanwhile, preheat oven to 350°F (180°C).

4. Bake for 18 to 20 minutes or until internal temperature of rolls registers 200°F (100°C) on an instant-read thermometer. Remove from the tin immediately and let cool completely on a rack.

Nutritional value per serving	
Calories	185
Fat, total	6 g
Fat, saturated	1 g
Cholesterol	25 mg
Sodium	262 mg
Carbohydrate	29 g
Fiber	3 g
Protein	4 g
Calcium	22 mg
Iron	1 mg

Rosemary Breadsticks

**Makes 24 breadsticks
(1 per serving)**

*Longing for a crunchy
breadstick with a
warm, golden brown,
crisp crust? Try this
twice-baked version.*

Tips

To ensure success, see page
178 for extra information
on using your bread
machine and page 179
for general tips on bread
machine baking.

For uniform breadsticks,
cut bread in half, then
lengthwise into quarters.
Finally, cut each quarter
lengthwise into 3 strips.

If breadsticks become
soft during storage, crisp
them in a toaster oven or
conventional oven at 350°F
(180°C) for a few minutes.

Nutritional value per serving	
Calories	87
Fat, total	3 g
Fat, saturated	1 g
Cholesterol	2 mg
Sodium	163 mg
Carbohydrate	12 g
Fiber	1 g
Protein	2 g
Calcium	39 mg
Iron	1 mg

- Two 9-inch (23 cm) square baking pans, lightly greased
- Baking sheets, ungreased

2 cups	water	500 mL
2 tbsp	extra virgin olive oil	25 mL
1 tsp	cider vinegar	5 mL
3½ cups	White Bread Mix for Bread Machine (pages 181–183)	875 mL
¼ cup	snipped fresh rosemary	50 mL
1 tsp	white (granulated) sugar	5 mL
½ tsp	freshly ground black pepper	2 mL
½ cup	freshly grated Parmesan cheese, divided	125 mL

1. Pour water, oil and vinegar into the bread machine baking pan.

2. Select the **Dough Cycle**. As the bread machine is mixing, gradually add the bread mix, rosemary, sugar and pepper, scraping bottom and sides of pan with a rubber spatula. Try to incorporate all the dry ingredients within 1 to 2 minutes. Stop bread machine as soon as the kneading portion of the cycle is complete. Do not let bread machine finish the cycle.

3. Sprinkle 2 tbsp (25 mL) of the Parmesan in the bottom of each prepared pan. Drop dough by spoonfuls over the Parmesan. Using a moistened rubber spatula, spread dough evenly to the edges of the pan. Sprinkle each with 2 tbsp (25 mL) Parmesan. Let rise, uncovered, in a warm, draft-free place for 30 minutes or until dough has risen to the top of the pans. Meanwhile, preheat oven to 400°F (200°C).

4. Bake for 12 to 15 minutes or until light brown. Remove from pan and transfer immediately to a cutting board. Reduce oven temperature to 350°F (180°C). Using a pizza wheel or a sharp knife, cut bread into 12 equal strips.

5. Arrange breadsticks, cut side up, at least ½ inch (1 cm) apart on baking sheets. Bake for 20 to 25 minutes or until dry, crisp and golden brown. Turn off oven and let breadsticks cool completely in oven.

6. Store in an airtight container at room temperature for up to 1 week.

Variation

Substitute thyme or tarragon, or a combination of herbs, for the rosemary.

Orange Chocolate Chip Loaf

This dessert bread is delightful when served warm. Enjoy for a quick snack.

Tip

To ensure success, see page 178 for extra information on using your bread machine and page 179 for general tips on bread machine baking.

¾ cup	water	175 mL
1 tbsp	grated orange zest	15 mL
¾ cup	freshly squeezed orange juice	175 mL
¼ cup	liquid honey	50 mL
2 tbsp	vegetable oil	25 mL
1 tsp	cider vinegar	5 mL
2	eggs, lightly beaten	2
1	egg white, lightly beaten	1
3½ cups	White Bread Mix for Bread Machine (pages 181–183)	875 mL
1 cup	jumbo or mini semisweet chocolate chips	250 mL

1. Pour water, orange zest, orange juice, honey, oil and vinegar into the bread machine baking pan. Add eggs and egg white.

2. Select the **Dough Cycle**. As the bread machine is mixing, gradually add the bread mix and chocolate chips, scraping bottom and sides of pan with a rubber spatula. Try to incorporate all the dry ingredients within 1 to 2 minutes. When the mixing and kneading are complete, remove the kneading blade, leaving the bread pan in the bread machine. Quickly smooth the top of the loaf. Allow the cycle to finish. Turn off the bread machine.

3. Select the **Bake Cycle**. Set time to 60 minutes and temperature to 350°F (180°C). Allow the cycle to finish. Do not turn machine off before taking the internal temperature of the loaf with an instant-read thermometer. It should be 200°F (100°C). If it's between 180°F (85°C) and 200°F (100°C), leave machine on the **Keep Warm Cycle** until baked. If it's below 180°F (85°C), turn on the **Bake Cycle** and check the internal temperature every 10 minutes. (Some bread machines are automatically set for 60 minutes; others need to be set by 10-minute intervals.)

4. Once the loaf has reached 200°F (100°C), remove it from the pan immediately and let cool completely on a rack.

Nutritional value per serving	
Calories	211
Fat, total	8 g
Fat, saturated	3 g
Cholesterol	27 mg
Sodium	219 mg
Carbohydrate	31 g
Fiber	3 g
Protein	4 g
Calcium	41 mg
Iron	1 mg

Tips

When oranges are in season, freeze extra zest and juice to have ready for recipes like this one.

Chocolate chips partially melt in most bread machines, giving a marbled effect to the bread.

Gluten-Free Cycle

If your bread machine has a Gluten-Free Cycle, you will need to make these adjustments:

1. Increase the water in the recipe to 1 cup (250 mL).

2. Warm the water to between 110°F and 115°F (43°C and 46°C).

3. Warm the eggs and egg white (see the Techniques Glossary, page 396).

4. Follow the recipe instructions, but select the **Gluten-Free Cycle** rather than the Dough Cycle and Bake Cycle.

5. At the end of the Gluten-Free Cycle, take the temperature of the loaf using an instant-read thermometer. It is baked at 200°F (100°C). If it's between 180°F (85°C) and 200°F (100°C), leave machine on the **Keep Warm Cycle** until baked. If it's below 180°F (85°C), turn on the **Bake Cycle** and check the internal temperature every 10 minutes. (Some bread machines are automatically set for 60 minutes; others need to be set by 10-minute intervals.)

Single-Loaf Brown Bread Mix for Bread Machine

Dairy-free
Lactose-free
Egg-free
White sugar–free

Makes about 3½ cups (875 mL), enough for 1 loaf

You asked us for a brown bread mix you could use to make a variety of nutritious loaves and rolls. We've done you one better and given you the recipe in two different batch sizes. Here's a single-loaf mix you can try before making the larger batch on page 191. You can use this nutritious mix to make Maritime (Boston) Brown Bread (page 192), Mock Bran Bread (page 194), Pumpernickel Bread (page 196) or Pizza Crust (page 212).

1¼ cups	sorghum flour	300 mL
⅔ cup	whole bean flour	150 mL
½ cup	brown rice flour	125 mL
2 tbsp	quinoa flour	25 mL
¼ cup + 1 tbsp	potato starch	65 mL
3 tbsp	tapioca starch	45 mL
2 tbsp	packed brown sugar	25 mL
1 tbsp	xanthan gum	15 mL
1½ tsp	bread machine or instant yeast	7 mL
1½ tsp	salt	7 mL

1. In a large bowl or plastic bag, combine sorghum flour, whole bean flour, brown rice flour, quinoa flour, potato starch, tapioca starch, brown sugar, xanthan gum, yeast and salt. Mix well.

2. Use right away or seal tightly in a plastic bag, removing as much air as possible. Store at room temperature for up to 3 days or in the freezer for up to 6 weeks.

Working with Bread Mix

Be sure the brown sugar is well distributed and any lumps are broken up; it clumps easily when mixed with other dry ingredients.

Label and date the package if not using bread mix immediately. We add the page number of the recipe to the label as a quick reference.

Let bread mix warm to room temperature, and mix well before using.

Nutritional value per serving (¹⁄₁₅ recipe)

Calories	94
Fat, total	1 g
Fat, saturated	0 g
Cholesterol	0 mg
Sodium	235 mg
Carbohydrate	20 g
Fiber	2 g
Protein	3 g
Calcium	10 mg
Iron	1 mg

Four-Loaf Brown Bread Mix for Bread Machine

Makes about 14 cups (3.5 L), enough for 4 loaves

Here's the four-loaf version of our bread machine brown bread mix, a nutritious mix that makes great whole-grain breads. Use it to make Maritime (Boston) Brown Bread (page 192), Mock Bran Bread (page 194), Pumpernickel Bread (page 196) and Pizza Crust (page 212).

Tips

For accuracy, use a 1-cup (250 mL) dry measure several times to measure each type of flour and starch. If you use a 4-cup (1 L) liquid measure, it's difficult to be accurate.

Nutritional value per serving (1/60 recipe)

Calories	96
Fat, total	1 g
Fat, saturated	0 g
Cholesterol	0 mg
Sodium	235 mg
Carbohydrate	21 g
Fiber	1 g
Protein	3 g
Calcium	10 mg
Iron	1 mg

5 cups	sorghum flour	1.25 L
2²⁄₃ cups	whole bean flour	650 mL
2 cups	brown rice flour	500 mL
½ cup	quinoa flour	125 mL
1¼ cups	potato starch	300 mL
¾ cup	tapioca starch	175 mL
½ cup	packed brown sugar	125 mL
¼ cup	xanthan gum	50 mL
2 tbsp	bread machine or instant yeast	25 mL
2 tbsp	salt	25 mL

1. In a very large container or roasting pan, combine sorghum flour, whole bean flour, brown rice flour, quinoa flour, potato starch, tapioca starch, brown sugar, xanthan gum, yeast and salt. Mix well.

2. Divide into four equal portions of about 3½ cups (875 mL) each. Seal tightly in plastic bags, removing as much air as possible. Store at room temperature for up to 3 days or in the freezer for up to 6 weeks.

Working with Bread Mix

Be sure the brown sugar is well distributed and any lumps are broken up; it clumps easily when mixed with other dry ingredients.

In step 2, stir the mix before spooning it very lightly into the dry measures. Do not pack.

Be sure to divide the mix into equal portions. Depending on how much air you incorporate into the mix, and the texture of the individual gluten-free flours, the total volume of the mix can vary slightly. The important thing is to make the number of portions specified in the recipe.

Label and date the packages before storing. We add the page number of the recipe to the labels as a quick reference.

Let bread mix warm to room temperature, and mix well before using.

Maritime (Boston) Brown Bread

**Makes 15 slices
(1 per serving)**

Here's a good basic brown bread for sandwiches and everyday use. It's especially good with homemade baked beans.

1¼ cups	water	300 mL
3 tbsp	vegetable oil	45 mL
2 tbsp	light (fancy) molasses	25 mL
1 tsp	cider vinegar	5 mL
2	eggs, lightly beaten	2
2	egg whites, lightly beaten	2
3½ cups	Brown Bread Mix for Bread Machine (pages 190–191)	875 mL

1. Pour water, oil, molasses and vinegar into the bread machine baking pan. Add eggs and egg whites.

2. Select the **Dough Cycle**. As the bread machine is mixing, gradually add the bread mix, scraping bottom and sides of pan with a rubber spatula. Try to incorporate all the bread mix within 1 to 2 minutes. When the mixing and kneading are complete, remove the kneading blade, leaving the bread pan in the bread machine. Quickly smooth the top of the loaf. Allow the cycle to finish. Turn off the bread machine.

3. Select the **Bake Cycle**. Set time to 60 minutes and temperature to 350°F (180°C). Allow the cycle to finish. Do not turn machine off before taking the internal temperature of the loaf with an instant-read thermometer. It should be 200°F (100°C). If it's between 180°F (85°C) and 200°F (100°C), leave machine on the **Keep Warm Cycle** until baked. If it's below 180°F (85°C), turn on the **Bake Cycle** and check the internal temperature every 10 minutes. (Some bread machines are automatically set for 60 minutes; others need to be set by 10-minute intervals.)

4. Once the loaf has reached 200°F (100°C), remove it from the pan immediately and let cool completely on a rack.

Variation
Add ½ cup (125 mL) raisins or chopped walnuts with the bread mix.

Nutritional value per serving

Calories	136
Fat, total	4 g
Fat, saturated	0 g
Cholesterol	25 mg
Sodium	251 mg
Carbohydrate	22 g
Fiber	2 g
Protein	4 g
Calcium	18 mg
Iron	1 mg

Tips

To ensure success, see page 178 for extra information on using your bread machine and page 179 for general tips on bread machine baking.

Measuring the oil before the molasses ensures that the molasses slides out of the measure. We enjoy using the OXO sloped ¼-cup (50 mL) measure for this. If the molasses is really thick or is straight out of the refrigerator, warm it slightly in the microwave before measuring.

Gluten-Free Cycle

If your bread machine has a Gluten-Free Cycle, you will need to make these adjustments:

1. Increase the water in the recipe to 1½ cups (375 mL).
2. Warm the water to between 110°F and 115°F (43°C and 46°C).
3. Warm the eggs and egg whites (see the Techniques Glossary, page 396).
4. Follow the recipe instructions, but select the **Gluten-Free Cycle** rather than the Dough Cycle and Bake Cycle.
5. At the end of the Gluten-Free Cycle, take the temperature of the loaf using an instant-read thermometer. It is baked at 200°F (100°C). If it's between 180°F (85°C) and 200°F (100°C), leave machine on the **Keep Warm Cycle** until baked. If it's below 180°F (85°C), turn on the **Bake Cycle** and check the internal temperature every 10 minutes. (Some bread machines are automatically set for 60 minutes; others need to be set by 10-minute intervals.)

Mock Bran Bread

**Makes 15 slices
(1 per serving)**

This is a sweeter, higher-fiber version of our basic Brown Sandwich Bread (page 198). You'll love using this bread for all of your sandwiches.

2 tbsp	rice bran	25 mL
3½ cups	Brown Bread Mix for Bread Machine (pages 190–191)	875 mL
1½ cups	water	375 mL
3 tbsp	vegetable oil	45 mL
1 tbsp	liquid honey	15 mL
1 tbsp	light (fancy) molasses	15 mL
1 tsp	cider vinegar	5 mL
2	eggs, lightly beaten	2
2	egg whites, lightly beaten	2

1. Add rice bran to the bread mix. Mix well and set aside.

2. Pour water, oil, honey, molasses and vinegar into the bread machine baking pan. Add eggs and egg whites.

3. Select the **Dough Cycle**. As the bread machine is mixing, gradually add the bread mix, scraping bottom and sides of pan with a rubber spatula. Try to incorporate all the bread mix within 1 to 2 minutes. When the mixing and kneading are complete, remove the kneading blade, leaving the bread pan in the bread machine. Quickly smooth the top of the loaf. Allow the cycle to finish. Turn off the bread machine.

4. Select the **Bake Cycle**. Set time to 60 minutes and temperature to 350°F (180°C). Allow the cycle to finish. Do not turn machine off before taking the internal temperature of the loaf with an instant-read thermometer. It should be 200°F (100°C). If it's between 180°F (85°C) and 200°F (100°C), leave machine on the **Keep Warm Cycle** until baked. If it's below 180°F (85°C), turn on the **Bake Cycle** and check the internal temperature every 10 minutes. (Some bread machines are automatically set for 60 minutes; others need to be set by 10-minute intervals.)

5. Once the loaf has reached 200°F (100°C), remove it from the pan immediately and let cool completely on a rack.

Variations

Add ½ cup (125 mL) raisins, chopped dates or chopped walnuts with the bread mix.

Substitute GF oat bran for the rice bran.

Nutritional value per serving	
Calories	140
Fat, total	4 g
Fat, saturated	0 g
Cholesterol	25 mg
Sodium	250 mg
Carbohydrate	23 g
Fiber	2 g
Protein	4 g
Calcium	16 mg
Iron	1 mg

Tips

To ensure success, see page 178 for extra information on using your bread machine and page 179 for general tips on bread machine baking.

Warm rice bran that has been stored in the refrigerator or freezer to room temperature.

Gluten-Free Cycle

If your bread machine has a Gluten-Free Cycle, you will need to make these adjustments:

1. Increase the water in the recipe to 1¾ cups (425 mL).

2. Warm the water to between 110°F and 115°F (43°C and 46°C).

3. Warm the eggs and egg whites (see the Techniques Glossary, page 396).

4. Follow the recipe instructions, but select the **Gluten-Free Cycle** rather than the Dough Cycle and Bake Cycle.

5. At the end of the Gluten-Free Cycle, take the temperature of the loaf using an instant-read thermometer. It is baked at 200°F (100°C). If it's between 180°F (85°C) and 200°F (100°C), leave machine on the **Keep Warm Cycle** until baked. If it's below 180°F (85°C), turn on the **Bake Cycle** and check the internal temperature every 10 minutes. (Some bread machines are automatically set for 60 minutes; others need to be set by 10-minute intervals.)

Pumpernickel Bread

**Makes 15 slices
(1 per serving)**

With all the hearty flavor of traditional pumpernickel, this version is great for sandwiches. Try it filled with sliced turkey, accompanied by a crisp garlic dill pickle.

1 tbsp	instant coffee granules	15 mL
1 tbsp	unsweetened cocoa powder, sifted	15 mL
½ tsp	ground ginger	2 mL
3½ cups	Brown Bread Mix for Bread Machine (pages 190–191)	875 mL
1½ cups	water	375 mL
3 tbsp	vegetable oil	45 mL
2 tbsp	light (fancy) molasses	25 mL
1 tsp	cider vinegar	5 mL
2	eggs, lightly beaten	2
2	egg whites, lightly beaten	2

1. Add coffee granules, cocoa and ginger to the bread mix. Mix well and set aside.

2. Pour water, oil, molasses and vinegar into the bread machine baking pan. Add eggs and egg whites.

3. Select the **Dough Cycle**. As the bread machine is mixing, gradually add the bread mix, scraping bottom and sides of pan with a rubber spatula. Try to incorporate all the bread mix within 1 to 2 minutes. When the mixing and kneading are complete, remove the kneading blade, leaving the bread pan in the bread machine. Quickly smooth the top of the loaf. Allow the cycle to finish. Turn off the bread machine.

4. Select the **Bake Cycle**. Set time to 60 minutes and temperature to 350°F (180°C). Allow the cycle to finish. Do not turn machine off before taking the internal temperature of the loaf with an instant-read thermometer. It should be 200°F (100°C). If it's between 180°F (85°C) and 200°F (100°C), leave machine on the **Keep Warm Cycle** until baked. If it's below 180°F (85°C), turn on the **Bake Cycle** and check the internal temperature every 10 minutes. (Some bread machines are automatically set for 60 minutes; others need to be set by 10-minute intervals.)

5. Once the loaf has reached 200°F (100°C), remove it from the pan immediately and let cool completely on a rack.

Nutritional value per serving

Calories	139
Fat, total	4 g
Fat, saturated	0 g
Cholesterol	25 mg
Sodium	251 mg
Carbohydrate	23 g
Fiber	2 g
Protein	4 g
Calcium	20 mg
Iron	1 mg

Tips

To ensure success, see page 178 for extra information on using your bread machine and page 179 for general tips on bread machine baking.

Sift cocoa just before using, as it lumps easily.

Variations

Add 2 tbsp (25 mL) caraway, fennel or anise seeds with the bread mix.

Substitute an equal quantity of strong brewed room-temperature coffee for the water.

Gluten-Free Cycle

If your bread machine has a Gluten-Free Cycle, you will need to make these adjustments:

1. Increase the water in the recipe to 1¾ cups (425 mL).

2. Warm the water to between 110°F and 115°F (43°C and 46°C).

3. Warm the eggs and egg whites (see the Techniques Glossary, page 396).

4. Follow the recipe instructions, but select the **Gluten-Free Cycle** rather than the Dough Cycle and Bake Cycle.

5. At the end of the Gluten-Free Cycle, take the temperature of the loaf using an instant-read thermometer. It is baked at 200°F (100°C). If it's between 180°F (85°C) and 200°F (100°C), leave machine on the **Keep Warm Cycle** until baked. If it's below 180°F (85°C), turn on the **Bake Cycle** and check the internal temperature every 10 minutes. (Some bread machines are automatically set for 60 minutes; others need to be set by 10-minute intervals.)

Brown Sandwich Bread

*For those who want
a rich, golden,
wholesome, nutritious
sandwich bread to
carry for lunch, this
is your loaf.*

1¼ cups	sorghum flour	300 mL
1 cup	pea flour	250 mL
½ cup	tapioca starch	125 mL
⅓ cup	rice bran	75 mL
2 tbsp	packed brown sugar	25 mL
1 tbsp	xanthan gum	15 mL
2 tsp	bread machine or instant yeast	10 mL
1½ tsp	salt	7 mL
1⅔ cups	water	400 mL
2 tbsp	vegetable oil	25 mL
2 tbsp	light (fancy) molasses	25 mL
1 tsp	cider vinegar	5 mL
2	eggs, lightly beaten	2
2	egg whites, lightly beaten	2

1. In a large bowl or plastic bag, combine sorghum flour, pea flour, tapioca starch, rice bran, brown sugar, xanthan gum, yeast and salt. Mix well and set aside.

2. Pour water, oil, molasses and vinegar into the bread machine baking pan. Add eggs and egg whites.

3. Select the **Dough Cycle**. As the bread machine is mixing, gradually add the dry ingredients, scraping bottom and sides of pan with a rubber spatula. Try to incorporate all the dry ingredients within 1 to 2 minutes. When the mixing and kneading are complete, remove the kneading blade, leaving the bread pan in the bread machine. Quickly smooth the top of the loaf. Allow the cycle to finish. Turn off the bread machine.

4. Select the **Bake Cycle**. Set time to 60 minutes and temperature to 350°F (180°C). Allow the cycle to finish. Do not turn machine off before taking the internal temperature of the loaf with an instant-read thermometer. It should be 200°F (100°C). If it's between 180°F (85°C) and 200°F (100°C), leave machine on the **Keep Warm Cycle** until baked. If it's below 180°F (85°C), turn on the **Bake Cycle** and check the internal temperature every 10 minutes. (Some bread machines are automatically set for 60 minutes; others need to be set by 10-minute intervals.)

5. Once the loaf has reached 200°F (100°C), remove it from the pan immediately and let cool completely on a rack.

Nutritional value per serving	
Calories	136
Fat, total	3 g
Fat, saturated	0 g
Cholesterol	25 mg
Sodium	251 mg
Carbohydrate	23 g
Fiber	3 g
Protein	5 g
Calcium	20 mg
Iron	2 mg

Tips

To ensure success, see page 178 for extra information on using your bread machine and page 179 for general tips on bread machine baking.

Pea flour, like soy flour, has a distinctive odor when wet that disappears with baking.

Variations

Any type of bean flour can be substituted for the pea flour.

Substitute GF oat bran for the rice bran.

For a slightly sweeter flavor, substitute liquid honey or packed brown sugar for the molasses.

Gluten-Free Cycle

If your bread machine has a Gluten-Free Cycle, you will need to make these adjustments:

1. Warm the water to between 110°F and 115°F (43°C and 46°C).

2. Warm the eggs and egg whites (see the Techniques Glossary, page 396).

3. Follow the recipe instructions, but select the **Gluten-Free Cycle** rather than the Dough Cycle and Bake Cycle.

4. At the end of the Gluten-Free Cycle, take the temperature of the loaf using an instant-read thermometer. It is baked at 200°F (100°C). If it's between 180°F (85°C) and 200°F (100°C), leave machine on the **Keep Warm Cycle** until baked. If it's below 180°F (85°C), turn on the **Bake Cycle** and check the internal temperature every 10 minutes. (Some bread machines are automatically set for 60 minutes; others need to be set by 10-minute intervals.)

Teff Bread

Makes 15 slices
(1 per serving)

Teff is a powerhouse of nutrition and makes a delicious bread.

Tip

To ensure success, see page 178 for extra information on using your bread machine and page 179 for general tips on bread machine baking.

¾ cup	brown rice flour	175 mL
¾ cup	teff flour	175 mL
½ cup	GF oat flour	125 mL
½ cup	potato starch	125 mL
¼ cup	teff grain	50 mL
2 tbsp	ground flaxseed	25 mL
1 tbsp	xanthan gum	15 mL
2 tsp	bread machine or instant yeast	10 mL
1½ tsp	salt	7 mL
2 tbsp	grated orange zest	25 mL
⅔ cup	dried blueberries	150 mL
1¼ cups	water	300 mL
¼ cup	vegetable oil	50 mL
¼ cup	liquid honey	50 mL
2 tsp	cider vinegar	10 mL
2	eggs, lightly beaten	2
2	egg whites, lightly beaten	2

1. In a large bowl or plastic bag, combine brown rice flour, teff flour, oat flour, potato starch, teff grain, flaxseed, xanthan gum, yeast, salt, orange zest and blueberries. Mix well and set aside.

2. Pour water, oil, honey and vinegar into the bread machine baking pan. Add eggs and egg whites.

3. Select the **Dough Cycle**. As the bread machine is mixing, gradually add the dry ingredients, scraping bottom and sides of pan with a rubber spatula. Try to incorporate all the dry ingredients within 1 to 2 minutes. When the mixing and kneading are complete, remove the kneading blade, leaving the bread pan in the bread machine. Quickly smooth the top of the loaf. Allow the cycle to finish. Turn off the bread machine.

4. Select the **Bake Cycle**. Set time to 60 minutes and temperature to 350°F (180°C). Allow the cycle to finish. Do not turn machine off before taking the internal temperature of the loaf with an instant-read thermometer. It should be 200°F (100°C). If it's between 180°F (85°C) and 200°F (100°C), leave machine on the **Keep Warm Cycle** until baked. If it's below 180°F (85°C), turn on the **Bake Cycle** and check the internal temperature every 10 minutes. (Some bread machines

Nutritional value per serving

Calories	179
Fat, total	6 g
Fat, saturated	1 g
Cholesterol	25 mg
Sodium	251 mg
Carbohydrate	29 g
Fiber	3 g
Protein	4 g
Calcium	36 mg
Iron	2 mg

See the Techniques Glossary, page 396, for information on grinding flaxseed.

You can use $\frac{1}{2}$ cup (125 mL) liquid whole eggs and $\frac{1}{4}$ cup (50 mL) liquid egg whites, if you prefer.

are automatically set for 60 minutes; others need to be set by 10-minute intervals.)

5. Once the loaf has reached 200°F (100°C), remove it from the pan immediately and let cool completely on a rack.

Variations

If you can't find teff grain, substitute $\frac{1}{4}$ cup (50 mL) poppy seeds or amaranth grain.

Substitute raisins or dried cranberries for the dried blueberries.

Gluten-Free Cycle

If your bread machine has a Gluten-Free Cycle, you will need to make these adjustments:

1. Warm the water to between 110°F and 115°F (43°C and 46°C).

2. Warm the eggs and egg whites (see the Techniques Glossary, page 396).

3. Follow the recipe instructions, but select the **Gluten-Free Cycle** rather than the Dough Cycle and Bake Cycle.

4. At the end of the Gluten-Free Cycle, take the temperature of the loaf using an instant-read thermometer. It is baked at 200°F (100°C). If it's between 180°F (85°C) and 200°F (100°C), leave machine on the **Keep Warm Cycle** until baked. If it's below 180°F (85°C), turn on the **Bake Cycle** and check the internal temperature every 10 minutes. (Some bread machines are automatically set for 60 minutes; others need to be set by 10-minute intervals.)

Historic Grains Bread

**Makes 15 slices
(1 per serving)**

Here's a quintet of healthy grains — sorghum, amaranth, quinoa, flaxseed and millet seeds — combined in a soft-textured, nutritious loaf that's perfect for sandwiches.

Tips

To ensure success, see page 178 for extra information on using your bread machine and page 179 for general tips on bread machine baking.

You can use either golden or brown flaxseed.

Nutritional value per serving

Calories	166
Fat, total	5 g
Fat, saturated	1 g
Cholesterol	25 mg
Sodium	212 mg
Carbohydrate	26 g
Fiber	4 g
Protein	5 g
Calcium	32 mg
Iron	3 mg

1¼ cups	sorghum flour	300 mL
1 cup	amaranth flour	250 mL
¼ cup	quinoa flour	50 mL
½ cup	cracked flaxseed	125 mL
¼ cup	millet seeds	50 mL
½ cup	tapioca starch	125 mL
1 tbsp	xanthan gum	15 mL
1¼ tsp	bread machine or instant yeast	6 mL
1¼ tsp	salt	6 mL
1¼ cups	water	300 mL
¼ cup	liquid honey	50 mL
2 tbsp	vegetable oil	25 mL
1 tsp	cider vinegar	5 mL
2	eggs, lightly beaten	2
2	egg whites, lightly beaten	2

1. In a large bowl or plastic bag, combine sorghum flour, amaranth flour, quinoa flour, flaxseed, millet seeds, tapioca starch, xanthan gum, yeast and salt. Mix well and set aside.

2. Pour water, honey, oil and vinegar into the bread machine baking pan. Add eggs and egg whites.

3. Select the **Dough Cycle**. As the bread machine is mixing, gradually add the dry ingredients, scraping bottom and sides of pan with a rubber spatula. Try to incorporate all the dry ingredients within 1 to 2 minutes. When the mixing and kneading are complete, remove the kneading blade, leaving the bread pan in the bread machine. Quickly smooth the top of the loaf. Allow the cycle to finish. Turn off the bread machine.

4. Select the **Bake Cycle**. Set time to 60 minutes and temperature to 350°F (180°C). Allow the cycle to finish. Do not turn machine off before taking the internal temperature of the loaf with an instant-read thermometer. It should be 200°F (100°C). If it's between 180°F (85°C) and 200°F (100°C), leave machine on the **Keep Warm Cycle** until baked. If it's below 180°F (85°C), turn on the **Bake Cycle** and check the internal temperature every 10 minutes. (Some bread machines are automatically set for 60 minutes; others need to be set by 10-minute intervals.)

See the Techniques Glossary, page 396, for information on cracking flaxseed.

You can use $\frac{1}{2}$ cup (125 mL) liquid whole eggs and $\frac{1}{4}$ cup (50 mL) liquid egg whites, if you prefer.

5. Once the loaf has reached 200°F (100°C), remove it from the pan immediately and let cool completely on a rack.

Variation
Substitute amaranth grain or whole flaxseed for the millet seeds.

Gluten-Free Cycle
If your bread machine has a Gluten-Free Cycle, you will need to make these adjustments:

1. Warm the water to between 110°F and 115°F (43°C and 46°C).

2. Warm the eggs and egg whites (see the Techniques Glossary, page 396).

3. Follow the recipe instructions, but select the **Gluten-Free Cycle** rather than the Dough Cycle and Bake Cycle.

4. At the end of the Gluten-Free Cycle, take the temperature of the loaf using an instant-read thermometer. It is baked at 200°F (100°C). If it's between 180°F (85°C) and 200°F (100°C), leave machine on the **Keep Warm Cycle** until baked. If it's below 180°F (85°C), turn on the **Bake Cycle** and check the internal temperature every 10 minutes. (Some bread machines are automatically set for 60 minutes; others need to be set by 10-minute intervals.)

Multigrain Bread

**Makes 15 slices
(1 per serving)**

*A celiac friend
suggested this variation
of our Whole-Grain
Amaranth Bread (The
Best Gluten-Free Family
Cookbook, page 72).
This soft-textured,
creamy, honey-colored
bread is so delicious
you won't even suspect
how nutritious it is.*

Tip

To ensure success, see page
178 for extra information
on using your bread
machine and page 179
for general tips on bread
machine baking.

¾ cup	amaranth flour	175 mL
¾ cup	brown rice flour	175 mL
½ cup	GF oat flour	125 mL
½ cup	potato starch	125 mL
¼ cup	amaranth grain	50 mL
2 tbsp	ground flaxseed	25 mL
1 tbsp	xanthan gum	15 mL
2 tsp	bread machine or instant yeast	10 mL
1½ tsp	salt	7 mL
1 cup	water	250 mL
¼ cup	vegetable oil	50 mL
¼ cup	liquid honey	50 mL
2 tsp	cider vinegar	10 mL
2	eggs, lightly beaten	2
2	egg whites, lightly beaten	2

1. In a large bowl or plastic bag, combine amaranth flour, brown rice flour, oat flour, potato starch, amaranth grain, flaxseed, xanthan gum, yeast and salt. Mix well and set aside.

2. Pour water, oil, honey and vinegar into the bread machine baking pan. Add eggs and egg whites.

3. Select the **Dough Cycle**. As the bread machine is mixing, gradually add the dry ingredients, scraping bottom and sides of pan with a rubber spatula. Try to incorporate all the dry ingredients within 1 to 2 minutes. When the mixing and kneading are complete, remove the kneading blade, leaving the bread pan in the bread machine. Quickly smooth the top of the loaf. Allow the cycle to finish. Turn off the bread machine.

4. Select the **Bake Cycle**. Set time to 60 minutes and temperature to 350°F (180°C). Allow the cycle to finish. Do not turn machine off before taking the internal temperature of the loaf with an instant-read thermometer. It should be 200°F (100°C). If it's between 180°F (85°C) and 200°F (100°C), leave machine on the **Keep Warm Cycle** until baked. If it's below 180°F (85°C), turn on the **Bake Cycle** and check the internal temperature every 10 minutes. (Some bread machines are automatically set for 60 minutes; others need to be set by 10-minute intervals.)

Nutritional value per serving

Calories	160
Fat, total	6 g
Fat, saturated	1 g
Cholesterol	25 mg
Sodium	250 mg
Carbohydrate	24 g
Fiber	2 g
Protein	4 g
Calcium	23 mg
Iron	2 mg

Tips

See the Techniques Glossary for information on making your own oat flour (page 398) and grinding flaxseed (page 396).

Amaranth is high in fiber, iron and calcium and lower in sodium than most grains. Store amaranth grain in an airtight container in the refrigerator for up to 6 months.

You can use $\frac{1}{2}$ cup (125 mL) liquid whole eggs and $\frac{1}{4}$ cup (50 mL) liquid egg whites, if you prefer.

5. Once the loaf has reached 200°F (100°C), remove it from the pan immediately and let cool completely on a rack.

Variations

Substitute millet seeds or poppy seeds for the amaranth grain.

Add $\frac{2}{3}$ cup (150 mL) dried cranberries and 2 tbsp (25 mL) grated orange zest with the dry ingredients.

Gluten-Free Cycle

If your bread machine has a Gluten-Free Cycle, you will need to make these adjustments:

1. Warm the water to between 110°F and 115°F (43°C and 46°C).

2. Warm the eggs and egg whites (see the Techniques Glossary, page 396).

3. Follow the recipe instructions, but select the **Gluten-Free Cycle** rather than the Dough Cycle and Bake Cycle.

4. At the end of the Gluten-Free Cycle, take the temperature of the loaf using an instant-read thermometer. It is baked at 200°F (100°C). If it's between 180°F (85°C) and 200°F (100°C), leave machine on the **Keep Warm Cycle** until baked. If it's below 180°F (85°C), turn on the **Bake Cycle** and check the internal temperature every 10 minutes. (Some bread machines are automatically set for 60 minutes; others need to be set by 10-minute intervals.)

Cranberry Pumpkin Seed Bread

Makes 15 slices
(1 per serving)

A CanolaInfo recipe

This attractive loaf is sure to bring compliments from guests. Pumpkin flavor, flecks of red cranberries and green pumpkin seeds make it the perfect accompaniment for turkey.

Tip

To ensure success, see page 178 for extra information on using your bread machine and page 179 for general tips on bread machine baking.

1½ cups	sorghum flour	375 mL
⅓ cup	flax flour	75 mL
¼ cup	quinoa flour	50 mL
½ cup	tapioca starch	125 mL
¼ cup	white (granulated) sugar	50 mL
2½ tsp	xanthan gum	12 mL
2 tsp	bread machine or instant yeast	10 mL
1½ tsp	salt	7 mL
¾ cup	dried cranberries	175 mL
½ cup	unsalted green pumpkin seeds, toasted	125 mL
1¼ cups	pumpkin purée (not pie filling)	300 mL
¼ cup	water	50 mL
¼ cup	vegetable oil	50 mL
2 tsp	cider vinegar	10 mL
2	eggs, lightly beaten	2
2	egg whites, lightly beaten	2

1. In a large bowl or plastic bag, combine sorghum flour, flax flour, quinoa flour, tapioca starch, sugar, xanthan gum, yeast, salt, cranberries and pumpkin seeds. Mix well and set aside.

2. Measure pumpkin purée, water, oil and vinegar into the bread machine baking pan. Add eggs and egg whites.

3. Select the **Dough Cycle**. As the bread machine is mixing, gradually add the dry ingredients, scraping bottom and sides of pan with a rubber spatula. Try to incorporate all the dry ingredients within 1 to 2 minutes. When the mixing and kneading are complete, remove the kneading blade, leaving the bread pan in the bread machine. Quickly smooth the top of the loaf. Allow the cycle to finish. Turn off the bread machine.

4. Select the **Bake Cycle**. Set time to 60 minutes and temperature to 350°F (180°C). Allow the cycle to finish. Do not turn machine off before taking the internal temperature of the loaf with an instant-read thermometer. It should be 200°F (100°C). If it's between 180°F (85°C) and 200°F (100°C), leave machine on the **Keep Warm Cycle** until baked. If it's below 180°F (85°C), turn on the **Bake Cycle** and check the internal

Nutritional value per serving

Calories	208
Fat, total	9 g
Fat, saturated	1 g
Cholesterol	25 mg
Sodium	252 mg
Carbohydrate	27 g
Fiber	4 g
Protein	7 g
Calcium	25 mg
Iron	3 mg

Tips

See the Techniques Glossary for information on grinding flaxseed to make flax flour (page 396) and toasting seeds (page 398).

We tried this bread with sprouted flax powder, flax meal and ground flaxseed in place of the flax flour. All yielded acceptable loaves.

Be sure to use pumpkin purée; pumpkin pie filling is too sweet.

temperature every 10 minutes. (Some bread machines are automatically set for 60 minutes; others need to be set by 10-minute intervals.)

5. Once the loaf has reached 200°F (100°C), remove it from the pan immediately and let cool completely on a rack.

Variations

Substitute halved dried cherries for the cranberries.

Substitute chopped pecans or unsalted sunflower seeds for the pumpkin seeds.

Gluten-Free Cycle

If your bread machine has a Gluten-Free Cycle, you will need to make these adjustments:

1. Warm the water to between 110°F and 115°F (43°C and 46°C).

2. Warm the eggs and egg whites (see the Techniques Glossary, page 396).

3. Follow the recipe instructions, but select the **Gluten-Free Cycle** rather than the Dough Cycle and Bake Cycle.

4. At the end of the Gluten-Free Cycle, take the temperature of the loaf using an instant-read thermometer. It is baked at 200°F (100°C). If it's between 180°F (85°C) and 200°F (100°C), leave machine on the **Keep Warm Cycle** until baked. If it's below 180°F (85°C), turn on the **Bake Cycle** and check the internal temperature every 10 minutes. (Some bread machines are automatically set for 60 minutes; others need to be set by 10-minute intervals.)

Honey Fig Loaf

**Makes 15 slices
(1 per serving)**

This sweet loaf is delicious spread with applesauce for a light dessert.

Tips

To ensure success, see page 178 for extra information on using your bread machine and page 179 for general tips on bread machine baking.

If using apple cider and applesauce from the refrigerator, warm them each in the microwave for 1 minute on High before measuring.

1²⁄₃ cups	sorghum flour	400 mL
½ cup	pea flour	125 mL
½ cup	tapioca starch	125 mL
1 tbsp	xanthan gum	15 mL
1 tbsp	bread machine or instant yeast	15 mL
1½ tsp	salt	7 mL
1 tsp	ground cardamom	5 mL
1 cup	dried figs, snipped	250 mL
1 cup	unsweetened apple cider, at room temperature	250 mL
¾ cup	unsweetened applesauce, at room temperature	175 mL
2 tbsp	liquid honey	25 mL
2 tbsp	vegetable oil	25 mL
2	eggs, lightly beaten	2
1	egg white, lightly beaten	1

1. In a large bowl or plastic bag, combine sorghum flour, pea flour, tapioca starch, xanthan gum, yeast, salt, cardamom and figs. Mix well and set aside.

2. Pour cider, applesauce, honey and oil into the bread machine baking pan. Add eggs and egg white.

3. Select the **Dough Cycle**. As the bread machine is mixing, gradually add the dry ingredients, scraping bottom and sides of pan with a rubber spatula. Try to incorporate all the dry ingredients within 1 to 2 minutes. When the mixing and kneading are complete, remove the kneading blade, leaving the bread pan in the bread machine. Quickly smooth the top of the loaf. Allow the cycle to finish. Turn off the bread machine.

4. Select the **Bake Cycle**. Set time to 60 minutes and temperature to 350°F (180°C). Allow the cycle to finish. Do not turn machine off before taking the internal temperature of the loaf with an instant-read thermometer. It should be 200°F (100°C). If it's between 180°F (85°C) and 200°F (100°C), leave machine on the **Keep Warm Cycle** until baked. If it's below 180°F (85°C), turn on the **Bake Cycle** and check the internal temperature every 10 minutes. (Some bread machines are automatically set for 60 minutes; others need to be set by 10-minute intervals.)

Nutritional value per serving

Calories	179
Fat, total	3 g
Fat, saturated	0 g
Cholesterol	25 mg
Sodium	250 mg
Carbohydrate	35 g
Fiber	4 g
Protein	5 g
Calcium	33 mg
Iron	2 mg

Tips

Snip the figs with sharp kitchen shears. When the blades become sticky, dip them in warm water.

If only sweetened apple cider and applesauce are available, decrease the honey to 1 tbsp (15 mL). If you can't find apple cider at all, purchase high-quality unsweetened apple juice, not sweetened apple drink.

5. Once the loaf has reached 200°F (100°C), remove it from the pan immediately and let cool completely on a rack.

Gluten-Free Cycle

If your bread machine has a Gluten-Free Cycle, you will need to make these adjustments:

1. Warm the water to between 110°F and 115°F (43°C and 46°C).

2. Warm the eggs and egg white (see the Techniques Glossary, page 396).

3. Follow the recipe instructions, but select the **Gluten-Free Cycle** rather than the Dough Cycle and Bake Cycle.

4. At the end of the Gluten-Free Cycle, take the temperature of the loaf using an instant-read thermometer. It is baked at 200°F (100°C). If it's between 180°F (85°C) and 200°F (100°C), leave machine on the **Keep Warm Cycle** until baked. If it's below 180°F (85°C), turn on the **Bake Cycle** and check the internal temperature every 10 minutes. (Some bread machines are automatically set for 60 minutes; others need to be set by 10-minute intervals.)

Swedish Wraps

**Makes 4 wraps
(1 per serving)**

*Use these to make
the ever-popular wrap
luncheon sandwich.*

Tips

Roll these wraps around
your favorite sandwich
fillings.

Dipping the spatula
repeatedly into warm
water makes it easier to
spread this dough thinly
and evenly.

- Preheat oven to 400°F (200°C)
- 15- by 10-inch (40 by 25 cm) jelly roll pan, lightly greased and lined with parchment paper

¼ cup	sorghum flour	50 mL
¼ cup	amaranth flour	50 mL
¼ cup	potato starch	50 mL
¼ cup	tapioca starch	50 mL
1 tsp	white (granulated) sugar	5 mL
2 tsp	xanthan gum	10 mL
1 tbsp	bread machine or instant yeast	15 mL
¾ tsp	salt	4 mL
1 tsp	anise seeds	5 mL
1 tsp	caraway seeds	5 mL
1 tsp	fennel seeds	5 mL
¾ cup	milk	175 mL
1 tsp	cider vinegar	5 mL
1 tsp	extra virgin olive oil	5 mL

1. In a large bowl or plastic bag, combine sorghum flour, amaranth flour, potato starch, tapioca starch, sugar, xanthan gum, yeast, salt, anise seeds, caraway seeds and fennel seeds. Mix well and set aside.

2. Pour milk, vinegar and oil into the bread machine baking pan. Select the **Dough Cycle**. As the bread machine is mixing, gradually add the dry ingredients, scraping bottom and sides of pan with a rubber spatula. Try to incorporate all the dry ingredients within 1 to 2 minutes. Stop bread machine as soon as the kneading portion of the cycle is complete. Do not let bread machine finish the cycle.

3. Remove dough to prepared pan. Using a moistened rubber spatula, spread dough evenly to the edges of the pan.

Nutritional value per serving	
Calories	165
Fat, total	3 g
Fat, saturated	0 g
Cholesterol	2 mg
Sodium	461 mg
Carbohydrate	31 g
Fiber	3 g
Protein	5 g
Calcium	86 mg
Iron	3 mg

To make this recipe dairy-free, use non-dairy powdered milk substitute and water.

4. Bake in preheated oven for 12 to 14 minutes or until edges are brown and top begins to brown. Let cool completely in pan on a rack. Remove from pan and cut into quarters.

Variation

Try adding dried herbs to the soft dough in place of the three varieties of seeds. To make a plainer variety, omit seeds and herbs.

Pizza Crust

**Makes 16 squares
(1 per serving)**

*You requested a
whole-grain pizza
crust recipe — here
it is.*

Tips

To ensure success, see page
178 for extra information
on using your bread
machine and page 179
for general tips on bread
machine baking.

To make pizza, add
your favorite topping
ingredients and bake until
crust is brown and crisp
and top is bubbly.

- Two 15- by 10-inch (40 by 25 cm) jelly roll pans,
  lightly greased

2 tsp	bread machine or instant yeast	10 mL
3½ cups	Brown Bread Mix for Bread Machine (pages 190–191)	875 mL
2¼ cups	water	550 mL
¼ cup	extra virgin olive oil	50 mL
1 tsp	cider vinegar	5 mL

1. Add yeast to the bread mix. Mix well and set aside.

2. Pour water, oil and vinegar into the bread machine baking pan.

3. Select the **Dough Cycle**. As the bread machine is mixing, gradually add the dry ingredients, scraping bottom and sides of pan with a rubber spatula. Try to incorporate all the dry ingredients within 1 to 2 minutes. Stop bread machine as soon as the kneading portion of the cycle is complete. Do not let bread machine finish the cycle.

4. Meanwhile, preheat oven to 400°F (200°C).

5. Divide dough in half. Place half the dough in each prepared pan and, using a moistened rubber spatula, spread evenly to the edges. Do not smooth tops.

6. Bake for 12 minutes or until bottom is golden and crust is partially baked.

7. Use right away to make pizza with your favorite toppings, or wrap airtight and store in the freezer for up to 1 month. Thaw in the refrigerator overnight before using.

Variations

If you like a thicker crust, leave the dough in one piece, spread it in the pan and let rise for 30 minutes before baking.

Add 1 to 2 tsp (5 to 10 mL) dried herbs or 1 to 2 tbsp (15 to 25 mL) chopped fresh herbs such as rosemary, oregano, basil or thyme with the bread mix.

Nutritional value per serving

Calories	121
Fat, total	4 g
Fat, saturated	1 g
Cholesterol	0 mg
Sodium	221 mg
Carbohydrate	19 g
Fiber	2
Protein	3 g
Calcium	9 mg
Iron	1 mg

Mixer
Yeast Breads

Tips for Mixer-Method Bread Baking

- Select a heavy-duty mixer with a paddle attachment (flat beater) for the best mixing of ingredients.
- Gradually add the dry ingredients to the liquids as the machine is mixing, then stop the machine to scrape the bottom and sides of the bowl. With the mixer set to medium speed, beat the dough for 4 minutes. Set a kitchen timer. You will be surprised how long 4 minutes seems when you are waiting.
- Fill the lightly greased pan only two-thirds full, then set, uncovered, in a warm, draft-free place until the dough reaches the top of the pan. This usually takes 60 to 75 minutes but may be shorter or longer depending on altitude, room temperature and humidity. Be patient: the loaf rises a lot in the last 15 minutes of the rising time. Do not let the loaf over-rise, or it could collapse during baking.
- After baking, take the temperature of the loaf using an instant-read thermometer. It should read 200°F (100°C). If it doesn't, continue baking until it does, even if loaf is golden brown and looks baked.
- Refer to How to Calibrate Your Thermometer (page 46).
- Remove loaf from pan and immediately place on a cooling rack to prevent a soggy loaf.
- During baking, if you notice that the loaf is as dark as desired but is not fully baked, tent it with foil for the remainder of the baking time.

Single-Loaf White Bread Mix for Mixer

Makes about 2¾ cups (675 mL), enough for 1 loaf

You asked us for a white bread mix you could use to make a variety of nutritious loaves and rolls. We've done you one better and given you the recipe in two different batch sizes. Here's a single-loaf mix you can try before making the larger batch on page 216. You can use this mix to make Sandwich Bread (page 217), Dinner Rolls (page 218), Rosemary Breadsticks (page 219) or Orange Chocolate Chip Loaf (page 220).

1 cup	brown rice flour	250 mL
½ cup	amaranth flour	125 mL
⅓ cup	almond flour	75 mL
⅓ cup	quinoa flour	75 mL
¼ cup	potato starch	50 mL
2 tbsp	tapioca starch	25 mL
1 tbsp	xanthan gum	15 mL
1 tbsp	bread machine or instant yeast	15 mL
1½ tsp	salt	7 mL

1. In a large bowl or plastic bag, combine brown rice flour, amaranth flour, almond flour, quinoa flour, potato starch, tapioca starch, xanthan gum, yeast and salt. Mix well.

2. Use right away or seal tightly in a plastic bag, removing as much air as possible. Store at room temperature for up to 3 days or in the freezer for up to 6 months.

Working with Bread Mix

Label and date the package if not using bread mix immediately. We add the page number of the recipe to the label as a quick reference.

Let bread mix warm to room temperature, and mix well before using.

Nutritional value per serving (¹⁄₁₅ recipe)	
Calories	93
Fat, total	2 g
Fat, saturated	0 g
Cholesterol	0 mg
Sodium	235 mg
Carbohydrate	16 g
Fiber	2 g
Protein	3 g
Calcium	14 mg
Iron	2 mg

Four-Loaf White Bread Mix for Mixer

Makes about 11 cups (2.75 L), enough for 4 loaves

Here's the four-loaf version of our mixer white bread mix. Use it to make Sandwich Bread (page 217), Dinner Rolls (page 218), Rosemary Breadsticks (page 219) or Orange Chocolate Chip Loaf (page 220).

Tips

For accuracy, use a 1-cup (250 mL) dry measure several times to measure each type of flour and starch. If you use a 4-cup (1 L) liquid measure, it's difficult to get an accurate volume and you'll end up with extra flour in the mix.

Nutritional value per serving ($\frac{1}{60}$ recipe)	
Calories	76
Fat, total	1 g
Fat, saturated	0 g
Cholesterol	0 mg
Sodium	234 mg
Carbohydrate	16 g
Fiber	1 g
Protein	2 g
Calcium	8 mg
Iron	1 mg

4 cups	brown rice flour	1 L
1½ cups	almond flour	375 mL
1½ cups	amaranth flour	375 mL
1½ cups	quinoa flour	375 mL
1 cup	potato starch	250 mL
½ cup	tapioca starch	125 mL
¼ cup	xanthan gum	50 mL
¼ cup	bread machine or instant yeast	50 mL
2 tbsp	salt	25 mL

1. In a very large container or roasting pan, combine brown rice flour, almond flour, amaranth flour, quinoa flour, potato starch, tapioca starch, xanthan gum, yeast and salt. Mix well.

2. Divide into four equal portions of about 2¾ cups (675 mL) each. Seal tightly in plastic bags, removing as much air as possible. Store at room temperature for up to 3 days or in the freezer for up to 6 weeks.

Working with Bread Mix

In step 2, stir the mix before spooning it very lightly into the dry measures. Do not pack.

Be sure to divide the mix into equal portions. Depending on how much air you incorporate into the mix, and the texture of the individual gluten-free flours, the total volume of the mix can vary slightly. The important thing is to make the number of portions specified in the recipe.

Label and date the packages before storing. We add the page number of the recipe to the labels as a quick reference.

Let bread mix warm to room temperature, and mix well before using.

Sandwich Bread

**Makes 15 slices
(1 per serving)**

This is sure to become your favorite nutritious white sandwich bread. It won't crumble in your packed lunch.

Tip

To ensure success, see page 214 for tips on mixer-method bread baking.

- 9- by 5-inch (23 by 12.5 cm) loaf pan, lightly greased

2	eggs, lightly beaten	2
1 cup	water	250 mL
2 tbsp	vegetable oil	25 mL
2 tbsp	liquid honey	25 mL
1 tsp	cider vinegar	5 mL
2¾ cups	White Bread Mix for Mixer (pages 215–216)	675 mL

1. In a bowl, using a heavy-duty electric mixer with paddle attachment, combine eggs, water, oil, honey and vinegar until well blended. With the mixer on its lowest speed, slowly add bread mix until combined. Stop the machine and scrape the bottom and sides of the bowl with a rubber spatula. With the mixer on medium speed, beat for 4 minutes.

2. Spoon into prepared pan. Let rise, uncovered, in a warm, draft-free place for 60 to 75 minutes or until dough has risen to the top of the pan. Meanwhile, preheat oven to 350°F (180°C).

3. Bake for 35 to 40 minutes or until internal temperature of loaf registers 200°F (100°C) on an instant-read thermometer. Remove from the pan immediately and let cool completely on a rack.

Variation

To turn this into a raisin loaf, add ½ cup (125 mL) raisins and 1 tsp (5 mL) ground cinnamon with the bread mix.

Nutritional value per serving	
Calories	126
Fat, total	4 g
Fat, saturated	1 g
Cholesterol	25 mg
Sodium	243 mg
Carbohydrate	19 g
Fiber	2 g
Protein	3 g
Calcium	18 mg
Iron	2 mg

Dinner Rolls

**Makes 12 rolls
(1 per serving)**

*Everyone loves a
golden brown dinner
roll, and they're so
easy to make from
our mix.*

Tips

To ensure success, see page
214 for tips on mixer-
method bread baking.

For a softer crust, brush it
with melted butter as soon
as you remove the rolls
from the oven.

You can use $\frac{1}{2}$ cup
(125 mL) liquid whole
eggs, if you prefer.

- **12-cup muffin tin, lightly greased**

2	eggs, lightly beaten	2
1 cup	water	250 mL
3 tbsp	vegetable oil	45 mL
2 tbsp	liquid honey	25 mL
1 tsp	cider vinegar	5 mL
2¾ cups	White Bread Mix for Mixer (pages 215–216)	675 mL

1. In a bowl, using a heavy-duty electric mixer with paddle attachment, combine eggs, water, oil, honey and vinegar until well blended. With the mixer on its lowest speed, slowly add bread mix until combined. Stop the machine and scrape the bottom and sides of the bowl with a rubber spatula. With the mixer on medium speed, beat for 4 minutes.

2. Using a ¼-cup (50 mL) scoop, drop dough into prepared muffin cups. Let rise, uncovered, in a warm, draft-free place for 60 to 75 minutes or until dough has risen to the top of the cups. Meanwhile, preheat oven to 350°F (180°C).

3. Bake for 18 to 20 minutes or until internal temperature of rolls registers 200°F (100°C) on an instant-read thermometer. Remove from the tin immediately and let cool completely on a rack.

Nutritional value per serving	
Calories	168
Fat, total	7 g
Fat, saturated	1 g
Cholesterol	31 mg
Sodium	304 mg
Carbohydrate	24 g
Fiber	3 g
Protein	4 g
Calcium	22 mg
Iron	2 mg

Rosemary Breadsticks

Makes 24 breadsticks (1 per serving)

Longing for a crunchy breadstick with a warm, golden brown, crisp crust? Try this twice-baked version.

Tips

To ensure success, see page 214 for tips on mixer-method bread baking.

For uniform breadsticks, cut bread in half, then lengthwise into quarters. Finally, cut each quarter lengthwise into 3 strips.

If breadsticks become soft during storage, crisp them in a toaster oven or conventional oven at 350°F (180°C) for a few minutes.

Nutritional value per serving

Calories	80
Fat, total	3 g
Fat, saturated	1 g
Cholesterol	2 mg
Sodium	186 mg
Carbohydrate	11 g
Fiber	1 g
Protein	3 g
Calcium	42 mg
Iron	1 mg

- Two 8-inch (20 cm) square baking pans, lightly greased
- Baking sheets, ungreased

1⅓ cups	water	325 mL
2 tbsp	extra virgin olive oil	25 mL
1 tsp	cider vinegar	5 mL
2¾ cups	White Bread Mix for Mixer (pages 215–216)	675 mL
¼ cup	snipped fresh rosemary	50 mL
1 tsp	white (granulated) sugar	5 mL
½ tsp	freshly ground black pepper	2 mL
½ cup	freshly grated Parmesan cheese, divided	125 mL

1. In a bowl, using a heavy-duty electric mixer with paddle attachment, combine water, oil and vinegar until well blended. With the mixer on its lowest speed, slowly add bread mix, rosemary, sugar and black pepper until combined. Stop the machine and scrape the bottom and sides of the bowl with a rubber spatula. With the mixer on medium speed, beat for 4 minutes.

2. Sprinkle 2 tbsp (25 mL) of the Parmesan in the bottom of each prepared pan. Drop dough by spoonfuls over the Parmesan. Using a moistened rubber spatula, spread dough evenly to the edges of the pan. Sprinkle each with 2 tbsp (25 mL) Parmesan. Let rise, uncovered, in a warm, draft-free place for 45 minutes or until dough has risen to the top of the pans. Meanwhile, preheat oven to 400°F (200°C).

3. Bake for 12 to 15 minutes or until light brown. Remove from pan and transfer immediately to a cutting board. Reduce oven temperature to 350°F (180°C). Using a pizza wheel or a sharp knife, cut bread into 12 equal strips.

4. Arrange breadsticks, cut side up, at least ½ inch (1 cm) apart on baking sheets. Bake for 20 to 25 minutes or until dry, crisp and golden brown. Turn off oven and let breadsticks cool completely in oven.

5. Store in an airtight container at room temperature for up to 1 week.

Variation

Substitute thyme or tarragon, or a combination of herbs, for the rosemary.

Orange Chocolate Chip Loaf

This dessert bread is delightful when served warm. Enjoy for a quick snack.

Tips

To ensure success, see page 214 for tips on mixer-method bread baking.

When oranges are in season, buy extra and freeze the zest and juice to have ready for recipes like this one.

Small chocolate chips tend to melt and produce a marbled effect. That's why we use the jumbos.

- 9- by 5-inch (23 by 12.5 cm) loaf pan, lightly greased

2	eggs, lightly beaten	2
1 tbsp	grated orange zest	15 mL
½ cup	freshly squeezed orange juice	125 mL
½ cup	water	125 mL
3 tbsp	liquid honey	45 mL
2 tbsp	vegetable oil	25 mL
1 tsp	cider vinegar	5 mL
2¾ cups	White Bread Mix for Mixer (pages 215–216)	675 mL
¾ cup	jumbo semisweet chocolate chips	175 mL

1. In a bowl, using a heavy-duty electric mixer with paddle attachment, combine eggs, orange zest, orange juice, water, honey, oil and vinegar until well blended. With the mixer on its lowest speed, slowly add bread mix until combined. Stop the machine and scrape the bottom and sides of the bowl with a rubber spatula. With the mixer on medium speed, beat for 4 minutes. With the mixer on its lowest speed, stir in chocolate chips.

2. Spoon into prepared pan. Let rise, uncovered, in a warm, draft-free place for 60 to 75 minutes or until dough has risen to the top of the pan. Meanwhile, preheat oven to 350°F (180°C).

3. Bake for 25 minutes. Tent with foil and bake for 20 to 25 minutes or until internal temperature of loaf registers 200°F (100°C) on an instant-read thermometer. Remove from the pan immediately and let cool completely on a rack.

Nutritional value per serving	
Calories	178
Fat, total	7 g
Fat, saturated	2 g
Cholesterol	27 mg
Sodium	250 mg
Carbohydrate	26 g
Fiber	2 g
Protein	4 g
Calcium	35 mg
Iron	2 mg

Single-Loaf Brown Bread Mix for Mixer

Makes about 2¾ cups (675 mL), enough for 1 loaf

You asked us for a brown bread mix you could use to make a variety of nutritious loaves and rolls. We've done you one better and given you the recipe in two different batch sizes. Here's a single-loaf mix you can try before making the larger batch on page 222. You can use this nutritious mix to make Maritime (Boston) Brown Bread (page 223), Mock Bran Bread (page 224), Pumpernickel Bread (page 225) or Pizza Crust (page 226).

1 cup	sorghum flour	250 mL
½ cup	whole bean flour	125 mL
⅓ cup	brown rice flour	75 mL
2 tbsp	quinoa flour	25 mL
¼ cup	potato starch	50 mL
2 tbsp	tapioca starch	25 mL
2 tbsp	packed brown sugar	25 mL
1 tbsp	xanthan gum	15 mL
1 tbsp	bread machine or instant yeast	15 mL
1½ tsp	salt	7 mL

1. In a large bowl or plastic bag, combine sorghum flour, whole bean flour, brown rice flour, quinoa flour, potato starch, tapioca starch, brown sugar, xanthan gum, yeast and salt. Mix well.

2. Use right away or seal tightly in a plastic bag, removing as much air as possible. Store at room temperature for up to 3 days or in the freezer for up to 6 weeks.

Working with Bread Mix

Be sure the brown sugar is well distributed and any lumps are broken up; it clumps easily when mixed with other dry ingredients

Label and date the package if not using bread mix immediately. We add the page number of the recipe to the label as a quick reference.

Let bread mix warm to room temperature, and mix well before using.

Nutritional value per serving (¹⁄₁₅ recipe)

Calories	77
Fat, total	1 g
Fat, saturated	0 g
Cholesterol	0 mg
Sodium	235 mg
Carbohydrate	17 g
Fiber	2 g
Protein	2 g
Calcium	9 mg
Iron	1 mg

Four-Loaf Brown Bread Mix for Mixer

Makes about 11 cups (2.75 L), enough for 4 loaves

Here's the four-loaf version of our bread machine brown bread mix. Use it to make Maritime (Boston) Brown Bread (page 223), Mock Bran Bread (page 224), Pumpernickel Bread (page 225) and Pizza Crust (page 226).

Tips

For accuracy, use a 1-cup (250 mL) dry measure several times to measure each type of flour and starch. If you use a 4 cup (1 L) liquid measure, it's difficult to get an accurate volume and you'll end up with extra flour in the mix.

Nutritional value per serving ($\frac{1}{60}$ recipe)

Calories	76
Fat, total	1 g
Fat, saturated	0 g
Cholesterol	0 mg
Sodium	234 mg
Carbohydrate	16 g
Fiber	1 g
Protein	2 g
Calcium	8 mg
Iron	1 mg

4 cups	sorghum flour	1 L
2 cups	whole bean flour	500 mL
1⅓ cups	brown rice flour	325 mL
½ cup	quinoa flour	125 mL
1 cup	potato starch	250 mL
½ cup	tapioca starch	125 mL
½ cup	packed brown sugar	125 mL
¼ cup	xanthan gum	50 mL
¼ cup	bread machine or instant yeast	50 mL
2 tbsp	salt	25 mL

1. In a very large container or roasting pan, combine sorghum flour, whole bean flour, brown rice flour, quinoa flour, potato starch, tapioca starch, brown sugar, xanthan gum, yeast and salt. Mix well.

2. Divide into four equal portions of about 2¾ cups (675 mL) each. Seal tightly in plastic bags, removing as much air as possible. Store at room temperature for up to 3 days or in the freezer for up to 6 weeks.

Working with Bread Mix

Be sure the brown sugar is well distributed and any lumps are broken up; it clumps easily when mixed with other dry ingredients.

In step 2, stir the mix before spooning it very lightly into the dry measures. Do not pack.

Be sure to divide the mix into equal portions. Depending on how much air you incorporate into the mix, and the texture of the individual gluten-free flours, the total volume of the mix can vary slightly. The important thing is to make the number of portions specified in the recipe.

Label and date the packages before storing. We add the page number of the recipe to the labels as a quick reference.

Let bread mix warm to room temperature, and mix well before using.

Maritime (Boston) Brown Bread

**Makes 15 slices
(1 per serving)**

Here's a good basic brown bread for sandwiches and everyday use. It's especially good with homemade baked beans.

Tips

To ensure success, see page 214 for tips on mixer-method bread baking.

Measuring the oil before the molasses ensures that the molasses slides out of the measure. We enjoy using the OXO sloped ¼-cup (50 mL) measure for this. If the molasses is really thick or is straight out of the refrigerator, warm it slightly in the microwave before measuring.

Nutritional value per serving	
Calories	122
Fat, total	4 g
Fat, saturated	0 g
Cholesterol	25 mg
Sodium	247 mg
Carbohydrate	23 g
Fiber	2 g
Protein	3 g
Calcium	17 mg
Iron	1 mg

• 9- by 5-inch (23 by 12.5 cm) loaf pan, lightly greased

2	eggs, lightly beaten	2
1	egg white, lightly beaten	1
1 cup	water	250 mL
3 tbsp	vegetable oil	45 mL
2 tbsp	light (fancy) molasses	25 mL
1 tbsp	liquid honey	15 mL
1 tsp	cider vinegar	5 mL
2¾ cups	Brown Bread Mix for Mixer (pages 221–222)	675 mL

1. In a bowl, using a heavy-duty electric mixer with paddle attachment, combine eggs, egg white, water, oil, molasses, honey and vinegar until well blended. With the mixer on its lowest speed, slowly add bread mix until combined. Stop the machine and scrape the bottom and sides of the bowl with a rubber spatula. With the mixer on medium speed, beat for 4 minutes.

2. Spoon into prepared pan. Let rise, uncovered, in a warm, draft-free place for 60 to 75 minutes or until dough has risen to the top of the pan. Meanwhile, preheat oven to 350°F (180°C).

3. Bake for 40 to 45 minutes or until internal temperature of loaf registers 200°F (100°C) on an instant-read thermometer. Remove from the pan immediately and let cool completely on a rack.

Variation
Add ½ cup (125 mL) raisins or chopped walnuts with the bread mix.

Mock Bran Bread

**Makes 15 slices
(1 per serving)**

This is a sweeter, higher-fiber version of our basic Brown Sandwich Bread (page 227). You'll love using this bread for all of your sandwiches.

Tips

To ensure success, see page 214 for tips on mixer-method bread baking.

Warm rice bran that has been stored in the refrigerator or freezer to room temperature.

- 9- by 5-inch (23 by 12.5 cm) loaf pan, lightly greased

2 tbsp	rice bran	25 mL
2¾ cups	Brown Bread Mix for Mixer (pages 221–222)	675 mL
2	eggs, lightly beaten	2
1	egg white, lightly beaten	1
1 cup	water	250 mL
3 tbsp	vegetable oil	45 mL
2 tbsp	liquid honey	25 mL
1 tbsp	light (fancy) molasses	15 mL
1 tsp	cider vinegar	5 mL

1. Add rice bran to the bread mix. Mix well and set aside.

2. In a bowl, using a heavy-duty electric mixer with paddle attachment, combine eggs, egg white, water, oil, honey, molasses and vinegar until well blended. With the mixer on its lowest speed, slowly add bread mix until combined. Stop the machine and scrape the bottom and sides of the bowl with a rubber spatula. With the mixer on medium speed, beat for 4 minutes.

3. Spoon into prepared pan. Let rise, uncovered, in a warm, draft-free place for 60 to 75 minutes or until dough has risen to the top of the pan. Meanwhile, preheat oven to 350°F (180°C).

4. Bake for 35 to 45 minutes or until internal temperature of loaf registers 200°F (100°C) on an instant-read thermometer. Remove from the pan immediately and let cool completely on a rack.

Variations

Add ½ cup (125 mL) raisins, chopped dates or chopped walnuts with the bread mix.

Substitute GF oat bran for the rice bran.

Nutritional value per serving

Calories	127
Fat, total	5 g
Fat, saturated	0 g
Cholesterol	25 mg
Sodium	250 mg
Carbohydrate	20 g
Fiber	2 g
Protein	4 g
Calcium	15 mg
Iron	1 mg

Pumpernickel Bread

**Makes 15 slices
(1 per serving)**

*With all the hearty
flavor of traditional
pumpernickel, this
version is great for
sandwiches. Try it
filled with sliced
turkey, accompanied
by a crisp garlic dill
pickle.*

Tips

To ensure success, see page
214 for tips on mixer-
method bread baking.

Sift cocoa just before using,
as it lumps easily.

Nutritional value per serving

Calories	125
Fat, total	4 g
Fat, saturated	0 g
Cholesterol	25 mg
Sodium	248 mg
Carbohydrate	20 g
Fiber	2 g
Protein	3 g
Calcium	22 mg
Iron	1 mg

• 9- by 5-inch (23 by 12.5 cm) loaf pan, lightly greased

1 tbsp	instant coffee granules	15 mL
1 tbsp	unsweetened cocoa powder, sifted	15 mL
¾ tsp	ground ginger	4 mL
2¾ cups	Brown Bread Mix for Mixer (pages 221–222)	675 mL
2	eggs, lightly beaten	2
1	egg white, lightly beaten	1
1 cup	water	250 mL
3 tbsp	vegetable oil	45 mL
3 tbsp	light (fancy) molasses	45 mL
1 tsp	cider vinegar	5 mL

1. Add coffee granules, cocoa and ginger to the bread mix. Mix well and set aside.

2. In a bowl, using a heavy-duty electric mixer with paddle attachment, combine eggs, egg white, water, oil, molasses and vinegar until well blended. With the mixer on its lowest speed, slowly add bread mix until combined. Stop the machine and scrape the bottom and sides of the bowl with a rubber spatula. With the mixer on medium speed, beat for 4 minutes.

3. Spoon into prepared pan. Let rise, uncovered, in a warm, draft-free place for 60 to 75 minutes or until dough has risen to the top of the pan. Meanwhile, preheat oven to 350°F (180°C).

4. Bake for 35 to 45 minutes or until internal temperature of loaf registers 200°F (100°C) on an instant-read thermometer. Remove from the pan immediately and let cool completely on a rack.

Variations

Add 2 tbsp (25 mL) caraway, fennel or anise seeds with the bread mix.

Substitute an equal quantity of strong brewed room-temperature coffee for the water.

Pizza Crust

**Makes 16 squares
(1 per serving)**

You requested a whole-grain pizza crust recipe — here it is.

Tips

To ensure success, see page 214 for tips on mixer-method bread baking.

To make pizza, add your favorite topping ingredients and bake until crust is brown and crisp and top is bubbly.

• Two 15- by 10-inch (40 by 25 cm) jelly roll pans, lightly greased

2 tsp	bread machine or instant yeast	10 mL
2¾ cups	Brown Bread Mix for Mixer (pages 221–222)	675 mL
2 cups	water	500 mL
3 tbsp	extra virgin olive oil	45 mL
1 tsp	cider vinegar	5 mL

1. Add yeast to the bread mix. Mix well and set aside.

2. In a bowl, using a heavy-duty electric mixer with paddle attachment, combine water, oil and vinegar until well blended. With the mixer on its lowest speed, slowly add bread mix until combined. Stop the machine and scrape the bottom and sides of the bowl with a rubber spatula. With the mixer on medium speed, beat for 4 minutes.

3. Meanwhile, preheat oven to 400°F (200°C).

4. Divide dough in half. Place half the dough in each prepared pan and, using a moistened rubber spatula, spread evenly to the edges. Do not smooth tops.

5. Bake for 12 minutes or until bottom is golden and crust is partially baked.

6. Use right away to make pizza with your favorite toppings, or wrap airtight and store in the freezer for up to 1 month. Thaw in the refrigerator overnight before using.

Variations

If you like a thicker crust, leave the dough in one piece, spread it in the pan and let rise for 30 minutes before baking.

Add 1 to 2 tsp (5 to 10 mL) dried herbs or 1 to 2 tbsp (15 to 25 mL) chopped fresh herbs such as rosemary, oregano, basil or thyme with the bread mix.

Nutritional value per serving

Calories	97
Fat, total	4 g
Fat, saturated	0 g
Cholesterol	0 mg
Sodium	221 mg
Carbohydrate	16 g
Fiber	2 g
Protein	2 g
Calcium	8 mg
Iron	1 mg

Brown Sandwich Bread

**Makes 15 slices
(1 per serving)**

A CanolaInfo recipe

For those who want a rich, golden, wholesome, nutritious sandwich bread to carry for lunch, this is your loaf.

Tips

To ensure success, see page 214 for tips on mixer-method bread baking.

Pea flour, like soy flour, has a distinctive odor when wet that disappears with baking.

Nutritional value per serving

Calories	116
Fat, total	4 g
Fat, saturated	1 g
Cholesterol	25 mg
Sodium	247 mg
Carbohydrate	18 g
Fiber	2 g
Protein	4 g
Calcium	17 mg
Iron	2 mg

- 9- by 5-inch (23 by 12.5 cm) loaf pan, lightly greased

1 cup	sorghum flour	250 mL
1/2 cup	pea flour	125 mL
1/3 cup	tapioca starch	75 mL
1/3 cup	rice bran	75 mL
2 tbsp	packed brown sugar	25 mL
1 tbsp	xanthan gum	15 mL
2 tsp	bread machine or instant yeast	10 mL
1 1/2 tsp	salt	7 mL
2	eggs, lightly beaten	2
1	egg white, lightly beaten	1
1 1/4 cups	water	300 mL
3 tbsp	vegetable oil	45 mL
2 tbsp	light (fancy) molasses	25 mL
1 tsp	cider vinegar	5 mL

1. In a large bowl or plastic bag, combine sorghum flour, pea flour, tapioca starch, rice bran, brown sugar, xanthan gum, yeast and salt. Mix well and set aside.

2. In a separate bowl, using a heavy-duty electric mixer with paddle attachment, combine eggs, egg white, water, oil, molasses and vinegar until well blended. With the mixer on its lowest speed, slowly add the dry ingredients until combined. Stop the machine and scrape the bottom and sides of the bowl with a rubber spatula. With the mixer on medium speed, beat for 4 minutes.

3. Spoon into prepared pan. Let rise, uncovered, in a warm, draft-free place for 60 to 75 minutes or until dough has risen to the top of the pan. Meanwhile, preheat oven to 350°F (180°C), with rack set in bottom third of oven.

4. Bake for 25 minutes. Tent loosely with foil (dull side out) and bake for 10 to 15 minutes or until internal temperature of loaf registers 200°F (100°C) on an instant-read thermometer. Remove from the pan immediately and let cool completely on a rack.

Variations

Any type of bean flour can be substituted for the pea flour.

Substitute GF oat bran for the rice bran.

Teff Bread

**Makes 15 slices
(1 per serving)**

*Teff is a powerhouse
of nutrition and makes
a delicious bread.*

- 9- by 5-inch (23 by 12.5 cm) loaf pan, lightly greased

⅔ cup	brown rice flour	150 mL
⅔ cup	teff flour	150 mL
½ cup	GF oat flour	125 mL
⅓ cup	potato starch	75 mL
3 tbsp	teff grain	45 mL
1 tbsp	ground flaxseed	15 mL
1 tbsp	xanthan gum	15 mL
2 tsp	bread machine or instant yeast	10 mL
1½ tsp	salt	7 mL
2 tbsp	grated orange zest	25 mL
⅔ cup	dried blueberries	150 mL
2	eggs, lightly beaten	2
2	egg whites, lightly beaten	2
¾ cup	water	175 mL
3 tbsp	vegetable oil	45 mL
3 tbsp	liquid honey	45 mL
2 tsp	cider vinegar	10 mL

1. In a large bowl or plastic bag, combine brown rice flour, teff flour, oat flour, potato starch, teff grain, flaxseed, xanthan gum, yeast, salt, orange zest and blueberries. Mix well and set aside.

2. In a separate bowl, using a heavy-duty electric mixer with paddle attachment, combine eggs, egg whites, water, oil, honey and vinegar until well blended. With the mixer on its lowest speed, slowly add the dry ingredients until combined. Stop the machine and scrape the bottom and sides of the bowl with a rubber spatula. With the mixer on medium speed, beat for 4 minutes.

3. Spoon into prepared pan. Let rise, uncovered, in a warm, draft-free place for 60 to 75 minutes or until dough has risen to the top of the pan. Meanwhile, preheat oven to 350°F (180°C).

**Nutritional value
per serving**

Calories	144
Fat, total	4 g
Fat, saturated	1 g
Cholesterol	25 mg
Sodium	250 mg
Carbohydrate	24 g
Fiber	3 g
Protein	4 g
Calcium	26 mg
Iron	2 mg

Tips

To ensure success, see page 214 for tips on mixer-method bread baking.

See the Techniques Glossary, page 396, for information on grinding flaxseed.

You can use ½ cup (125 mL) liquid whole eggs and ¼ cup (50 mL) liquid egg whites, if you prefer.

4. Bake for 35 to 40 minutes or until internal temperature of loaf registers 200°F (100°C) on an instant-read thermometer. Remove from the pan immediately and let cool completely on a rack.

Variations

If you can't find teff grain, substitute ¼ cup (50 mL) poppy seeds or amaranth grain.

Substitute raisins or dried cranberries for the dried blueberries.

Historic Grains Bread

**Makes 15 slices
(1 per serving)**

Here's a quintet of healthy grains — sorghum, amaranth, quinoa, flaxseed and millet seeds — combined in a soft-textured, nutritious loaf that's perfect for sandwiches.

Tips

To ensure success, see page 214 for tips on mixer-method bread baking.

You can use either golden or brown flaxseed.

See the Techniques Glossary, page 396, for information on cracking flaxseed.

You can use ½ cup (125 mL) liquid whole eggs and ¼ cup (50 mL) liquid egg whites, if you prefer.

Nutritional value per serving	
Calories	134
Fat, total	5 g
Fat, saturated	0 g
Cholesterol	25 mg
Sodium	2 mg
Carbohydrate	20 g
Fiber	3 g
Protein	4 g
Calcium	24 mg
Iron	211 mg

• **9- by 5-inch (23 by 12.5 cm) loaf pan, lightly greased**

1 cup	sorghum flour	250 mL
¾ cup	amaranth flour	175 mL
¼ cup	quinoa flour	50 mL
⅓ cup	cracked flaxseed	75 mL
¼ cup	millet seeds	50 mL
⅓ cup	tapioca starch	75 mL
1 tbsp	xanthan gum	15 mL
2 tsp	bread machine or instant yeast	10 mL
1¼ tsp	salt	6 mL
2	eggs, lightly beaten	2
2	egg whites, lightly beaten	2
1 cup	water	250 mL
3 tbsp	liquid honey	45 mL
2 tbsp	vegetable oil	25 mL
1 tsp	cider vinegar	5 mL

1. In a large bowl or plastic bag, combine sorghum flour, amaranth flour, quinoa flour, flaxseed, millet seeds, tapioca starch, xanthan gum, yeast and salt. Mix well and set aside.

2. In a separate bowl, using a heavy-duty electric mixer with paddle attachment, combine eggs, egg whites, water, honey, oil and vinegar until well blended. With the mixer on its lowest speed, slowly add the dry ingredients until combined. Stop the machine and scrape the bottom and sides of the bowl with a rubber spatula. With the mixer on medium speed, beat for 4 minutes.

3. Spoon into prepared pan. Let rise, uncovered, in a warm, draft-free place for 60 to 75 minutes or until dough has risen to the top of the pan. Meanwhile, preheat oven to 350°F (180°C).

4. Bake for 40 to 45 minutes or until internal temperature of loaf registers 200°F (100°C) on an instant-read thermometer. Remove from the pan immediately and let cool completely on a rack.

Variation

Substitute amaranth grain or whole flaxseed for the millet seeds.

Honey Fig Loaf

**Makes 15 slices
(1 per serving)**

This sweet loaf is delicious spread with applesauce for a light dessert.

Tips

To ensure success, see page 214 for tips on mixer-method bread baking.

If using apple cider and applesauce from the refrigerator, warm them each in the microwave for 1 minute on High before measuring.

Chop the figs with sharp kitchen shears. When the blades become sticky, dip them in warm water.

If only sweetened apple cider and applesauce are available, decrease the honey to 1 tbsp (15 mL). If you can't find apple cider at all, purchase high-quality unsweetened apple juice, not sweetened apple drink.

Nutritional value per serving

Calories	154
Fat, total	3 g
Fat, saturated	0 g
Cholesterol	25 mg
Sodium	169 mg
Carbohydrate	30 g
Fiber	3 g
Protein	4 g
Calcium	27 mg
Iron	1 mg

- 9- by 5-inch (23 by 12.5 cm) loaf pan, lightly greased

1¼ cups	sorghum flour	300 mL
½ cup	pea flour	125 mL
⅓ cup	tapioca starch	75 mL
1 tbsp	xanthan gum	15 mL
1 tbsp	bread machine or instant yeast	15 mL
1 tsp	salt	5 mL
¾ tsp	ground cardamom	4 mL
2	eggs, lightly beaten	2
¾ cup	unsweetened apple cider, at room temperature	175 mL
½ cup	unsweetened applesauce, at room temperature	125 mL
2 tbsp	vegetable oil	25 mL
2 tbsp	liquid honey	25 mL
¾ cup	dried figs, chopped	175 mL

1. In a large bowl or plastic bag, combine sorghum flour, pea flour, tapioca starch, xanthan gum, yeast, salt and cardamom. Mix well and set aside.

2. In a separate bowl, using a heavy-duty electric mixer with paddle attachment, combine eggs, cider, applesauce, oil and honey until well blended. With the mixer on its lowest speed, slowly add the dry ingredients until combined. Stop the machine and scrape the bottom and sides of the bowl with a rubber spatula. With the mixer on medium speed, beat for 4 minutes. With the mixer on its lowest speed, stir in figs.

3. Spoon into prepared pan. Let rise, uncovered, in a warm, draft-free place for 60 to 75 minutes or until dough has risen to the top of the pan. Meanwhile, preheat oven to 350°F (180°C).

4. Bake for 35 to 40 minutes or until internal temperature of loaf registers 200°F (100°C) on an instant-read thermometer. Remove from the pan immediately and let cool completely on a rack.

Multigrain Bread

**Makes 15 slices
(1 per serving)**

*A celiac friend suggested this variation of our Whole-Grain Amaranth Bread (*The Best Gluten-Free Family Cookbook*, page 72). This soft-textured, creamy, honey-colored bread is so delicious you won't even suspect how nutritious it is.*

Tips

To ensure success, see page 214 for tips on mixer-method bread baking.

See the Techniques Glossary for information on making your own oat flour (page 398) and grinding flaxseed (page 396).

Nutritional value per serving

Calories	132
Fat, total	5 g
Fat, saturated	1 g
Cholesterol	25 mg
Sodium	211 mg
Carbohydrate	20 g
Fiber	2 g
Protein	4 g
Calcium	20 mg
Iron	2 mg

- 9- by 5-inch (23 by 12.5 cm) loaf pan, lightly greased

½ cup	brown rice flour	125 mL
½ cup	GF oat flour	125 mL
⅔ cup	amaranth flour	150 mL
½ cup	potato starch	125 mL
3 tbsp	amaranth grain	45 mL
1 tbsp	ground flaxseed	15 mL
1 tbsp	xanthan gum	15 mL
2 tsp	bread machine or instant yeast	10 mL
1¼ tsp	salt	6 mL
2	eggs, lightly beaten	2
2	egg whites, lightly beaten	2
¾ cup	water	175 mL
3 tbsp	vegetable oil	45 mL
3 tbsp	liquid honey	45 mL
2 tsp	cider vinegar	10 mL

1. In a large bowl or plastic bag, combine brown rice flour, oat flour, amaranth flour, potato starch, amaranth grain, flaxseed, xanthan gum, yeast and salt. Mix well and set aside.

2. In a separate bowl, using a heavy-duty electric mixer with paddle attachment, combine eggs, egg whites, water, oil, honey and vinegar until well blended. With the mixer on its lowest speed, slowly add the dry ingredients until combined. Stop the machine and scrape the bottom and sides of the bowl with a rubber spatula. With the mixer on medium speed, beat for 4 minutes.

3. Spoon into prepared pan. Let rise, uncovered, in a warm, draft-free place for 60 to 75 minutes or until dough has risen to the top of the pan. Meanwhile, preheat oven to 350°F (180°C).

Tips

Amaranth is high in fiber, iron and calcium and lower in sodium than most grains. Store amaranth grain in an airtight container in the refrigerator for up to 6 months

You can use $\frac{1}{2}$ cup (125 mL) liquid whole eggs and $\frac{1}{4}$ cup (50 mL) liquid egg whites, if you prefer.

4. Bake for 35 to 40 minutes or until internal temperature of loaf registers 200°F (100°C) on an instant-read thermometer. Remove from the pan immediately and let cool completely on a rack.

Variations

Substitute millet seeds or poppy seeds for the amaranth grain.

Add $\frac{2}{3}$ cup (150 mL) dried cranberries and 2 tbsp (25 mL) grated orange zest with the dry ingredients.

Cranberry Pumpkin Seed Bread

Makes 15 slices
(1 per serving)

A CanolaInfo recipe

This attractive loaf is sure to bring compliments from guests. Pumpkin flavor, flecks of red cranberries and green pumpkin seeds make it the perfect accompaniment for turkey.

Tip

To ensure success, see page 214 for tips on mixer-method bread baking.

- 9- by 5-inch (23 by 12.5 cm) loaf pan, lightly greased

1 cup	sorghum flour	250 mL
1/4 cup	flax flour	50 mL
1/4 cup	quinoa flour	50 mL
1/3 cup	tapioca starch	75 mL
3 tbsp	white (granulated) sugar	45 mL
2 1/2 tsp	xanthan gum	12 mL
2 tsp	bread machine or instant yeast	10 mL
1 1/4 tsp	salt	6 mL
1/2 cup	dried cranberries	125 mL
1/3 cup	unsalted green pumpkin seeds, toasted	75 mL
2	eggs, lightly beaten	2
1	egg white, lightly beaten	1
1 cup	pumpkin purée (not pie filling)	250 mL
1/4 cup	water	50 mL
1/4 cup	vegetable oil	50 mL
2 tsp	cider vinegar	10 mL

1. In a large bowl or plastic bag, combine sorghum flour, flax flour, quinoa flour, tapioca starch, sugar, xanthan gum, yeast, salt, cranberries and pumpkin seeds. Mix well and set aside.

2. In a separate bowl, using a heavy-duty electric mixer with paddle attachment, combine eggs, egg white, pumpkin purée, water, oil and vinegar until well blended. With the mixer on its lowest speed, slowly add the dry ingredients until combined. Stop the machine and scrape the bottom and sides of the bowl with a rubber spatula. With the mixer on medium speed, beat for 4 minutes.

3. Spoon into prepared pan. Let rise, uncovered, in a warm, draft-free place for 60 to 75 minutes or until dough has risen to the top of the pan. Meanwhile, preheat oven to 350°F (180°C).

Tip

See the Techniques Glossary for information on grinding flaxseed to make flax flour (page 396) and toasting seeds (page 399).

We tried this bread with sprouted flax powder, flax meal and ground flaxseed in place of the flax flour. All yielded acceptable loaves.

Be sure to use pumpkin purée; pumpkin pie filling is too sweet.

4. Bake for 35 to 40 minutes or until internal temperature of loaf registers 200°F (100°C) on an instant-read thermometer. Remove from the pan immediately and let cool completely on a rack.

Variations

Substitute halved dried cherries for the cranberries.

Substitute chopped pecans or unsalted sunflower seeds for the pumpkin seeds.

Swedish Wraps

*Use these to make
the ever-popular wrap
luncheon sandwich.*

Tip

Roll these wraps around
your favorite sandwich
fillings.

Dipping the spatula
repeatedly into warm
water makes it easier to
spread this dough thinly
and evenly.

To make this recipe
dairy-free, use non-dairy
powdered milk substitute
and water.

- Preheat oven to 400°F (200°C)
- 15- by 10-inch (40 by 25 cm) jelly roll pan, lightly greased and lined with parchment paper

1/4 cup	sorghum flour	50 mL
1/4 cup	amaranth flour	50 mL
1/4 cup	potato starch	50 mL
1/4 cup	tapioca starch	50 mL
1 tsp	white (granulated) sugar	5 mL
2 tsp	xanthan gum	10 mL
1 tbsp	bread machine or instant yeast	15 mL
3/4 tsp	salt	4 mL
1 tsp	anise seeds	5 mL
1 tsp	caraway seeds	5 mL
1 tsp	fennel seeds	5 mL
3/4 cup	milk	175 mL
1 tsp	cider vinegar	5 mL
1 tsp	extra virgin olive oil	5 mL

1. In a large bowl or plastic bag, combine sorghum flour, amaranth flour, potato starch, tapioca starch, sugar, xanthan gum, yeast, salt, anise seeds, caraway seeds and fennel seeds. Mix well and set aside.

2. In a separate bowl, using a heavy-duty electric mixer with paddle attachment, combine milk, vinegar and oil until well blended. With the mixer on its lowest speed, slowly add the dry ingredients until combined. Stop the machine and scrape the bottom and sides of the bowl with a rubber spatula. With the mixer on medium speed, beat for 4 minutes.

3. Remove dough to prepared pan. Using a moistened rubber spatula, spread dough evenly to the edges of the pan.

4. Bake in preheated oven for 12 to 14 minutes or until edges are brown and top begins to brown. Let cool completely on pan on a rack. Remove from pan and cut into quarters.

Variation

Try adding dried herbs to the soft dough in place of the three varieties of seeds. To make a plainer variety, omit seeds and herbs.

Nutritional value per serving

Calories	165
Fat, total	3 g
Fat, saturated	0 g
Cholesterol	2 mg
Sodium	461 mg
Carbohydrate	31 g
Fiber	3 g
Protein	5 g
Calcium	86 mg
Iron	3 mg

Yeast-Free Loaves, Biscuits and Muffins

Blueberry Cornbread

Makes 10 servings

Moist, flavorful — perfect with chili or stew.

Tip

Use cooked fresh, thawed frozen or well-drained canned corn.

• 9-inch (23 cm) pie plate, lightly greased

1¼ cups	cornmeal	300 mL
¾ cup	amaranth flour	175 mL
¼ cup	cornstarch	50 mL
¼ cup	packed brown sugar	50 mL
1½ tsp	xanthan gum	7 mL
1 tbsp	GF baking powder	15 mL
1 tsp	baking soda	5 mL
½ tsp	salt	2 mL
2	eggs	2
1 cup	corn kernels	250 mL
1 cup	buttermilk	250 mL
½ cup	butter, melted and cooled	125 mL
1¼ cups	blueberries	300 mL

1. In a large bowl, whisk together cornmeal, amaranth flour, cornstarch, brown sugar xanthan gum, baking powder, baking soda and salt. Set aside.

2. In a food processor, purée eggs, corn, buttermilk and butter for 5 seconds or until combined. Add to dry ingredients and mix until combined. Gently fold in blueberries.

3. Spoon into prepared pie plate, smoothing top. Let stand for 30 minutes. Meanwhile, preheat oven to 350°F (180°C).

4. Bake for 35 to 40 minutes or until deep golden and a cake tester inserted in the center comes out clean. Let cool in pan on a rack for 5 minutes. Remove from pan and serve warm.

Variations

For added crunch, sprinkle the top with ½ tsp (2 mL) white (granulated) sugar just before baking.

For blue cornbread, choose blue cornmeal.

Nutritional value per serving

Calories	267
Fat, total	11 g
Fat, saturated	6 g
Cholesterol	63 mg
Sodium	448 mg
Carbohydrate	37 g
Fiber	3 g
Protein	5 g
Calcium	120 mg
Iron	3 mg

Sun-Dried Tomato Green Onion Cornbread

Serve this moist, savory cornbread, flavored with salty bursts of sun-dried tomatoes, with beef stew, chili, cioppino or a bowl of soup.

Tips

Use dry, not oil-packed, sun-dried tomatoes in this recipe.

To keep your cast-iron skillet from rusting, set it in a warm oven to dry completely before storing. Be careful: the handle gets hot.

We prefer to use low-fat soy flour in this recipe, but the higher-fat variety works well too. Remember, it browns quickly, so the cornbread may need to be tented with foil partway through the baking time.

Nutritional value per serving	
Calories	161
Fat, total	6 g
Fat, saturated	1 g
Cholesterol	32 mg
Sodium	298 mg
Carbohydrate	22 g
Fiber	1 g
Protein	6 g
Calcium	73 mg
Iron	1 mg

- **10-inch (25 cm) cast-iron skillet, 2 inches (5 cm) deep**

1⅓ cups	buttermilk	325 mL
1 cup	cornmeal	250 mL
	Vegetable oil	
¾ cup	low-fat soy flour	175 mL
¼ cup	tapioca starch	50 mL
¼ cup	white (granulated) sugar	50 mL
1½ tsp	xanthan gum	7 mL
1 tsp	GF baking powder	5 mL
1 tsp	baking soda	5 mL
1 tsp	salt	5 mL
2	eggs	2
¼ cup	vegetable oil	50 mL
⅔ cup	snipped sun-dried tomatoes	150 mL
½ cup	thinly sliced green onions	125 mL

1. In a bowl, combine buttermilk and cornmeal; set aside for 20 minutes. Meanwhile, preheat oven to 400°F (200°C).

2. Lightly brush bottom and sides of skillet with oil. Heat pan for 10 minutes in preheated oven.

3. In a large bowl or plastic bag, combine soy flour, tapioca starch, sugar, xanthan gum, baking powder, baking soda and salt. Mix well and set aside.

4. In a separate bowl, using an electric mixer, beat eggs and ¼ cup (50 mL) oil. Stir in buttermilk mixture. Add dry ingredients and mix until just combined. Stir in sun-dried tomatoes and green onions.

5. Carefully spoon batter into hot skillet. Bake for 20 to 25 minutes or until a cake tester inserted in the center comes out clean. Let cool in pan on a rack for 10 minutes. Cut into wedges and serve warm.

Variation

Add 6 slices of GF bacon, cooked crisp and crumbled, with the dry ingredients.

Mini Fruit 'n' Nut Loaves

**Makes 3 loaves,
6 slices each
(1 slice per serving)**

Sometimes you want just enough for you and a friend. Freeze the extras for another time.

- Three 5¾- by 3¼-inch (14 by 8 cm) loaf pans, lightly greased

1 cup	diced dried apricots	250 mL
1 cup	raisins	250 mL
1 tbsp	grated orange zest	15 mL
⅔ cup	freshly squeezed orange juice	150 mL
1¼ cups	sorghum flour	300 mL
⅓ cup	teff flour	75 mL
¼ cup	tapioca starch	50 mL
1½ tsp	xanthan gum	7 mL
2 tsp	GF baking powder	10 mL
1 tsp	baking soda	5 mL
½ tsp	salt	2 mL
½ cup	coarsely chopped walnuts	125 mL
⅓ cup	vegetable oil	75 mL
⅔ cup	packed brown sugar	150 mL
3	eggs	3
1 tsp	vanilla extract	5 mL

1. In a microwave-safe bowl, combine apricots, raisins, orange zest and orange juice. Microwave on High for 2 to 3 minutes or until steaming. Let cool to room temperature.

2. In a large bowl or plastic bag, combine sorghum flour, teff flour, tapioca starch, xanthan gum, baking powder, baking soda, salt and walnuts. Mix well and set aside.

3. In a separate bowl, using an electric mixer, beat oil, brown sugar, eggs and vanilla until combined. Stir in the apricot mixture. Add dry ingredients and stir just until combined.

4. Spoon batter into prepared pans, dividing evenly. Using a moistened rubber spatula, spread to edges and smooth tops. Let stand for 30 minutes. Meanwhile, preheat oven to 350°F (180°C).

Nutritional value per serving

Calories	196
Fat, total	7 g
Fat, saturated	1 g
Cholesterol	31 mg
Sodium	150 mg
Carbohydrate	31 g
Fiber	2 g
Protein	3 g
Calcium	52 mg
Iron	1 mg

Tent the loaves with foil
for the last 10 minutes if
they are getting too dark.

5. Bake for 35 to 40 minutes or until a tester inserted in
   the center comes out clean. Let cool in pan on a rack for
   10 minutes. Remove from pan and let cool completely
   on rack.

Variations

Substitute brandy for the orange juice and brandy extract
for the vanilla.

Make 12 muffins: Spoon batter into a lightly greased 12-cup
muffin tin. Bake for 20 minutes or until deep brown.

You could also make one larger loaf in a 9- by 5-inch (23 by
12.5 cm) loaf pan and bake for 50 to 60 minutes, or make
4 muffins and 2 mini loaves.

Cranberry Orange Drop Biscuits

**Makes 12 biscuits
(1 per serving)**

This is the favorite flavor combination of one of Donna's daughters-in-law. Now it's so popular you can even buy orange-flavored dried cranberries.

Tips

To make a drop biscuit, spoon the dough onto a large serving spoon and push it off onto the baking sheet with the back of another large spoon.

Biscuits should all be the same size, to bake in the same length of time.

Nutritional value per serving

Calories	143
Fat, total	10 g
Fat, saturated	4 g
Cholesterol	8 mg
Sodium	53 mg
Carbohydrate	13 g
Fiber	1 g
Protein	2 g
Calcium	74 mg
Iron	2 mg

- Preheat oven to 350°F (180°C)
- Baking sheet, lightly greased

¾ cup	amaranth flour	175 mL
½ cup	low-fat soy flour	125 mL
¼ cup	tapioca starch	50 mL
¼ cup	white (granulated) sugar	50 mL
1 tbsp	GF baking powder	15 mL
1 tsp	baking soda	5 mL
1½ tsp	xanthan gum	7 mL
¼ tsp	salt	1 mL
1 tbsp	grated orange zest	15 mL
¼ cup	cold butter, cut into 1-inch (2.5 cm) cubes	50 mL
½ cup	freshly squeezed orange juice	125 mL
½ cup	dried cranberries	125 mL

Food Processor Method

1. In a food processor, pulse amaranth flour, soy flour, tapioca starch, sugar, baking powder, baking soda, xanthan gum, salt and orange zest 3 or 4 times to combine. Add butter and pulse for 3 to 5 seconds or until mixture resembles coarse crumbs about the size of small peas. Add orange juice and cranberries all at once; process until dough holds together.

Traditional Method

1. In a large bowl, combine amaranth flour, soy flour, tapioca starch, sugar, baking powder, baking soda, xanthan gum, salt and orange zest. Using a pastry blender or two knives, cut in butter until mixture resembles coarse crumbs about the size of small peas. Add orange juice and cranberries all at once, stirring with a fork to make a thick dough.

For Both Methods

2. Drop dough by large spoonfuls 2 inches (5 cm) apart on prepared baking sheet. Bake in preheated oven for 11 to 13 minutes or until tops are golden. Serve immediately.

Variation

Substitute flavored dried cranberries for the plain ones.

White Chocolate Macadamia Drop Biscuits

**Makes 18 biscuits
(1 per serving)**

Here's the ultimate in decadent enjoyment. Forget about the guilt — just go ahead and enjoy. We could suggest alternative ingredients, but why bother? You can't improve on the combination of white chocolate and macadamia nuts.

Tips

Spoon the dough onto a large serving spoon and push it off onto the baking sheet with the back of another large spoon.

Watch carefully — 1 to 2 extra minutes can burn these sweet biscuits.

Nutritional value per serving

Calories

Fat, total

Fat, saturated

Cholesterol

Sodium

Carbohydrate

Fiber

Protein

Calcium

Iron

- **Preheat oven to 350°F (180°C)**
- **Baking sheet, lightly greased**

2/3 cup	macadamia nuts	150 mL
3/4 cup	amaranth flour	175 mL
1/3 cup	almond flour	75 mL
1/4 cup	tapioca starch	50 mL
1/4 cup	white (granulated) sugar	50 mL
1 tbsp	GF baking powder	15 mL
1 1/2 tsp	xanthan gum	7 mL
1/8 tsp	salt	0.5 mL
1/4 cup	cold butter, cut into 1-inch (2.5 cm) cubes	50 mL
2/3 cup	white chocolate chips	150 mL
1/2 cup	milk	125 mL

Food Processor Method

1. In a food processor, pulse nuts until coarsely chopped. Add amaranth flour, almond flour, tapioca starch, sugar, baking powder, xanthan gum and salt; pulse 3 or 4 times to combine. Add butter and chocolate chips; pulse for 5 to 10 seconds or until mixture resembles coarse crumbs about the size of small peas. Add milk all at once and process until dough begins to hold together.

Traditional Method

1. Coarsely chop nuts and set aside. In a large bowl, combine amaranth flour, almond flour, tapioca starch, sugar, baking powder, xanthan gum and salt. Using a pastry blender or two knives, cut in butter until mixture resembles coarse crumbs about the size of small peas. Stir in nuts and chocolate chips. Add milk all at once, stirring with a fork to make a thick dough.

For Both Methods

2. Drop dough by spoonfuls onto prepared baking sheet. Bake in top third of preheated oven for 10 minutes or until tops are golden. Serve immediately.

Hazelnut Scones

*Enjoy these nutty,
crunchy scones hot
from the oven — they
are truly addictive!*

- Preheat oven to 350°F (180°C)
- 9-inch (23 cm) round baking pan, lightly greased and lined with parchment paper

1	egg	1
½ cup	buttermilk	125 mL
1 tsp	vanilla extract	5 mL
1 cup	hazelnuts, toasted	250 mL
¾ cup	amaranth flour	175 mL
½ cup	hazelnut flour	125 mL
¼ cup	tapioca starch	50 mL
¼ cup	white (granulated) sugar	50 mL
1 tbsp	GF baking powder	15 mL
1 tsp	baking soda	5 mL
1½ tsp	xanthan gum	7 mL
¼ tsp	salt	1 mL
¼ cup	cold butter, cut into 1-inch (2.5 cm) cubes	50 mL

Food Processor Method

1. In a small bowl, whisk together egg, buttermilk and vanilla. Set aside.

2. In a food processor, pulse nuts until coarsely chopped. Add amaranth flour, hazelnut flour, tapioca starch, sugar, baking powder, baking soda, xanthan gum and salt; pulse 3 or 4 times to combine. Add butter and pulse for 3 to 5 seconds or until mixture resembles coarse crumbs about the size of small peas. Add egg mixture all at once and process until dough holds together.

Traditional Method

1. In a small bowl, whisk together egg, buttermilk and vanilla. Set aside.

2. Coarsely chop nuts. In a large bowl, combine amaranth flour, hazelnut flour, tapioca starch, sugar, baking powder, baking soda, xanthan gum, salt and nuts. Using a pastry blender or two knives, cut in butter until mixture resembles coarse crumbs about the size of small peas. Add egg mixture all at once, stirring with a fork to make a thick dough.

Nutritional value per serving	
Calories	193
Fat, total	13 g
Fat, saturated	3 g
Cholesterol	26 mg
Sodium	210 mg
Carbohydrate	15 g
Fiber	2 g
Protein	4 g
Calcium	98 mg
Iron	3 mg

Tips

See the Techniques Glossary, page 398, for information on toasting nuts. Don't skip this step, as the added flavor makes a big difference.

For information on making your own hazelnut flour, see the Techniques Glossary, page 397.

For Both Methods

3. Spoon dough into prepared pan, leaving the top rough. Bake in preheated oven for 24 to 28 minutes or until top is deep golden. Cut into wedges and serve immediately.

Variation

To turn this into a dessert scone, increase the white sugar to $\frac{1}{3}$ cup (75 mL) and add 2 tbsp (25 mL) grated orange zest.

Greek Pesto Scones

**Makes 12 wedges
(1 per serving)**

*Here's a savory biscuit
to serve alongside
soup, stew or salad.*

- Preheat oven to 350°F (180°C)
- 9-inch (23 cm) round baking pan, lightly greased and lined with parchment paper

1	egg	1
¾ cup	plain yogurt	175 mL
¼ cup	Greek Pesto (page 73)	50 mL
¾ cup	sorghum flour	175 mL
½ cup	teff flour	125 mL
¼ cup	tapioca starch	50 mL
1 tbsp	white (granulated) sugar	15 mL
1 tbsp	GF baking powder	15 mL
1 tsp	baking soda	5 mL
1½ tsp	xanthan gum	7 mL
¼ tsp	salt	1 mL
¼ cup	cold butter, cut into 1-inch (2.5 cm) cubes	50 mL
½ cup	cubed feta cheese (1-inch/2.5 cm cubes)	125 mL

Food Processor Method

1. In a small bowl, whisk together egg, yogurt and pesto. Set aside.

2. In a food processor, pulse sorghum flour, teff flour, tapioca starch, sugar, baking powder, baking soda, xanthan gum and salt 3 or 4 times to combine. Add butter and pulse for 3 to 5 seconds or until mixture resembles coarse crumbs about the size of small peas. Add egg mixture and feta all at once; process until dough holds together.

Traditional Method

1. In a small bowl, whisk together egg, yogurt and pesto. Set aside.

2. In a large bowl, combine sorghum flour, teff flour, tapioca starch, sugar, baking powder, baking soda, xanthan gum and salt. Using a pastry blender or two knives, cut in butter until mixture resembles coarse crumbs about the size of small peas. Add egg mixture and feta all at once, stirring with a fork to make a thick dough.

**Nutritional value
per serving**

Calories	135
Fat, total	7 g
Fat, saturated	4 g
Cholesterol	33 mg
Sodium	290 mg
Carbohydrate	16 g
Fiber	2 g
Protein	4 g
Calcium	134 mg
Iron	1 mg

Tip

The pesto darkens on the top and edges during storage in the refrigerator. Stir before using.

For Both Methods

3. Spoon dough into prepared pan, leaving the top rough. Bake in preheated oven for 24 to 26 minutes or until top is deep golden. Cut into wedges and serve immediately.

Variations

Add $\frac{1}{2}$ cup (125 mL) sliced kalamata olives with the feta.

Use any commercial GF pesto in place of the Greek.

Scottish Oatmeal Scones

**Makes 8 wedges
(1 per serving)**

Served hot from the oven and drizzled with honey, these scones add the perfect homemade touch to any meal.

Tip

To enjoy these scones warm the next day, split them in half and warm them in a toaster oven.

- Preheat oven to 375°F (190°C)
- 8-inch (20 cm) round baking pan, lightly greased

1	egg	1
¾ cup	buttermilk	175 mL
1 cup	brown rice flour	250 mL
⅔ cup	GF oats	150 mL
½ cup	GF oat flour	125 mL
¼ cup	tapioca starch	50 mL
1½ tsp	GF baking powder	7 mL
1½ tsp	xanthan gum	7 mL
½ tsp	salt	2 mL
⅓ cup	cold butter, cut into 1-inch (2.5 cm) cubes	75 mL

Food Processor Method

1. In a small bowl, whisk together egg and buttermilk. Set aside.

2. In a food processor, pulse brown rice flour, oats, oat flour, tapioca starch, baking powder, xanthan gum and salt 3 or 4 times to combine. Add butter and pulse for 3 to 5 seconds or until mixture resembles coarse crumbs about the size of small peas. Add egg mixture all at once and process, stopping to scrape the bottom and sides once or twice, until dough begins to hold together.

Traditional Method

1. In a small bowl, whisk together egg and buttermilk. Set aside.

2. In a large bowl, combine brown rice flour, oats, oat flour, tapioca starch, baking powder, xanthan gum and salt. Using a pastry blender or two knives, cut in butter until mixture resembles coarse crumbs about the size of small peas. Add egg mixture all at once, stirring with a fork to make a thick dough.

For Both Methods

3. Press dough into prepared pan. With a sharp knife, lightly score the top into 8 wedges. Bake in preheated oven for 20 to 25 minutes or until a cake tester inserted in the center comes out clean. Let cool in pan on a rack for 5 minutes. Cut into wedges and serve hot.

Variation

For a heavier, more traditional oatmeal biscuit, omit the butter.

Nutritional value per serving	
Calories	233
Fat, total	10 g
Fat, saturated	5 g
Cholesterol	43 mg
Sodium	252 mg
Carbohydrate	31 g
Fiber	3 g
Protein	5 g
Calcium	85 mg
Iron	2 mg

Make-Your-Own Muffin Mix

Makes about 3¾ cups (925 mL) mix, enough for 3 batches of 6 muffins

We continually receive special requests for a soy-free muffin mix that will make just a half-dozen muffins. This recipe answers those requests.

Tips

Stir the mix before spooning very lightly into the dry measures. Do not pack.

Be sure to divide the mix into three equal portions. Depending on how much air you incorporate into the mix and the texture of the individual gluten-free flours, the total volume of the mix can vary. The portions will be about 1¼ cups (300 mL) each.

1¼ cups	sorghum flour	300 mL
⅔ cup	amaranth flour	150 mL
⅔ cup	brown rice flour	150 mL
¼ cup	quinoa flour	50 mL
2 tbsp	potato starch	25 mL
2 tbsp	tapioca starch	25 mL
⅓ cup	white (granulated) sugar	75 mL
1 tbsp	GF baking powder	15 mL
1½ tsp	baking soda	7 mL
¾ tsp	xanthan gum	4 mL
¾ tsp	salt	4 mL

1. In a large bowl, combine sorghum flour, amaranth flour, brown rice flour, quinoa flour, potato starch, tapioca starch, sugar, baking powder, baking soda, xanthan gum and salt. Mix well.

2. Divide into three equal portions of about 1¼ cups (300 mL) each. Seal tightly in plastic bags, removing as much air as possible. Store at room temperature for up to 3 days or in the freezer for up to 3 months. Let warm to room temperature and mix well before using.

Nutritional value per serving

Calories	99
Fat, total	1 g
Fat, saturated	0 g
Cholesterol	0 mg
Sodium	204 mg
Carbohydrate	21 g
Fiber	2 g
Protein	2 g
Calcium	47 mg
Iron	2 mg

Apricot Prune Muffins

**Makes 6 muffins
(1 per serving)**

Looking for a delicious way to add fiber to your diet? Here it is.

Tips

Instead of chopping with a knife, snip dried apricots and prunes with kitchen shears. Dip the blades in hot water when they become sticky.

To make a dozen muffins, double all ingredients.

- 6-cup muffin tin, lightly greased

1	egg	1
$\frac{2}{3}$ cup	freshly squeezed orange juice	150 mL
2 tbsp	vegetable oil	25 mL
1$\frac{1}{4}$ cups	Make-Your-Own Muffin Mix (page 249)	300 mL
$\frac{1}{4}$ tsp	ground allspice	1 mL
$\frac{1}{2}$ cup	snipped dried apricots	125 mL
$\frac{1}{2}$ cup	snipped pitted prunes	125 mL

1. In a bowl, using an electric mixer, beat egg, orange juice and oil until combined. Add muffin mix and allspice; mix until just combined. Stir in apricots and prunes.

2. Spoon batter evenly into prepared muffin cups. Let stand for 30 minutes. Meanwhile, preheat oven to 350°F (180°C).

3. Bake for 18 to 20 minutes or until firm to the touch. Remove from pan immediately and let cool completely on a rack.

Variations

Try using snipped dates instead of the prunes.

Substitute ground ginger for the ground allspice.

Nutritional value per serving

Calories	233
Fat, total	6 g
Fat, saturated	1 g
Cholesterol	31 mg
Sodium	215 mg
Carbohydrate	42 g
Fiber	3 g
Protein	4 g
Calcium	69 mg
Iron	3 mg

Blueberry Blast Muffins

**Makes 6 muffins
(1 per serving)**

*This blueberry-studded
muffin is sure to
please even the most
discriminating palates.*

Tips

We defrosted small frozen
blueberries in a single
layer on a microwave-safe
plate in the microwave for
45 seconds on High. For
large blueberries, double
the microwave time and
check for partially thawed.

To make a dozen muffins,
double all ingredients.

For a more pronounced
banana flavor, serve warm
from the oven.

- **6-cup muffin tin, lightly greased**

1	egg	1
1 cup	mashed bananas	250 mL
2 tbsp	vegetable oil	25 mL
1 tbsp	freshly squeezed lemon juice	15 mL
1¼ cups	Make-Your-Own Muffin Mix (page 249)	300 mL
⅓ cup	GF oats	75 mL
2 tbsp	GF oat bran	25 mL
¾ cup	fresh or partially thawed frozen blueberries	175 mL

1. In a bowl, using an electric mixer, beat egg, bananas, oil and lemon juice until combined. Add muffin mix, oats and oat bran; mix until just combined. Stir in blueberries.

2. Spoon batter evenly into prepared muffin cups. Let stand for 30 minutes. Meanwhile, preheat oven to 350°F (180°C).

3. Bake for 20 to 23 minutes or until firm to the touch. Remove from pan immediately and let cool completely on a rack.

Variations

Substitute rice bran for the GF oat bran.
Substitute chopped plums for the blueberries.

Nutritional value per serving

Calories	228
Fat, total	7 g
Fat, saturated	1 g
Cholesterol	31 mg
Sodium	214 mg
Carbohydrate	38 g
Fiber	4 g
Protein	5 g
Calcium	59 mg
Iron	3 mg

Blueberry Peach Muffins

**Makes 6 muffins
(1 per serving)**

As pleasing to the eye as they are to the palate, these attractive muffins make a sweet treat to serve in summer, at the height of peach and blueberry season.

Tips

We defrosted small frozen blueberries in a single layer on a microwave-safe plate in the microwave for 45 seconds on High. For large blueberries, double the microwave time and check for partially thawed.

To make a dozen muffins, double all ingredients.

- Preheat oven to 350°F (180°C)
- 6-cup muffin tin, lightly greased

1	egg	1
2/3 cup	plain yogurt	150 mL
2 tbsp	vegetable oil	25 mL
1 tbsp	freshly squeezed lemon juice	15 mL
1¼ cups	Make-Your-Own Muffin Mix (page 249)	300 mL
½ tsp	ground cardamom	2 mL
½ cup	chopped peaches	125 mL
¼ cup	fresh or partially thawed frozen blueberries	50 mL

1. In a bowl, using an electric mixer, beat egg, yogurt, oil and lemon juice until combined. Add muffin mix and cardamom; mix until just combined. Stir in peaches and blueberries.

2. Spoon batter evenly into prepared muffin cups. Bake for 20 to 23 minutes or until firm to the touch. Remove from pan immediately and let cool completely on a rack.

Variations

For a milder spice flavor, use ground mace or nutmeg instead of the cardamom.

Substitute chopped plums for the blueberries.

Nutritional value per serving	
Calories	183
Fat, total	7 g
Fat, saturated	1 g
Cholesterol	33 mg
Sodium	233 mg
Carbohydrate	27 g
Fiber	2 g
Protein	5 g
Calcium	103 mg
Iron	2 mg

Cranberry Hazelnut Muffins

**Makes 6 muffins
(1 per serving)**

The colors in this recipe are perfect for the holidays, but the muffins are so good, you may want to serve them all year round.

Tips

Use your favorite type of marmalade — lemon, orange or three-fruit.

Purchase fresh cranberries when they're in season and freeze them in their original package for later use.

We defrosted the frozen cranberries in a single layer on a microwave-safe plate in the microwave for 1 minute on High.

To make a dozen muffins, double all ingredients.

- **6-cup muffin tin, lightly greased**

1	egg	1
1/3 cup	milk	75 mL
1/4 cup	marmalade (see tip, at left)	50 mL
2 tbsp	vegetable oil	25 mL
1 1/4 cups	Make-Your-Own Muffin Mix (page 249)	300 mL
1/2 tsp	ground cardamom	2 mL
1/4 cup	chopped hazelnuts	50 mL
3/4 cup	fresh or partially thawed frozen cranberries	175 mL

1. In a bowl, using an electric mixer, beat egg, milk, marmalade and oil until combined. Add muffin mix and cardamom; mix until just combined. Stir in nuts and cranberries.

2. Spoon batter evenly into prepared muffin cups. Let stand for 30 minutes. Meanwhile, preheat oven to 350°F (180°C).

3. Bake for 20 to 23 minutes or until firm to the touch. Remove from pan immediately and let cool completely on a rack.

Nutritional value per serving	
Calories	226
Fat, total	9 g
Fat, saturated	1 g
Cholesterol	32 mg
Sodium	228 mg
Carbohydrate	33 g
Fiber	3 g
Protein	4 g
Calcium	79 mg
Iron	2 mg

Date Orange Muffins

**Makes 6 muffins
(1 per serving)**

As attractive as they are healthy, these golden, date-studded muffins are unbelievably moist and flavorful.

Tips

Instead of chopping with a knife, snip dates with kitchen shears. Dip the blades in hot water when they become sticky.

Be sure to use freshly squeezed orange juice. The flavor makes all the difference.

To make a dozen muffins, double all ingredients.

● **6-cup muffin tin, lightly greased**

⅔ cup	coarsely snipped dates	150 mL
⅓ cup	boiling water	75 mL
1	egg	1
1 tbsp	grated orange zest	15 mL
¼ cup	freshly squeezed orange juice	50 mL
2 tbsp	vegetable oil	25 mL
1¼ cups	Make-Your-Own Muffin Mix (page 249)	300 mL

1. In a small bowl, combine dates and water. Let cool to room temperature.

2. In a bowl, using an electric mixer, beat egg, orange juice and oil until combined. Stir in date mixture. Add muffin mix and orange zest; mix until just combined.

3. Spoon batter evenly into prepared muffin cups. Let stand for 30 minutes. Meanwhile, preheat oven to 350°F (180°C).

4. Bake for 18 to 20 minutes or until firm to the touch. Remove from pan immediately and let cool completely on a rack.

Variation

Substitute lemon zest for the orange zest and 2 tbsp (25 mL) each freshly squeezed lemon juice and water for the orange juice.

Nutritional value per serving	
Calories	210
Fat, total	6 g
Fat, saturated	1 g
Cholesterol	16 mg
Sodium	214 mg
Carbohydrate	37 g
Fiber	3 g
Protein	4 g
Calcium	60 mg
Iron	2 mg

Yogurt Plum Muffins

With moist, tender plums popping to the surface, these muffins would have Little Jack Horner warming up his thumb.

Tips

For attractive contrast in color and flavor, use both yellow and dark plums.

Two large plums yield 1 cup (250 mL) chopped. No need to peel the plums.

To make a dozen muffins, double all ingredients.

- 6-cup muffin tin, lightly greased

1	egg	1
⅔ cup	plain yogurt	150 mL
2 tbsp	vegetable oil	25 mL
1¼ cups	Make-Your-Own Muffin Mix (page 249)	300 mL
1 tbsp	grated orange zest	15 mL
1 cup	diced fresh plums	250 mL

1. In a bowl, using an electric mixer, beat egg, yogurt and oil until combined. Add muffin mix and orange zest; mix until just combined. Stir in plums.

2. Spoon batter evenly into prepared muffin cups. Let stand for 30 minutes. Meanwhile, preheat oven to 350°F (180°C).

3. Bake for 20 to 23 minutes or until firm to the touch. Remove from pan immediately and let cool completely on a rack.

Variation

Try apricot- or peach-flavored yogurt (regular, low-fat or fat-free) instead of the plain.

Nutritional value per serving

Calories	187
Fat, total	7 g
Fat, saturated	1 g
Cholesterol	33 mg
Sodium	233 mg
Carbohydrate	28 g
Fiber	2 g
Protein	5 g
Calcium	103 mg
Iron	2 mg

Crunchy Peanut Butter Muffins

**Makes 12 muffins
(1 per serving)**

Follow one of these kid-pleasing muffins with a banana and a frosty glass of milk.

Tips

Don't substitute dry-roasted peanuts — they may contain gluten.

For information on toasting nuts, see the Techniques Glossary, page 398.

We like to use low-fat soy flour for baking.

Nutritional value per serving	
Calories	181
Fat, total	11 g
Fat, saturated	2 g
Cholesterol	16 mg
Sodium	109 mg
Carbohydrate	15 g
Fiber	1 g
Protein	8 g
Calcium	89 mg
Iron	1 mg

• **12-cup muffin tin, lightly greased**

¾ cup	low-fat soy flour	175 mL
⅓ cup	whole bean flour	75 mL
¼ cup	tapioca starch	50 mL
1½ tsp	xanthan gum	7 mL
1 tbsp	GF baking powder	15 mL
½ tsp	salt	2 mL
1	egg	1
½ cup	GF crunchy peanut butter, at room temperature	125 mL
⅓ cup	packed brown sugar	75 mL
1 tbsp	vegetable oil	15 mL
1¼ cups	water	300 mL
1 tsp	cider vinegar	5 mL
¾ cup	toasted coarsely chopped peanuts	175 mL

1. In a large bowl or plastic bag, combine soy flour, whole bean flour, tapioca starch, xanthan gum, baking powder and salt. Mix well and set aside.

2. In a separate bowl, using an electric mixer, beat egg, peanut butter, brown sugar and oil until combined. Add water and vinegar; mix until just combined. Add dry ingredients and peanuts; mix until just combined.

3. Spoon batter evenly into prepared muffin cups. Let stand for 30 minutes. Meanwhile, preheat oven to 350°F (180°C).

4. Bake for 18 to 20 minutes or until firm to the touch. Remove from pan immediately and let cool completely on a rack.

Variation
Substitute pea flour for the whole bean flour.

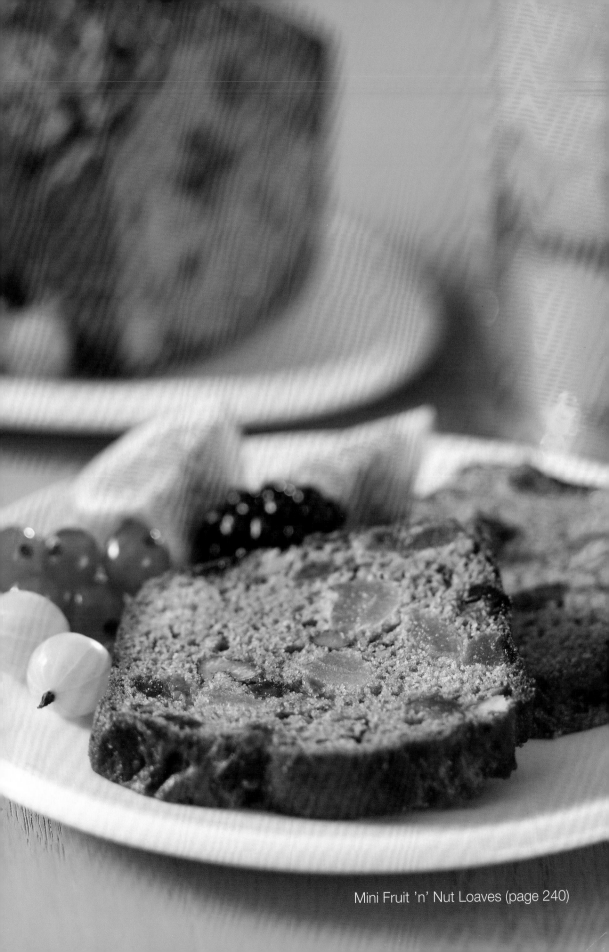

Mini Fruit 'n' Nut Loaves (page 240)

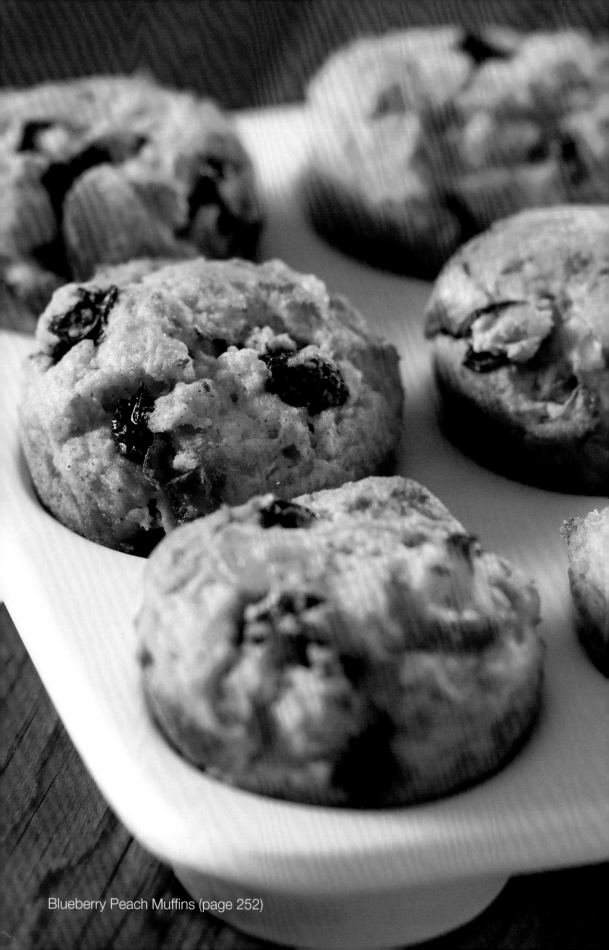

Blueberry Peach Muffins (page 252)

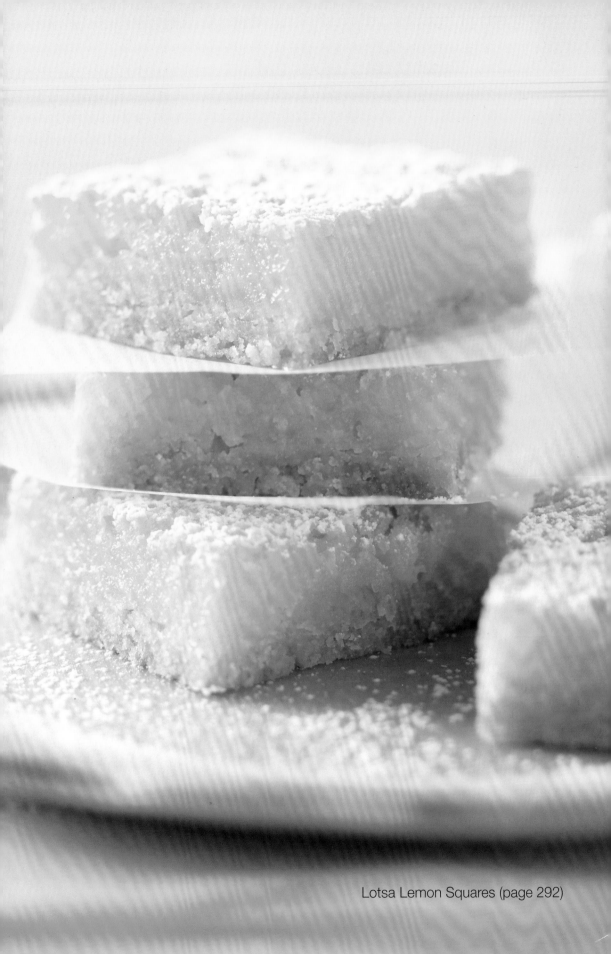

Lotsa Lemon Squares (page 292)

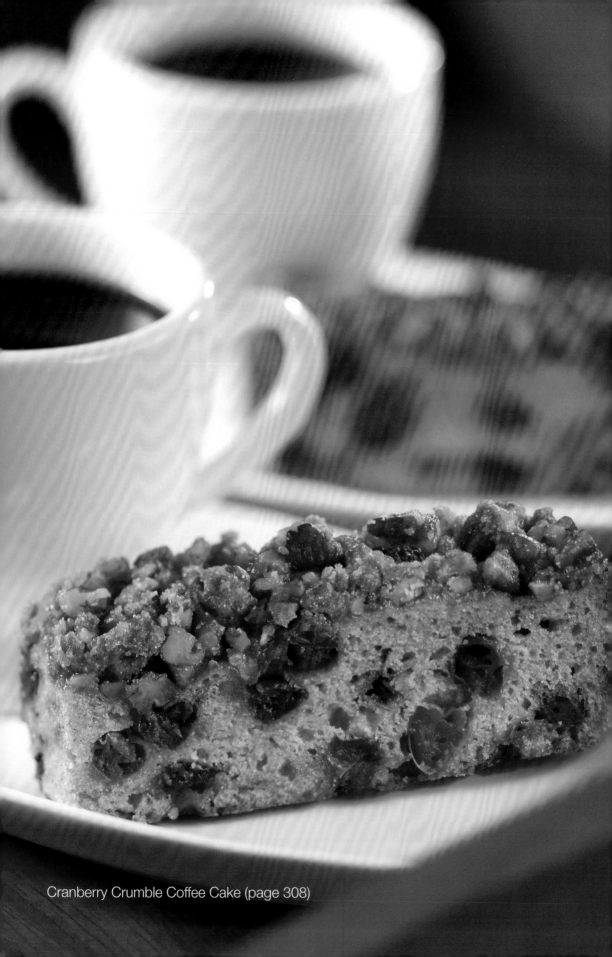

Cranberry Crumble Coffee Cake (page 308)

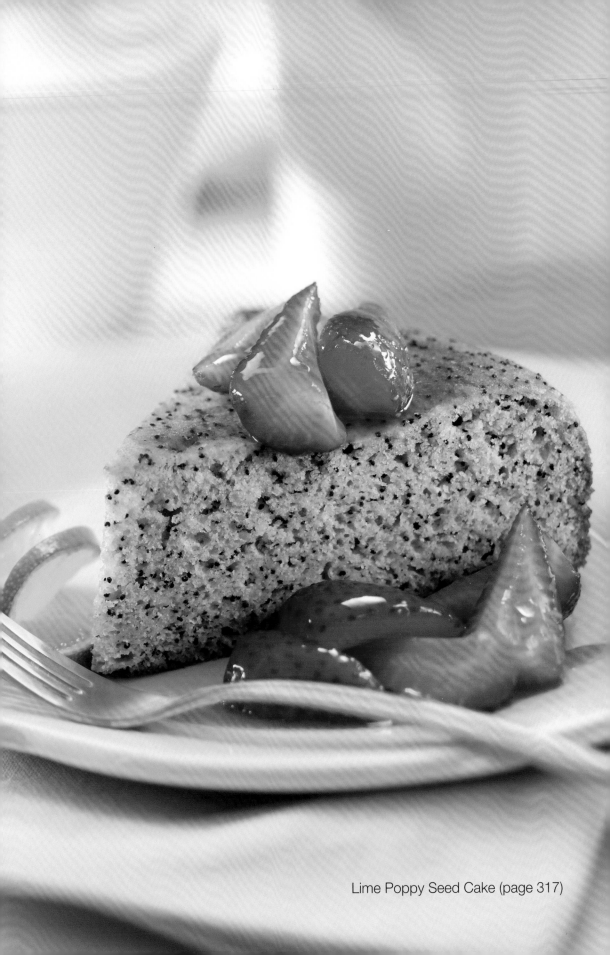

Lime Poppy Seed Cake (page 317)

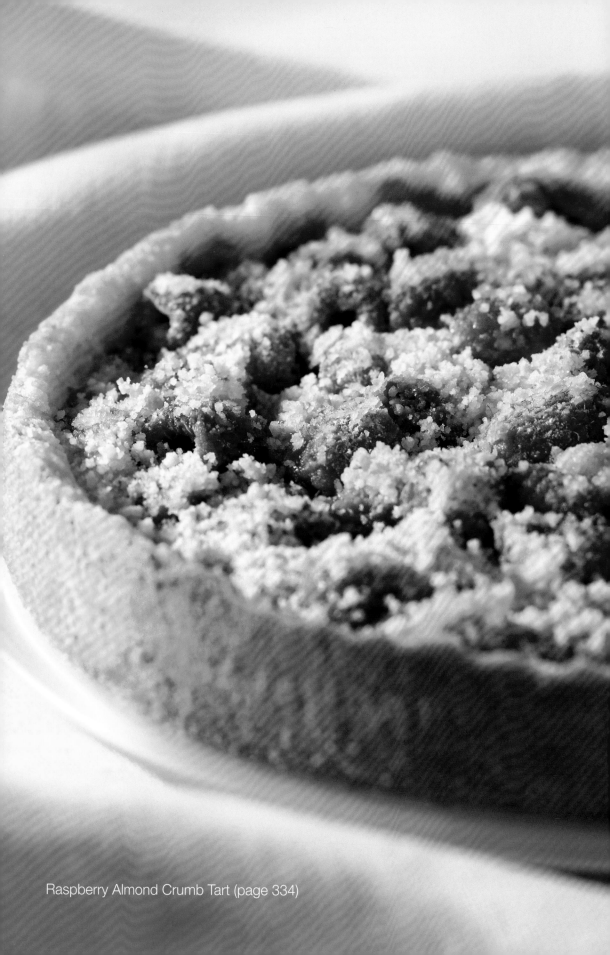

Raspberry Almond Crumb Tart (page 334)

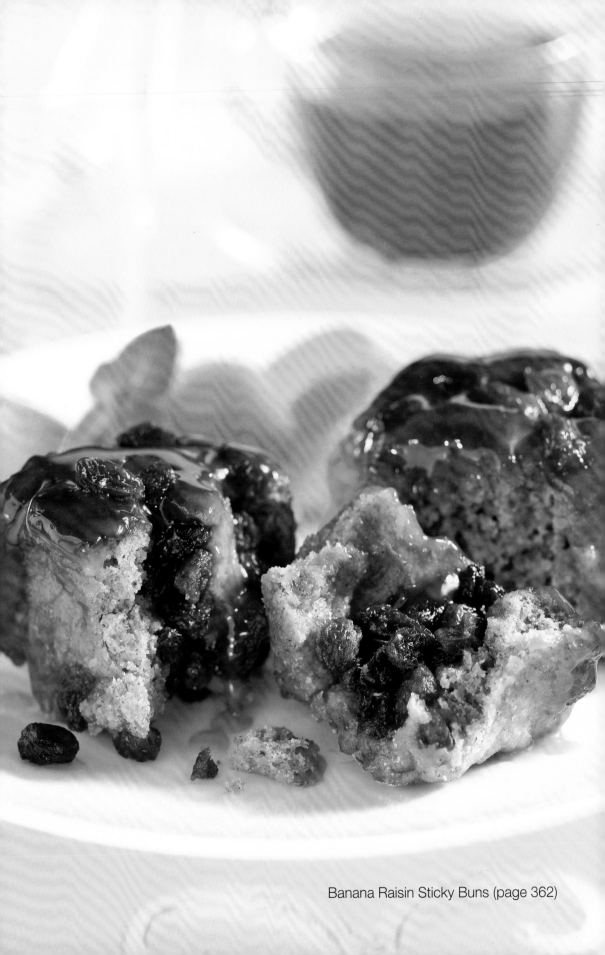

Banana Raisin Sticky Buns (page 362)

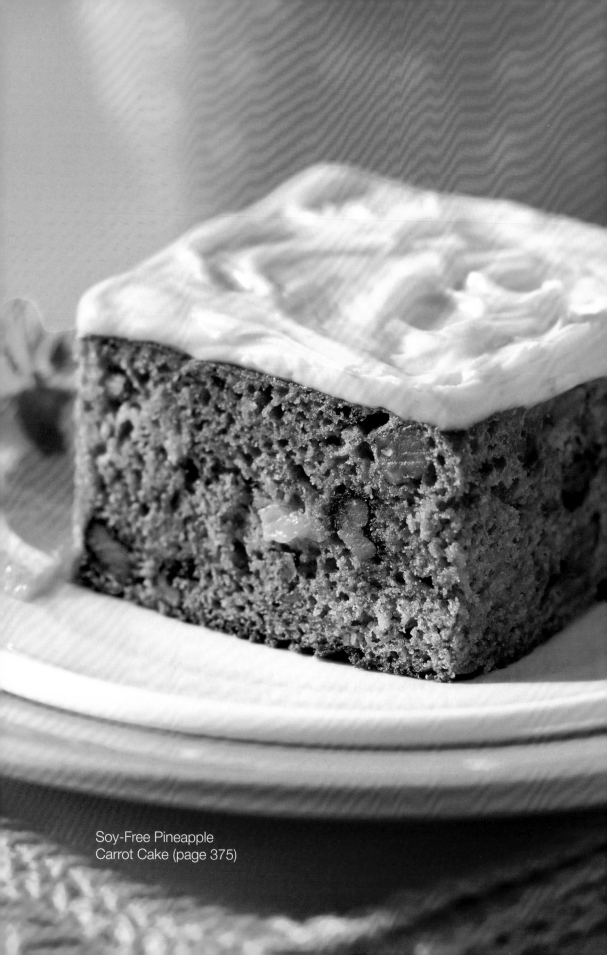

Soy-Free Pineapple
Carrot Cake (page 375)

Peanut Butter Banana Granola Muffins

**Makes 12 muffins
(1 per serving)**

*The answer to
breakfast on the go!*

Tips

If your version of
Heather's Granola is quite
sweet, decrease the brown
sugar to 2 tbsp (25 mL).

You can use a commercial
gluten-free granola instead
of the homemade one.

- 12-cup muffin tin, lightly greased

¾ cup	sorghum flour	175 mL
¼ cup	quinoa flour	50 mL
¼ cup	tapioca starch	50 mL
1½ tsp	xanthan gum	7 mL
1 tbsp	GF baking powder	15 mL
½ tsp	salt	2 mL
1 cup	Heather's Granola (page 50)	250 mL
1	egg	1
1¼ cups	mashed bananas	300 mL
⅓ cup	GF crunchy peanut butter, at room temperature	75 mL
¼ cup	packed brown sugar	50 mL
1 tbsp	vegetable oil	15 mL
1 tsp	cider vinegar	5 mL

1. In a large bowl or plastic bag, combine sorghum flour, quinoa flour, tapioca starch, xanthan gum, baking powder, salt and granola. Mix well and set aside.

2. In a separate bowl, using an electric mixer, beat egg, bananas, peanut butter, brown sugar, oil and vinegar until combined. Add dry ingredients and mix until just combined.

3. Spoon batter evenly into prepared muffin cups. Let stand for 30 minutes. Meanwhile, preheat oven to 350°F (180°C).

4. Bake for 18 to 20 minutes or until firm to the touch. Remove from pan immediately and let cool completely on a rack.

Nutritional value per serving

Calories	193
Fat, total	8 g
Fat, saturated	1 g
Cholesterol	16 mg
Sodium	108 mg
Carbohydrate	29 g
Fiber	3 g
Protein	5 g
Calcium	80 mg
Iron	2 mg

Oatmeal Raisin Muffins

Makes 12 muffins (1 per serving)

The hearty goodness of high-fiber oatmeal and the sweet moistness of raisins make this an ideal breakfast muffin.

Tips

If you can't tolerate GF oats, substitute amaranth, buckwheat or quinoa flakes.

Use an ice cream scoop to portion an even amount of batter into each muffin cup.

• **12-cup muffin tin, lightly greased**

1¼ cups	sorghum flour	300 mL
¼ cup	brown rice flour	50 mL
¾ cup	GF oats	175 mL
¼ cup	tapioca starch	50 mL
⅓ cup	packed brown sugar	75 mL
1½ tsp	xanthan gum	7 mL
1 tbsp	GF baking powder	15 mL
1 tsp	salt	5 mL
1 tsp	ground cinnamon	5 mL
2	eggs	2
1 cup	milk	250 mL
⅓ cup	vegetable oil	75 mL
2 tsp	freshly squeezed lemon juice	10 mL
1¼ cups	raisins	300 mL

1. In a large bowl or plastic bag, combine sorghum flour, brown rice flour, oats, tapioca starch, brown sugar, xanthan gum, baking powder, salt and cinnamon. Mix well and set aside.

2. In a separate bowl, using an electric mixer, beat eggs, milk, oil and lemon juice until combined. Add dry ingredients and mix until just combined. Stir in raisins.

3. Spoon batter evenly into prepared muffin cups. Let stand for 30 minutes. Meanwhile, preheat oven to 350°F (180°C).

4. Bake for 22 to 25 minutes or until firm to the touch. Remove from pan immediately and let cool completely on a rack.

Variations

Substitute snipped dates or figs or dried cranberries for half or all of the raisins.

To make mini loaves, spoon batter into 2 lightly greased 5¾- by 3¼-inch (14 by 8 cm) loaf pans. Let stand for 30 minutes. Meanwhile, preheat oven to 350°F (180°C). Bake for 40 to 50 minutes or until a cake tester inserted in the center comes out clean. Let cool in pan on a rack for 10 minutes. Remove from pan and let cool completely on rack.

Nutritional value per serving	
Calories	248
Fat, total	8 g
Fat, saturated	1 g
Cholesterol	32 mg
Sodium	219 mg
Carbohydrate	41 g
Fiber	3 g
Protein	5 g
Calcium	108 mg
Iron	3 mg

Sunrise Muffins

**Makes 12 muffins
(1 per serving)**

You don't have to see the sunrise to enjoy these sweet, moist, golden muffins. Pack them in your lunch for a mid-morning snack.

Tips

If muffins stick to the pan, let stand for 2 to 3 minutes, then try again to remove them.

As soon as muffins cool to room temperature, wrap individually in plastic wrap or a small freezer bag and freeze for up to 1 month for a grab-and-go breakfast or lunch.

Nutritional value per serving

Calories	191
Fat, total	3 g
Fat, saturated	0 g
Cholesterol	16 mg
Sodium	163 mg
Carbohydrate	38 g
Fiber	2 g
Protein	3 g
Calcium	85 mg
Iron	3 mg

- 12-cup muffin tin, lightly greased

¾ cup	amaranth flour	175 mL
¾ cup	sorghum flour	175 mL
⅓ cup	millet seeds	75 mL
⅓ cup	tapioca starch	75 mL
½ cup	packed brown sugar	125 mL
1 tbsp	GF baking powder	15 mL
½ tsp	baking soda	2 mL
1½ tsp	xanthan gum	7 mL
½ tsp	salt	2 mL
1	egg	1
1¼ cups	canned crushed pineapple, including juice	300 mL
1 tbsp	grated lemon zest	15 mL
2 tbsp	vegetable oil	25 mL
½ cup	raisins	125 mL
½ cup	snipped dried apricots	125 mL

1. In a large bowl or plastic bag, combine amaranth flour, sorghum flour, millet seeds, tapioca starch, brown sugar, baking powder, baking soda, xanthan gum and salt. Mix well and set aside.

2. In a separate bowl, using an electric mixer, beat egg, pineapple, lemon zest and oil until combined. Add dry ingredients and mix just until combined. Stir in raisins and apricots.

3. Spoon batter evenly into prepared muffin cups. (The cups will be fuller than in most other muffin recipes.) Let stand for 30 minutes. Meanwhile, preheat oven to 350°F (180°C).

4. Bake for 20 to 23 minutes or until firm to the touch. Remove from pan immediately and let cool completely on a rack.

Variations

Substitute dried papaya, mango or pear for the apricots.

To make a loaf, spoon batter into a lightly greased 9- by 5-inch (23 by 12.5 cm) loaf pan. Let stand for 30 minutes. Meanwhile, preheat oven to 350°F (180°C). Bake for 55 to 65 minutes or until a cake tester inserted in the center comes out clean. Let cool in pan on a rack for 10 minutes. Remove from pan and let cool completely on rack.

Lemon Blueberry Almond Muffins

**Makes 12 muffins
(1 per serving)**

As the name promises, these muffins deliver an extra-refreshing burst of lemon in every bite.

Tips

Keep a lemon in the freezer. Zest while frozen, then juice after warming in the microwave.

For information on toasting nuts, see the Techniques Glossary, page 398.

Gently fold in the blueberries, rather than vigorously stirring them in; otherwise, you'll end up with blue muffins.

Nutritional value per serving

Calories	208
Fat, total	9 g
Fat, saturated	1 g
Cholesterol	32 mg
Sodium	169 mg
Carbohydrate	28 g
Fiber	3 g
Protein	6 g
Calcium	115 mg
Iron	3 mg

- 12-cup muffin tin, lightly greased

¾ cup	amaranth flour	175 mL
¾ cup	sorghum flour	175 mL
½ cup	almond flour	125 mL
⅓ cup	tapioca starch	75 mL
1½ tsp	xanthan gum	7 mL
1 tbsp	GF baking powder	15 mL
½ tsp	baking soda	2 mL
½ tsp	salt	2 mL
¾ cup	toasted slivered almonds	175 mL
2	eggs	2
½ cup	milk	125 mL
⅓ cup	liquid honey	75 mL
2 tbsp	grated lemon zest	25 mL
⅓ cup	freshly squeezed lemon juice	75 mL
2 tbsp	vegetable oil	25 mL
½ tsp	almond extract	2 mL
1 cup	fresh or partially thawed frozen blueberries	250 mL

1. In a large bowl or plastic bag, combine amaranth flour, sorghum flour, almond flour, tapioca starch, xanthan gum, baking powder, baking soda, salt and almonds. Mix well and set aside.

2. In a separate bowl, using an electric mixer, beat eggs, milk, honey, lemon zest, lemon juice, oil and almond extract until combined. Add dry ingredients and mix until just combined. Carefully fold in blueberries.

3. Spoon batter evenly into prepared muffin cups. Let stand for 30 minutes. Meanwhile, preheat oven to 350°F (180°C).

4. Bake for 18 to 20 minutes or until firm to the touch. Remove from pan immediately and let cool completely on a rack.

Variation

Substitute cranberries for the blueberries and chopped walnuts or pecans for the almonds.

Blueberry Lemon Pea Fiber Muffins

**Makes 12 muffins
(1 per serving)**

This tasty high-fiber muffin has the added benefit of antioxidants!

Tips

Pea fiber, when wet, has a pungent aroma that disappears during baking. For more information about pea fiber, see page 31.

Gently folding in blueberries reduces the amount of blue color in the batter.

- 12-cup muffin tin, lightly greased

1 cup	pea fiber	250 mL
1/2 cup	brown rice flour	125 mL
1/4 cup	tapioca starch	50 mL
3/4 cup	white (granulated) sugar	175 mL
1 1/2 tsp	xanthan gum	7 mL
1 tbsp	GF baking powder	15 mL
1 tsp	baking soda	5 mL
1/2 tsp	salt	2 mL
1	egg	1
1 1/2 cups	milk	375 mL
1/2 cup	vegetable oil	125 mL
2 tbsp	grated lemon zest	25 mL
1/4 cup	freshly squeezed lemon juice	50 mL
1 cup	fresh or partially thawed frozen blueberries	250 mL

1. In a large bowl or plastic bag, combine pea fiber, brown rice flour, tapioca starch, sugar, xanthan gum, baking powder, baking soda and salt. Mix well and set aside.

2. In a separate bowl, using an electric mixer, beat egg, milk, oil, lemon zest and lemon juice until combined. Add dry ingredients and mix until just combined. Carefully fold in blueberries.

3. Spoon batter evenly into prepared muffin cups. Let stand for 30 minutes. Meanwhile, preheat oven to 350°F (180°C).

4. Bake for 18 to 20 minutes or until firm to the touch. Remove from pan immediately and let cool completely on a rack.

Variation
Substitute any pea or bean flour for the pea fiber.

Nutritional value per serving

Calories	225
Fat, total	10 g
Fat, saturated	1 g
Cholesterol	17 mg
Sodium	226 mg
Carbohydrate	30 g
Fiber	2 g
Protein	5 g
Calcium	102 mg
Iron	1 mg

Blueberry Poppy Muffins

**Makes 12 muffins
(1 per serving)**

*Our friend Patti loves
this combination. You
will too.*

Tips

For information on
toasting nuts, see the
Techniques Glossary,
page 398.

If using partially thawed
frozen blueberries, gently
pat dry with paper towels.

- **12-cup muffin tin, lightly greased**

¾ cup	amaranth flour	175 mL
½ cup	sorghum flour	125 mL
⅓ cup	almond flour	75 mL
¼ cup	tapioca starch	50 mL
½ cup	packed brown sugar	125 mL
1½ tsp	xanthan gum	7 mL
1 tbsp	GF baking powder	15 mL
½ tsp	baking soda	2 mL
½ tsp	salt	2 mL
¼ cup	poppy seeds	50 mL
1 cup	toasted slivered almonds	250 mL
2	eggs	2
1¼ cups	GF sour cream	300 mL
1 tbsp	grated lemon zest	15 mL
2 tbsp	freshly squeezed lemon juice	25 mL
2 tbsp	vegetable oil	25 mL
1 cup	fresh or partially thawed frozen blueberries	250 mL

1. In a large bowl or plastic bag, combine amaranth flour, sorghum flour, almond flour, tapioca starch, brown sugar, xanthan gum, baking powder, baking soda, salt, poppy seeds and almonds. Mix well and set aside.

2. In a separate bowl, using an electric mixer, beat eggs, sour cream, lemon zest, lemon juice and oil until combined. Add dry ingredients and mix until just combined. Carefully fold in blueberries.

3. Spoon batter evenly into prepared muffin cups. Let stand for 30 minutes. Meanwhile, preheat oven to 350°F (180°C).

4. Bake for 22 to 24 minutes or until firm to the touch. Remove from pan immediately and let cool completely on a rack.

Variations

Substitute plain yogurt for the sour cream.

Substitute fresh or partially thawed frozen cranberries for the blueberries.

Nutritional value per serving

Calories	258
Fat, total	14 g
Fat, saturated	4 g
Cholesterol	48 mg
Sodium	149 mg
Carbohydrate	30 g
Fiber	3 g
Protein	6 g
Calcium	168 mg
Iron	3 mg

Cranberry Flax Muffins

**Makes 12 muffins
(1 per serving)**

The freshness of the orange flavor and warmth of the golden flaxseed contrasts with the deep rich red of the dried cranberries in these muffins.

Tip

For information on cracking flaxseed, see the Techniques Glossary, page 396.

- 12-cup muffin tin, lightly greased

¾ cup	sorghum flour	175 mL
¼ cup	flax flour	50 mL
¼ cup	quinoa flour	50 mL
¼ cup	tapioca starch	50 mL
⅓ cup	packed brown sugar	75 mL
1½ tsp	xanthan gum	7 mL
1 tbsp	GF baking powder	15 mL
½ tsp	salt	2 mL
⅓ cup	golden flaxseed, cracked	75 mL
1	egg	1
2 tbsp	grated orange zest	25 mL
1 cup	freshly squeezed orange juice	250 mL
2 tbsp	vegetable oil	25 mL
¾ cup	dried cranberries	175 mL

1. In a large bowl or plastic bag, combine sorghum flour, flax flour, quinoa flour, tapioca starch, brown sugar, xanthan gum, baking powder, salt and flaxseed. Mix well and set aside.

2. In a separate bowl, using an electric mixer, beat egg, orange zest, orange juice and oil until combined. Add dry ingredients and mix until just combined. Stir in cranberries.

3. Spoon batter evenly into prepared muffin cups. Let stand for 30 minutes. Meanwhile, preheat oven to 350°F (180°C).

4. Bake for 22 to 25 minutes or until firm to the touch. Remove from pan immediately and let cool completely on a rack.

Variation
Substitute ground flaxseed for the flax flour and brown flaxseed for the golden.

Nutritional value per serving	
Calories	165
Fat, total	6 g
Fat, saturated	1 g
Cholesterol	16 mg
Sodium	109 mg
Carbohydrate	27 g
Fiber	4 g
Protein	3 g
Calcium	93 mg
Iron	1 mg

Orange Coconut Muffins

**Makes 12 muffins
(1 per serving)**

*We love these moist
muffins, along with
a piece of fruit, for
dessert.*

Tips

Use either flaked or
shredded coconut in this
recipe. If you can only
find sweetened coconut,
decrease the sugar by 1 or
2 tbsp (15 or 25 mL).

For this recipe, you'll be
filling the muffin cups
almost level with the top.

Freeze these easy-to-carry
muffins individually and
include one in your lunch.

- **12-cup muffin tin, lightly greased**

²⁄₃ cup	sorghum flour	150 mL
²⁄₃ cup	amaranth flour	150 mL
¹⁄₃ cup	tapioca starch	75 mL
¹⁄₂ cup	white (granulated) sugar	125 mL
1 tbsp	GF baking powder	15 mL
1 tsp	xanthan gum	5 mL
¹⁄₄ tsp	salt	1 mL
³⁄₄ cup	unsweetened coconut (see tip, at left)	175 mL
1	egg	1
1	egg white	1
¹⁄₄ cup	vegetable oil	50 mL
2 tbsp	grated orange zest	25 mL
1 cup	freshly squeezed orange juice	250 mL

1. In a large bowl or plastic bag, combine sorghum flour, amaranth flour, tapioca starch, sugar, baking powder, xanthan gum, salt and coconut. Mix well and set aside.

2. In a separate bowl, using an electric mixer, beat egg, egg white, oil, orange zest and orange juice until combined. Add dry ingredients and mix until just combined.

3. Spoon batter evenly into prepared muffin cups. Let stand for 30 minutes. Meanwhile, preheat oven to 350°F (180°C).

4. Bake for 20 to 25 minutes or until a tester inserted in the center of a muffin comes out clean. Let cool in pan on a rack for 5 minutes. Remove from pan and let cool completely on rack.

Variation

For an orange glaze, place muffins on a piece of parchment paper. In a small bowl, combine 1 cup (250 mL) sifted GF confectioner's (icing) sugar and 2 to 3 tbsp (25 to 45 mL) freshly squeezed orange juice to make a thin glaze. Dip cooled muffins in glaze.

Nutritional value per serving	
Calories	194
Fat, total	9 g
Fat, saturated	4 g
Cholesterol	16 mg
Sodium	62 mg
Carbohydrate	26 g
Fiber	2 g
Protein	3 g
Calcium	74 mg
Iron	2 mg

Banana Fig Muffins

**Makes 12 muffins
(1 per serving)**

*These look just like
bran muffins and are
delicious, warm from
the oven, with cream
cheese, honey or jam.*

Tip

You'll need about 7 oz
(210 g) dried figs for 1 cup
(250 mL) coarsely snipped.

• **12-cup muffin tin, lightly greased**

1 cup	sorghum flour	250 mL
¼ cup	quinoa flour	50 mL
⅓ cup	tapioca starch	75 mL
⅓ cup	packed brown sugar	75 mL
1½ tsp	xanthan gum	7 mL
1 tbsp	GF baking powder	15 mL
1 tsp	baking soda	5 mL
¼ tsp	salt	1 mL
½ tsp	ground cinnamon	2 mL
2	egg whites	2
1	egg	1
1¼ cups	mashed bananas	300 mL
¼ cup	vegetable oil	50 mL
1 tsp	cider vinegar	5 mL
1 cup	coarsely snipped dried figs	250 mL

1. In a large bowl or plastic bag, combine sorghum flour, quinoa flour, tapioca starch, brown sugar, xanthan gum, baking powder, baking soda, salt and cinnamon. Mix well and set aside.

2. In a separate bowl, using an electric mixer, beat egg whites, egg, bananas, oil and vinegar until combined. Add dry ingredients and mix until just combined. Stir in figs.

3. Spoon batter evenly into prepared muffin cups. Let stand for 30 minutes. Meanwhile, preheat oven to 350°F (180°C).

4. Bake for 18 to 20 minutes or until firm to the touch. Remove from pan immediately and let cool completely on a rack.

Variations

Substitute dates, raisins or apricots for the figs.
Substitute ground cardamom for the cinnamon.

Nutritional value per serving

Calories	200
Fat, total	6 g
Fat, saturated	1 g
Cholesterol	16 mg
Sodium	175 mg
Carbohydrate	37 g
Fiber	4 g
Protein	3 g
Calcium	93 mg
Iron	2 mg

Banana Chocolate Chip Muffins

These muffins cater to the child in all of us. All you need to accompany them is a tall glass of cold milk.

Tips

You'll need about 3 bananas for 1¼ cups (300 mL) mashed. Do not add extra.

You can use any size chocolate chips, from mini chips to chunks. We like to use half mini and half regular size.

• 12-cup muffin tin, lightly greased

1 cup	sorghum flour	250 mL
½ cup	amaranth flour	125 mL
¼ cup	tapioca starch	50 mL
1½ tsp	xanthan gum	7 mL
2 tsp	GF baking powder	10 mL
1 tsp	baking soda	5 mL
¼ tsp	salt	1 mL
2	eggs	2
1¼ cups	mashed bananas	300 mL
¼ cup	liquid honey	50 mL
3 tbsp	vegetable oil	45 mL
1 tsp	freshly squeezed lemon juice	5 mL
¾ cup	semisweet chocolate chips	175 mL

1. In a large bowl or plastic bag, combine sorghum flour, amaranth flour, tapioca starch, xanthan gum, baking powder, baking soda and salt. Mix well and set aside.

2. In a separate bowl, using an electric mixer, beat eggs, bananas, honey, oil and lemon juice until combined. Add dry ingredients and mix until just combined. Stir in chocolate chips.

3. Spoon batter evenly into prepared muffin cups. Let stand for 30 minutes. Meanwhile, preheat oven to 350°F (180°C).

4. Bake for 22 to 24 minutes or until firm to the touch. Remove from pan immediately and let cool completely on a rack.

Variations

Substitute coarsely chopped walnuts or pecans for half of the chocolate chips.

To make a loaf, spoon batter into a lightly greased 9- by 5-inch (23 by 12.5 cm) loaf pan. Let stand for 30 minutes. Meanwhile, preheat oven to 350°F (180°C). Bake for 55 to 65 minutes or until a cake tester inserted in the center comes out clean. Let cool in pan on a rack for 10 minutes. Remove from pan and let cool completely on rack.

Nutritional value per serving	
Calories	207
Fat, total	8 g
Fat, saturated	3 g
Cholesterol	34 mg
Sodium	173 mg
Carbohydrate	32 g
Fiber	2 g
Protein	4 g
Calcium	72 mg
Iron	2 mg

Carrot Yogurt Muffins

**Makes 12 muffins
(1 per serving)**

*Carrots give these
muffins a great color,
flavor and texture.
They are even moister
the next day.*

Tips

Shred the carrots just
before using; exposure to
air causes them to darken.

For information on
toasting nuts, see the
Techniques Glossary,
page 398.

• 12-cup muffin tin, lightly greased

1¼ cups	sorghum flour	300 mL
⅓ cup	brown rice flour	75 mL
¼ cup	tapioca starch	50 mL
1½ tsp	xanthan gum	7 mL
1 tbsp	GF baking powder	15 mL
½ tsp	baking soda	2 mL
½ tsp	salt	2 mL
¾ tsp	ground nutmeg	4 mL
1 cup	toasted chopped pecans	250 mL
1	egg	1
1½ cups	shredded carrots	375 mL
¾ cup	plain yogurt	175 mL
½ cup	liquid honey	125 mL
¼ cup	vegetable oil	50 mL

1. In a large bowl or plastic bag, combine sorghum flour, brown rice flour, tapioca starch, xanthan gum, baking powder, baking soda, salt, nutmeg and pecans. Mix well and set aside.

2. In a separate bowl, using an electric mixer, beat egg, carrots, yogurt, honey and oil until combined. Add dry ingredients and mix until just combined.

3. Spoon batter evenly into prepared muffin cups. Let stand for 30 minutes. Meanwhile, preheat oven to 350°F (180°C).

4. Bake for 18 to 20 minutes or until firm to the touch. Remove from pan immediately and let cool completely on a rack.

Variation
For a stronger flavor, increase the amount of nutmeg or substitute ground ginger.

Nutritional value per serving

Calories	251
Fat, total	13 g
Fat, saturated	1 g
Cholesterol	17 mg
Sodium	172 mg
Carbohydrate	33 g
Fiber	3 g
Protein	4 g
Calcium	101 mg
Iron	1 mg

Carrot Cranberry Muffins

**Makes 12 muffins
(1 per serving)**

*What a great way
to include fruit and
vegetables in your
kids' diet. Teff adds
a powerhouse of
nutrients, especially
iron and calcium.*

Tip
Shred the carrots just
before using; exposure to
air causes them to darken.

- 12-cup muffin tin, lightly greased

1⅓ cups	sorghum flour	325 mL
¼ cup	teff flour	50 mL
¼ cup	tapioca starch	50 mL
1½ tsp	xanthan gum	7 mL
1 tbsp	GF baking powder	15 mL
½ tsp	baking soda	2 mL
½ tsp	salt	2 mL
¾ tsp	ground allspice	4 mL
1 cup	dried cranberries	250 mL
2	eggs	2
1½ cups	shredded carrots	375 mL
2 tbsp	grated orange zest	25 mL
¾ cup	freshly squeezed orange juice	175 mL
⅓ cup	liquid honey	75 mL
¼ cup	vegetable oil	50 mL

1. In a large bowl or plastic bag, combine sorghum flour, teff flour, tapioca starch, xanthan gum, baking powder, baking soda, salt, allspice and cranberries. Mix well and set aside.

2. In a separate bowl, using an electric mixer, beat eggs, carrots, orange zest, orange juice, honey and oil until combined. Add dry ingredients and mix until just combined.

3. Spoon batter evenly into prepared muffin cups. Let stand for 30 minutes. Meanwhile, preheat oven to 350°F (180°C).

4. Bake for 18 to 20 minutes or until firm to the touch. Remove from pan immediately and let cool completely on a rack.

Variations
Add ½ cup (125 mL) raisins or chopped walnuts with the cranberries.

Substitute quinoa flour for the teff flour.

Nutritional value per serving

Calories	205
Fat, total	6 g
Fat, saturated	1 g
Cholesterol	31 mg
Sodium	167 mg
Carbohydrate	36 g
Fiber	3 g
Protein	4 g
Calcium	83 mg
Iron	1 mg

Pumpkin Millet Muffins

**Makes 12 muffins
(1 per serving)**

These colorful muffins, with the added crunch of millet seeds and pumpkin seeds, carry well for lunch or a snack in any season.

Tips

For instructions on toasting seeds, see the Techniques Glossary, page 399.

If you substitute pumpkin pie spice for the cinnamon, cloves and nutmeg, watch for hidden gluten.

Purchase unroasted, unsalted pumpkin seeds.

Nutritional value per serving

Calories	247
Fat, total	14 g
Fat, saturated	3 g
Cholesterol	38 mg
Sodium	237 mg
Carbohydrate	26 g
Fiber	2 g
Protein	9 g
Calcium	82 mg
Iron	3 mg

* **12-cup muffin tin, lightly greased**

¾ cup	sorghum flour	175 mL
¾ cup	whole bean flour	175 mL
¼ cup	tapioca starch	50 mL
1½ tsp	xanthan gum	7 mL
2 tsp	GF baking powder	10 mL
1 tsp	baking soda	5 mL
½ tsp	salt	2 mL
½ tsp	ground cinnamon	2 mL
¼ tsp	ground cloves	1 mL
¼ tsp	ground nutmeg	1 mL
½ cup	millet seeds	125 mL
¾ cup	green pumpkin seeds, toasted	175 mL
2	eggs	2
1 cup	pumpkin purée (not pie filling)	250 mL
½ cup	milk	125 mL
½ cup	GF sour cream	125 mL
⅓ cup	liquid honey	75 mL
¼ cup	vegetable oil	50 mL

1. In a large bowl or plastic bag, combine sorghum flour, whole bean flour, tapioca starch, xanthan gum, baking powder, baking soda, salt, cinnamon, cloves, nutmeg, millet seeds and pumpkin seeds. Mix well and set aside.

2. In a separate bowl, using an electric mixer, beat eggs, pumpkin purée, milk, sour cream, honey and oil until combined. Add dry ingredients and mix until just combined.

3. Spoon batter evenly into prepared muffin cups. Let stand for 30 minutes. Meanwhile, preheat oven to 350°F (180°C).

4. Bake for 18 to 20 minutes or until firm to the touch. Remove from pan immediately and let cool completely on a rack.

Variation
Substitute plain yogurt for the sour cream.

Spinach Feta Muffins

**Makes 12 muffins
(1 per serving)**

*Prefer a savory muffin
to a sweet one? This
tangy, colorful option
will complement any
soup or salad.*

- 12-cup muffin tin, lightly greased

1	package (10 oz/300 g) frozen spinach	1
1¼ cups	sorghum flour	300 mL
½ cup	quinoa flour	125 mL
⅓ cup	tapioca starch	75 mL
2 tbsp	packed brown sugar	25 mL
1½ tsp	xanthan gum	7 mL
1 tbsp	GF baking powder	15 mL
¼ tsp	salt	1 mL
2 tsp	dried oregano	10 mL
2	eggs	2
1 cup	water	250 mL
3 tbsp	vegetable oil	45 mL
1 tsp	cider vinegar	5 mL
1 cup	snipped dry-packed sun-dried tomatoes	250 mL
½ cup	cubed feta cheese	125 mL

1. In a microwave-safe bowl, defrost spinach on High for 1 minute. Break apart and defrost on High for 1 to 2 minutes or until thawed. Drain and squeeze out excess moisture. Coarsely chop and set aside.

2. In a large bowl or plastic bag, combine sorghum flour, quinoa flour, tapioca starch, brown sugar, xanthan gum, baking powder, salt and oregano. Mix well and set aside.

3. In a separate bowl, using an electric mixer, beat eggs, water, oil, vinegar and spinach until combined. Add dry ingredients and mix until just combined. Stir in sun-dried tomatoes and feta.

4. Spoon batter evenly into prepared muffin cups. Let stand for 30 minutes. Meanwhile, preheat oven to 350°F (180°C).

5. Bake for 22 to 25 minutes or until firm to the touch. Remove from pan immediately and serve warm.

Nutritional value per serving	
Calories	169
Fat, total	6 g
Fat, saturated	1 g
Cholesterol	37 mg
Sodium	243 mg
Carbohydrate	24 g
Fiber	3 g
Protein	6 g
Calcium	133 mg
Iron	2 mg

Tip

Oil-packed sun-dried tomatoes are not suited to this recipe. For the best results, look for soft, pliable dry-packed sun-dried tomatoes.

Variations

Substitute 1 cup (250 mL) cooked fresh spinach for the frozen.

Substitute cooked chopped kale for the spinach.

Vary the herb — try basil, marjoram or rosemary.

Extra Baking Tips for Loaves, Biscuits and Muffins

- The batters should be the same consistency as wheat flour batters, but you can mix them more without producing tough products, full of tunnels.
- Use a portion scoop to quickly divide the batter into muffin cups to ensure muffins are equal in size and bake in the same length of time.
- When baking one of the recipes that yields 6 muffins, if you don't have a 6-cup muffin tin, use a 12-cup tin and half-fill the empty cups with water before baking.
- Bake in muffin tins of a different size. Mini muffins take 12 to 15 minutes to bake, while jumbo muffins bake in 20 to 40 minutes. Check jumbo muffins for doneness after 20 minutes, then again every 5 to 10 minutes. Keep in mind that the baking time will vary with the amount of batter in each muffin cup.

Chunky Jalapeño Corn Muffins

Summer brings juicy sweet ears of fresh corn to the farmers' market, but these muffins can be a year-round treasure.

Nutritional value per serving

Calories	191
Fat, total	6 g
Fat, saturated	1 g
Cholesterol	32 mg
Sodium	206 mg
Carbohydrate	30 g
Fiber	2 g
Protein	4 g
Calcium	103 mg
Iron	3 mg

- **12-cup muffin tin, lightly greased**

1 cup	amaranth flour	250 mL
1 cup	cornmeal	250 mL
1/4 cup	cornstarch	50 mL
1 tbsp	GF baking powder	15 mL
1/2 tsp	baking soda	2 mL
1 1/2 tsp	xanthan gum	7 mL
1/2 tsp	salt	2 mL
2	eggs	2
1 1/4 cups	buttermilk	300 mL
1/3 cup	liquid honey	75 mL
1/4 cup	vegetable oil	50 mL
1/2 cup	well-drained canned corn kernels	125 mL
1/3 cup	chopped red bell pepper (1/4-inch/0.5 cm pieces)	75 mL
1 to 2	jalapeño peppers, chopped	1 to 2

1. In a large bowl or plastic bag, combine amaranth flour, cornmeal, cornstarch, baking powder, baking soda, xanthan gum and salt. Mix well and set aside.

2. In a separate bowl, using an electric mixer, beat eggs, buttermilk, honey and oil until combined. Add dry ingredients and mix until just combined. Stir in corn, red pepper and jalapeños to taste.

3. Spoon batter evenly into prepared muffin cups. Let stand for 30 minutes. Meanwhile, preheat oven to 350°F (180°C).

4. Bake for 18 to 20 minutes or until firm to the touch. Remove from pan immediately and let cool completely on a rack.

Tips

A chile pepper with a pointed tip will be hotter than one that is rounded.

In place of buttermilk, mix together the same amount of milk and 1 tsp (5 mL) freshly squeezed lemon juice.

Variation

To make a loaf, spoon batter into a lightly greased 9- by 5-inch (23 by 12.5 cm) loaf pan. Let stand for 30 minutes. Meanwhile, preheat oven to 350°F (180°C). Bake for 55 to 65 minutes or until a cake tester inserted in the center comes out clean. Let cool in pan on a rack for 10 minutes. Remove from pan and let cool completely on rack.

Extra Baking Tips for Loaves, Biscuits and Muffins

- Fill muffin tins and loaf pans no more than three-quarters full. Let batter-filled pans stand for 30 minutes for a more tender product. It's worth the wait. We set a timer for 20 minutes, then preheat the oven so both the oven and the batter are ready at the same time.

- If muffins stick to the lightly greased tins, let stand for a minute or two and try again. Loosen with a spatula, if necessary.

- Muffins and biscuits can be reheated in the microwave, wrapped in a paper towel, for a few seconds on Medium (50%) power.

- To freeze, place individual muffins or loaf slices in small freezer bags, then place all in a large airtight freezer plastic bag. Freeze for up to 1 month.

Texas-Style Cheese Muffins

**Makes 8 muffins
(1 per serving)**

This warm brown muffin stays moist, so it is a perfect addition to your lunch bag.

Tips

Pea flour, when wet, has a pungent aroma that disappears during baking.

Use care when removing the muffins from the oven, so you don't spill the hot water in the empty cups and burn yourself.

- 12-cup muffin tin, lightly greased

½ cup	pea flour	125 mL
⅓ cup	sorghum flour	75 mL
2 tbsp	tapioca starch	25 mL
1 tsp	xanthan gum	5 mL
2 tsp	GF baking powder	10 mL
1 tsp	baking soda	5 mL
⅛ tsp	dry mustard	0.5 mL
⅛ tsp	cayenne pepper	0.5 mL
1	egg	1
¾ cup	milk	175 mL
2 tbsp	vegetable oil	25 mL
¾ cup	shredded aged Cheddar cheese	175 mL
½ cup	diced onion	125 mL

1. In a large bowl or plastic bag, combine pea flour, sorghum flour, tapioca starch, xanthan gum, baking powder, baking soda, dry mustard and cayenne. Mix well and set aside.

2. In a separate bowl, using an electric mixer, beat egg, milk and oil until combined. Add dry ingredients and mix until just combined. Stir in cheese and onion.

3. Spoon batter evenly into 8 prepared muffin cups. Fill the empty cups half-full with water. Let stand for 30 minutes. Meanwhile, preheat oven to 350°F (180°C).

4. Bake for 22 to 24 minutes or until firm to the touch. Remove from pan immediately and let cool completely on a rack.

Variations

Substitute any bean flour for the pea flour.

For a milder flavor, substitute paprika for the cayenne pepper, or omit it.

Nutritional value per serving	
Calories	129
Fat, total	5 g
Fat, saturated	1 g
Cholesterol	26 mg
Sodium	262 mg
Carbohydrate	15 g
Fiber	2 g
Protein	7 g
Calcium	132 mg
Iron	1 mg

Cookies, Bars and Squares

Sugar Cookies

**Makes 30 cookies
(1 per serving)**

Everybody's favorite variety of cookie! No need to wait for holiday baking time to enjoy these.

Tips

To bake 2 baking sheets at once, bake in the top and bottom thirds of the oven, rotating and switching baking sheets halfway through.

Diet margarine cannot be substituted for the butter, as it has too high a water content.

If the dough sticks to the cookie cutter, dip the cutter in a saucer of sweet rice flour, or place the dough back in the refrigerator until thoroughly chilled.

Sprinkle hot cookies with sugar or decorate cooled cookies with colored icing.

Nutritional value per serving	
Calories	108
Fat, total	5 g
Fat, saturated	3 g
Cholesterol	18 mg
Sodium	67 mg
Carbohydrate	15 g
Fiber	1 g
Protein	1 g
Calcium	11 mg
Iron	1 mg

- 2-inch (5 cm) cookie cutter
- Baking sheets, lightly greased and lined with parchment paper

1 cup	amaranth flour	250 mL
1/4 cup	brown rice flour	50 mL
1/2 cup	GF confectioner's (icing) sugar	125 mL
3/4 cup	cornstarch	175 mL
2 tsp	xanthan gum	10 mL
1/2 tsp	GF baking powder	2 mL
1/4 tsp	salt	1 mL
1 cup	white (granulated) sugar	250 mL
3/4 cup	butter, softened	175 mL
1	egg	1
1 tsp	vanilla extract	5 mL

1. In a bowl or plastic bag, combine amaranth flour, brown rice flour, confectioner's sugar, cornstarch, xanthan gum, baking powder and salt. Mix well and set aside.

2. In a separate bowl, using an electric mixer, beat sugar and butter until light and fluffy. Beat in egg and vanilla until combined. Slowly beat in dry ingredients until just combined.

3. Divide dough in half. Wrap each half in plastic wrap. Flatten slightly and refrigerate at least 1 hour or overnight. Meanwhile, preheat oven to 375°F (190°C).

4. On a lightly floured surface, roll out each half to 1/4-inch (0.5 cm) thickness. Using the cookie cutter, cut out shapes, rerolling scraps. Place 1 inch (2.5 cm) apart on prepared baking sheets.

5. Bake for 10 minutes or until light golden on the bottom. Let cool on pans on racks for 1 minute. Transfer to racks and let cool completely.

Crunchy Chocolate Chip Cookies

**Makes 24 cookies
(1 per serving)**

*Can't tolerate nuts but
still like a cookie with
crunch? Try these!*

Tips

Select good-quality
chocolate chips. Read the
label: chocolate liquor and
cocoa butter should come
before sugar in the list of
ingredients.

Mini chips or jumbo chips
can be used in this recipe.

- Preheat oven to 350°F (180°C)
- Baking sheets, lightly greased

¾ cup	sorghum flour	175 mL
½ cup	GF oat flour	125 mL
⅓ cup	tapioca starch	75 mL
1 tsp	xanthan gum	5 mL
2 tsp	GF baking powder	10 mL
¼ tsp	salt	1 mL
¼ cup	ground flaxseed	50 mL
¼ cup	GF oat bran	50 mL
2 tsp	ground cinnamon	10 mL
1 cup	semisweet chocolate chips	250 mL
½ cup	millet seeds	125 mL
1	egg	1
¾ cup	packed brown sugar	175 mL
⅔ cup	butter, softened	150 mL

1. In a large bowl or plastic bag, combine sorghum flour, oat flour, tapioca starch, xanthan gum, baking powder, salt, ground flaxseed, oat bran, cinnamon, chocolate chips and millet seeds. Mix well and set aside.

2. In a separate bowl, using an electric mixer, beat egg, brown sugar and butter for 2 to 3 minutes or until smooth. Slowly beat in dry ingredients until just combined.

3. Drop dough by rounded spoonfuls 2 inches (5 cm) apart on prepared baking sheets. Flatten slightly with a fork.

4. Bake in preheated oven for 14 to 16 minutes or until set. Transfer to a rack and let cool completely.

5. Store in an airtight container at room temperature for up to 5 days or in the freezer for up to 2 months.

Variation

Substitute rice bran and rice flour for the oat bran and oat flour.

Nutritional value per serving

Calories	152
Fat, total	8 g
Fat, saturated	5 g
Cholesterol	22 mg
Sodium	85 mg
Carbohydrate	20 g
Fiber	2 g
Protein	2 g
Calcium	52 mg
Iron	1 mg

White Chocolate Oatmeal Cookies with Cranberries

**Makes 30 cookies
(1 per serving)**

Colorful and attractive, this recipe turns an oatmeal cookie into a Christmas treat.

Tips

To make into bars, press or pat dough into a lightly greased 9-inch (23 cm) baking pan and bake in a 350°F (180°C) oven for 25 minutes.

Underbake for a chewy cookie. Bake longer for a crisp one. Watch carefully, as cookies burn within an extra 1 to 2 minutes.

- Preheat oven to 350°F (180°C)
- Baking sheets, lightly greased

1 1/2 cups	GF oats	375 mL
1 cup	amaranth flour	250 mL
1/4 cup	tapioca starch	50 mL
1/2 tsp	xanthan gum	2 mL
1/2 tsp	GF baking powder	2 mL
1/2 tsp	baking soda	2 mL
1/4 tsp	salt	1 mL
1	egg	1
3/4 cup	packed brown sugar	175 mL
2/3 cup	butter, softened	150 mL
2 tbsp	milk	25 mL
1 tsp	vanilla extract	5 mL
1 cup	dried cranberries	250 mL
1 cup	white chocolate chips	250 mL

1. In a bowl or plastic bag, combine oats, amaranth flour, tapioca starch, xanthan gum, baking powder, baking soda and salt. Mix well and set aside.

2. In a separate bowl, using an electric mixer, beat egg, brown sugar, butter, milk and vanilla until light and fluffy. Slowly beat in dry ingredients until just combined. Stir in cranberries and chocolate chips.

3. Drop dough by rounded spoonfuls 2 inches (5 cm) apart on prepared baking sheets. Flatten slightly.

4. Bake in preheated oven for 12 to 14 minutes or until lightly browned and just set. Let cool on baking sheets on a rack for 2 to 3 minutes. Carefully transfer to rack and let cool completely.

5. Store in an airtight container at room temperature for up to 5 days or in the freezer for up to 2 months.

Variations

Try flavored dried cranberries.

Chop chocolate squares or wafers into chunks and use instead of the white chocolate chips.

Nutritional value per serving

Calories	139
Fat, total	6 g
Fat, saturated	4 g
Cholesterol	18 mg
Sodium	89 mg
Carbohydrate	19 g
Fiber	1 g
Protein	2 g
Calcium	31 mg
Iron	2 mg

Brandy Tuiles

Egg-free

**Makes 12 cookies
(1 per serving)**

"Tuile" (pronounced twee) is the French word for "tile" and describes a thin, crisp wafer cookie traditionally shaped while still hot around a curved object such as a rolling pin.

Tips

Be patient — bake only one baking sheet at a time. Be sure to let the baking sheet cool between batches.

Don't worry if the wafers spread together during baking; just wait 1 minute, until they cool slightly, and cut apart.

Nutritional value per serving	
Calories	89
Fat, total	4 g
Fat, saturated	2 g
Cholesterol	10 mg
Sodium	50 mg
Carbohydrate	11 g
Fiber	0 g
Protein	2 g
Calcium	10 mg
Iron	0 mg

- Preheat oven to 350°F (180°C)
- Baking sheet, lined with parchment paper

¼ cup	white (granulated) sugar	50 mL
¼ cup	butter	50 mL
¼ cup	corn syrup	50 mL
⅓ cup	low-fat soy flour	75 mL
⅓ cup	pecan flour	75 mL
2 tbsp	brandy	25 mL

1. In a small saucepan, combine sugar, butter and corn syrup. Bring to a boil over medium heat, stirring constantly. Remove from heat and stir in soy flour, pecan flour and brandy until combined.

2. Working in batches of 4 at a time, drop dough by tablespoonfuls (15 mL) at least 5 inches (12.5 cm) apart on prepared baking sheet. Spread with the back of a spoon to a 3-inch (7.5 cm) circle. Return saucepan to low heat between batches to prevent mixture from becoming too thick.

3. Bake in center of preheated oven for 5 to 7 minutes or until a dark caramel color, bubbly and lacy. (Watch carefully, as they brown quickly.)

4. Let baked tuiles cool for 30 seconds. Then, while they're still warm and pliable, loosely roll each around the handle of a wooden spoon or rolling pin. Slip off and place on paper towels to cool completely. If cookies become too crisp before all are rolled, place back in hot but turned-off oven just until soft and pliable.

5. Store between layers of waxed paper in an airtight container at room temperature for up to 3 days.

Variations

To make flat tuiles, use a metal spatula to transfer cookies from baking sheets to paper towels. Cover with additional paper towels. Pat gently. Let cool completely.

Drop batter by teaspoonfuls (5 mL) and spread to make 36 mini tuiles. Bake them 6 at a time, reducing the baking time to 4 to 5 minutes, and watch carefully.

Substitute unsweetened apple juice for the brandy.

Fruitcake Cookies

White sugar–free

**Makes 36 cookies
(1 per serving)**

*No time to make a
fruitcake? Try these
miniature versions.*

- Preheat oven to 350°F (180°C)
- Baking sheets, lightly greased

½ cup	whole bean flour	125 mL
½ cup	sorghum flour	125 mL
2 tbsp	cornstarch	25 mL
½ tsp	xanthan gum	2 mL
¼ tsp	GF baking powder	1 mL
¼ tsp	baking soda	1 mL
½ tsp	salt	2 mL
½ tsp	ground cinnamon	2 mL
½ tsp	ground ginger	2 mL
½ tsp	ground nutmeg	2 mL
¼ tsp	ground allspice	1 mL
1	egg	1
½ cup	packed brown sugar	125 mL
¼ cup	butter, softened	50 mL
2 tbsp	dark rum	25 mL
2 tbsp	water	25 mL
1 tsp	vanilla extract	5 mL
2 cups	coarsely chopped red and green glacé cherries	500 mL
1 cup	coarsely chopped pecans	250 mL
½ cup	chopped candied peel	125 mL

1. In a large bowl or plastic bag, combine whole bean flour, sorghum flour, cornstarch, xanthan gum, baking powder, baking soda, salt, cinnamon, ginger, nutmeg and allspice. Mix well and set aside.

2. In a separate bowl, using an electric mixer, beat egg, brown sugar and butter until combined. Beat in rum, water and vanilla until combined. Slowly beat in dry ingredients until just combined. Stir in cherries, pecans and peel.

3. Drop dough by heaping spoonfuls 2 inches (5 cm) apart on prepared baking sheets.

Nutritional value per serving

Calories	55
Fat, total	2 g
Fat, saturated	1 g
Cholesterol	9 mg
Sodium	61 mg
Carbohydrate	10 g
Fiber	0 g
Protein	1 g
Calcium	7 mg
Iron	0 mg

Tips

For the candied peel, you can use orange or lemon, or a combination.

The batter may appear to be curdled, but will blend when the dry ingredients are added.

Be sure to let baking sheets cool between batches.

4. Bake in preheated oven for 13 to 15 minutes or until deep golden brown. Transfer to a rack and let cool completely.

5. Store in an airtight container at room temperature for up to 5 days or in the freezer for up to 2 months.

Variations

Substitute ½ cup (125 mL) semisweet chocolate chips for an equal amount of the glacé cherries.

Substitute unsweetened apple juice for the rum.

Mock (Peanut-Free) Peanut Brittle

**Makes 12 cookies
(1 per serving)**

The flavor of these cookies is like peanut brittle, but the texture is like that of tuiles.

Tip

Purchase unroasted, unsalted pumpkin seeds.

- Preheat oven to 350°F (180°C)
- Baking sheet, lined with parchment paper

1/3 cup	white (granulated) sugar	75 mL
1/4 cup	corn syrup	50 mL
1/4 cup	butter	50 mL
1/2 cup	whole bean flour	125 mL
1/2 cup	green pumpkin seeds, toasted	125 mL
Pinch	ground ginger	Pinch

1. In a small saucepan, combine sugar, corn syrup and butter. Bring to a boil over medium heat, stirring constantly. Remove from heat and stir in whole bean flour, pumpkin seeds and ginger until combined.

2. Working in batches of 4 at a time, drop dough by tablespoonfuls (15 mL) at least 5 inches (12.5 cm) apart on prepared baking sheet. Spread with the back of a spoon to a 3-inch (7.5 cm) circle. Return saucepan to low heat between batches to prevent mixture from becoming too thick.

3. Bake in center of preheated oven for 7 to 8 minutes or until a light caramel color, bubbly and lacy. (Watch carefully, as they brown quickly and darken further upon cooling.) Let cool on baking sheet on a rack for 2 minutes. Using a metal spatula, remove from baking sheet and place on parchment paper. Cover with paper towels. Pat gently and remove paper towels. Let cool completely.

4. Store between layers of waxed paper in an airtight container at room temperature for up to 3 days.

Nutritional value per serving	
Calories	131
Fat, total	8 g
Fat, saturated	3 g
Cholesterol	10 mg
Sodium	51 mg
Carbohydrate	13 g
Fiber	1 g
Protein	4 g
Calcium	9 mg
Iron	2 mg

Tips

Bake only 4 at a time, or you'll end up with one piece with baked edges but a gummy center.

See the Techniques Glossary, page 399, for information on toasting seeds.

Variations

For cookies the shape of tuiles, let baked cookies cool for 1 minute. Then, while they're still warm and pliable, loosely roll each around the handle of a wooden spoon or rolling pin. Slip off and place on parchment paper to cool completely. If cookies become too crisp before all are rolled, place back in hot but turned-off oven just until soft and pliable.

Drop batter by teaspoonfuls (5 mL) and spread to make 36 mini cookies. Bake them 6 at a time, reducing the baking time to 5 to 7 minutes, and watch carefully.

Chocolate Pecan Biscotti

**Makes 24 cookies
(1 per serving)**

Biscotti, traditional Italian cookies, have become part of North American cuisine. This chocolate version is delicious dipped in a cup of espresso.

Tip

Recipe can be doubled. Use a 13- by 9- inch (33 by 23 cm) baking pan and increase the baking time in step 4 by about 5 minutes, or use two 8-inch (20 cm) baking pans (the baking time will stay the same).

- Preheat oven to 325°F (160°C)
- 8-inch (20 cm) square baking pan, lightly greased
- Baking sheets, ungreased

¾ cup	brown rice flour	175 mL
¼ cup	pecan flour	50 mL
3 tbsp	tapioca starch	45 mL
2 tbsp	potato starch	25 mL
¾ tsp	xanthan gum	4 mL
½ tsp	GF baking powder	2 mL
Pinch	salt	Pinch
½ cup	unsweetened cocoa powder, sifted	125 mL
2	eggs	2
⅔ cup	white (granulated) sugar	150 mL
½ tsp	orange extract	2 mL
¾ cup	semisweet chocolate chips	175 mL
¾ cup	toasted chopped pecans	175 mL

1. In a large bowl or plastic bag, combine brown rice flour, pecan flour, tapioca starch, potato starch, xanthan gum, baking powder, salt and cocoa. Mix well and set aside.

2. In a separate bowl, using an electric mixer, beat eggs, sugar and orange extract until combined. Slowly beat in dry ingredients until just combined. Stir in chocolate chips and pecans.

3. Spoon batter into prepared pan. Using a moistened rubber spatula, spread to edges and smooth top.

4. Bake in preheated oven for 30 to 35 minutes or until firm to the touch. Let cool in pan for 5 minutes. Remove from pan and let cool on a cutting board for 5 minutes. Reduce oven temperature to 300°F (150°C).

5. Using a very sharp knife, carefully cut into quarters, then cut each quarter into 6 slices. Arrange slices upright (with both cut sides exposed) at least ½ inch (1 cm) apart on baking sheets.

Nutritional value per serving

Calories	88
Fat, total	5 g
Fat, saturated	2 g
Cholesterol	17 mg
Sodium	22 mg
Carbohydrate	10 g
Fiber	2 g
Protein	2 g
Calcium	22 mg
Iron	1 mg

Tips

For information on toasting nuts, see the Techniques Glossary, page 398.

Biscotti will be medium-firm and crunchy. For softer, chewier biscotti, bake for only 10 minutes in step 6; for very firm biscotti, bake for 20 minutes.

6. Bake for 15 minutes or until dry and crisp. Transfer to a rack and let cool completely.

7. Store in an airtight container at room temperature for up to 3 weeks or in the freezer for up to 2 months.

Variation

Substitute almond or hazelnut flour for the pecan flour and toasted slivered almonds or chopped hazelnuts for the pecans.

Pecan Amaretti

**Makes 24 cookies
(1 per serving)**

*Amaretti are airy
Italian macaroons
traditionally made
with bitter almond or
apricot kernel paste.
These melt in your
mouth.*

Tips

See the Techniques
Glossary, page 396, for
information on warming
egg whites.

Add the sugar gradually,
beating constantly, or the
beaten egg whites will
become gritty, smooth
and shiny.

• **Preheat oven to 300°F (150°C)**
• **Baking sheets, lined with parchment paper**

2	egg whites, at room temperature	2
¼ tsp	cream of tartar	1 mL
1 cup	white (granulated) sugar	250 mL
½ tsp	vanilla extract	2 mL
2½ cups	pecan flour	625 mL

1. In a bowl, using an electric mixer with wire whisk attachment, beat egg whites and cream of tartar until soft peaks form. Gradually beat in sugar, 1 to 2 tbsp (15 to 25 mL) at a time. Continue beating until mixture is very stiff and glossy but not dry. Beat in vanilla. Gently fold in one-quarter of the pecan flour at a time, making sure each addition is well blended before adding the next.

2. Drop by tablespoonfuls (15 mL) 2 inches (5 cm) apart on prepared baking sheets.

3. Bake in preheated oven for 20 minutes or until crisp and firm to the touch. Transfer to a rack and let cool completely.

4. Store between layers of waxed paper in an airtight container at room temperature for up to 3 days.

Variation

Substitute almond flour for the pecan flour and almond extract for the vanilla.

Nutritional value per serving

Calories	55
Fat, total	0 g
Fat, saturated	0 g
Cholesterol	0 mg
Sodium	5 mg
Carbohydrate	12 g
Fiber	0 g
Protein	2 g
Calcium	2 mg
Iron	0 mg

Hazelnut Macaroons

**Makes 30 cookies
(1 per serving)**

These melt-in-your-mouth cookies are quick and easy to make with ingredients you have on hand.

Tips

When the macaroons are cooked, they lift cleanly off the parchment paper.

Use light-colored baking sheets, as dark baking sheets tend to make macaroons too dark.

See the Techniques Glossary, page 396, for information on warming egg whites.

Add the sugar very gradually, beating constantly, or the macaroons will be small and grainy.

- Preheat oven to 275°F (140°C)
- Baking sheets, lined with parchment paper

1/2 cup	hazelnut flour	125 mL
1 tbsp	amaranth flour	15 mL
3	egg whites, at room temperature	3
1/2 tsp	white vinegar	2 mL
1/2 tsp	vanilla extract	2 mL
2/3 cup	white (granulated) sugar	150 mL

1. In a small bowl or plastic bag, combine hazelnut flour and amaranth flour. Mix well and set aside.

2. In a large bowl, using an electric mixer with wire whisk attachment, beat egg whites until foamy. Beat in vinegar and vanilla. Continue beating until egg whites form stiff peaks. Gradually beat in sugar. Continue beating until mixture is very stiff and glossy but not dry. Gently fold in dry ingredients.

3. Drop by heaping spoonfuls 2 inches (5 cm) apart on prepared baking sheets.

4. Bake in preheated oven for 20 to 25 minutes or until light brown and tops are crisp. Let cool on baking sheets on a rack for 2 minutes. Transfer to rack and let cool completely.

5. Store in an airtight container at room temperature for up to 2 weeks.

Variation

To turn these macaroons into amaretti, substitute almond flour for the hazelnut flour and almond extract for the vanilla.

Nutritional value per serving

Calories	32
Fat, total	1 g
Fat, saturated	0 g
Cholesterol	0 mg
Sodium	6 mg
Carbohydrate	5 g
Fiber	0 g
Protein	1 g
Calcium	3 mg
Iron	0 mg

Cranberry White Chocolate Chip Blondies

Makes 16 blondies (1 per serving)

A CanolaInfo recipe

Wrap these bars individually to freeze, then take them directly from the freezer and pack for a mid-morning or mid-afternoon pick-me-up.

- 9-inch (23 cm) square baking pan, lightly greased and lined with parchment paper

⅔ cup	low-fat soy flour	150 mL
½ cup	brown rice flour	125 mL
¼ cup	tapioca starch	50 mL
1½ tsp	xanthan gum	7 mL
1 tbsp	GF baking powder	15 mL
2	eggs	2
½ cup	packed brown sugar	125 mL
½ cup	unsweetened applesauce	125 mL
¼ cup	vegetable oil	50 mL
1 tsp	vanilla extract	5 mL
½ cup	dried cranberries	125 mL
½ cup	white chocolate chips	125 mL

1. In a small bowl or plastic bag, combine soy flour, brown rice flour, tapioca starch, xanthan gum and baking powder. Mix well and set aside.

2. In a large bowl, using an electric mixer, beat eggs, brown sugar, applesauce, oil and vanilla until well blended. Slowly beat in dry ingredients until just combined. Stir in cranberries and chocolate chips.

3. Spoon batter into prepared pan. Using a moistened rubber spatula, spread to edges and smooth top. Let stand for 30 minutes. Meanwhile, preheat oven to 350°F (180°C).

4. Bake for 25 to 30 minutes or until a cake tester inserted in the center comes out clean. Let cool in pan on a rack for 10 minutes. Remove to rack and let cool completely, then cut into bars.

Nutritional value per serving

Calories	149
Fat, total	6 g
Fat, saturated	2 g
Cholesterol	25 mg
Sodium	17 mg
Carbohydrate	21 g
Fiber	1 g
Protein	3 g
Calcium	71 mg
Iron	1 mg

Tip

Letting the batter stand for 30 minutes yields a better texture. However, if you're short on time, you can bake right away.

5. Store in an airtight container at room temperature for up to 4 days or individually wrapped in the freezer for up to 1 month.

Variation

Substitute flavored dried cranberries and flavored chocolate chips. Try strawberry-, orange- or cherry-flavored cranberries and raspberry-flavored chocolate chips.

Three-Fruit Energy Bars

**Makes 18 bars
(1 per serving)**

Choose these moist, colorful, nutritious bars for a make-and-take snack.

Tips

We like to snip dried fruit with kitchen shears. Dip the blades in hot water when they get sticky.

Check for gluten if you use a dried fruit mix.

- Preheat oven to 325°F (160°C)
- 13- by 9-inch (33 by 23 cm) baking pan, lightly greased and lined with parchment paper

1	can (14 oz or 300 mL) sweetened condensed milk	1
2 tbsp	butter, melted	25 mL
2 cups	GF cereal flakes	500 mL
1/2 cup	GF oats	125 mL
1/2 cup	slivered almonds	125 mL
1/3 cup	snipped dried apricots	75 mL
1/3 cup	snipped pitted dates	75 mL
1/3 cup	snipped dried mango	75 mL
1/4 cup	unroasted green pumpkin seeds	50 mL

1. In a large bowl, using an electric mixer, combine condensed milk and butter. Add cereal flakes, oats, almonds, apricots, dates, mango and pumpkin seeds. Stir until all is well coated. Press evenly into prepared pan.

2. Bake in preheated oven for 30 to 35 minutes or until golden brown. Let cool completely in pan on a rack, then cut into bars.

3. Store in an airtight container at room temperature for up to 1 week or individually wrapped in the freezer for up to 1 month.

Variation

Substitute any dried fruit, in varying amounts, but keep to a total of 1 cup (250 mL). Try cranberries, blueberries, papaya, raisins and prunes.

Nutritional value per serving	
Calories	195
Fat, total	7 g
Fat, saturated	2 g
Cholesterol	11 mg
Sodium	46 mg
Carbohydrate	31 g
Fiber	2 g
Protein	5 g
Calcium	77 mg
Iron	1 mg

Peanut Butter Chocolate Squares

Need a crowd-pleasing sweet treat in a hurry? Here's the answer. Make these ahead and freeze for holiday entertaining.

Tips

Double the recipe and bake in a 13- by 9-inch (33 by 23 cm) baking pan. Increase the baking time in step 4 by about 5 minutes.

The base tends to crumble if cut while still warm. It will cut more easily if you refrigerate it overnight first.

No food processor? Use a pastry blender or two knives to cut the butter into the dry ingredients. Add the egg and mix until a soft dough forms.

Nutritional value per serving	
Calories	310
Fat, total	21 g
Fat, saturated	7 g
Cholesterol	50 mg
Sodium	92 mg
Carbohydrate	28 g
Fiber	2 g
Protein	8 g
Calcium	20 mg
Iron	1 mg

- Preheat oven to 350°F (180°C)
- 9-inch (23 cm) square baking pan, lightly greased and lined with parchment paper

Base

¼ cup	brown rice flour	50 mL
¾ cup	potato starch	175 mL
3 tbsp	tapioca starch	45 mL
1 tsp	xanthan gum	5 mL
¼ cup	packed brown sugar	50 mL
Pinch	salt	Pinch
½ cup	cold butter, cut into 1-inch (2.5 cm) cubes	125 mL
1	egg, lightly beaten	1

Topping

2	eggs, lightly beaten	2
1½ cups	GF crunchy peanut butter	375 mL
½ cup	white (granulated) sugar	125 mL
4 oz	milk chocolate, finely chopped	125 g

1. *Base:* In a food processor, pulse brown rice flour, potato starch, tapioca starch, xanthan gum, brown sugar and salt to combine. Add butter and pulse for 5 to 10 seconds or until mixture resembles coarse crumbs about the size of small peas. With the motor running, through the feed tube, add egg and process until dough forms a ball.

2. Spread evenly in bottom of prepared pan, smoothing with a moistened rubber spatula. Bake in preheated oven for 12 to 15 minutes or until browned.

3. *Topping:* Meanwhile, in a bowl, using an electric mixer, beat eggs, peanut butter and sugar. Spread over the hot base. Sprinkle with chocolate.

4. Bake for 20 to 25 minutes or until center is almost firm. Spread the now melted chocolate evenly over top. Let cool completely in pan on a rack, then cut into squares.

5. Store in an airtight container at room temperature for up to 3 days or individually wrapped in the freezer for up to 1 month.

Lotsa Lemon Squares

**Makes 36 squares
(1 per serving)**

A CanolaInfo recipe

*Temptingly tart,
amazingly addictive —
you're going to want a
second or third piece.
You'll be so glad this
recipe is gluten-free.*

- Preheat oven to 350°F (180°C)
- 9-inch (23 cm) square baking pan, lightly greased and lined with parchment paper

Base

1/4 cup	brown rice flour	50 mL
3/4 cup	cornstarch	175 mL
3 tbsp	tapioca starch	45 mL
1 tsp	xanthan gum	5 mL
1/4 cup	packed brown sugar	50 mL
Pinch	salt	Pinch
1/3 cup	vegetable oil	75 mL
1	egg	1

Topping

4	eggs	4
1 1/2 cups	white (granulated) sugar	375 mL
2 tbsp	grated lemon zest	25 mL
1/2 cup	freshly squeezed lemon juice	125 mL
1/4 cup	cornstarch	50 mL
1 tsp	GF baking powder	5 mL

1. *Base:* In a food processor, pulse brown rice flour, cornstarch, tapioca starch, xanthan gum, brown sugar and salt to combine. In a small bowl, whisk together oil and egg. With the motor running, through the feed tube, add egg mixture in a slow, steady stream and process for 5 to 10 seconds or until mixture resembles coarse crumbs.

2. Press evenly into bottom of prepared pan. Bake in preheated oven for 12 to 15 minutes or until set. Reduce oven temperature to 325°F (160°C).

3. *Topping:* Meanwhile, in a bowl, using an electric mixer, beat eggs, sugar, lemon zest, lemon juice, cornstarch and baking powder until blended. Pour over the hot base.

Nutritional value per serving

Calories	86
Fat, total	3 g
Fat, saturated	0 g
Cholesterol	26 mg
Sodium	17 mg
Carbohydrate	15 g
Fiber	0 g
Protein	1 g
Calcium	11 mg
Iron	0 mg

If your baking pan has a light-colored finish, bake the base for an extra 3 minutes and the topping for up to an extra 5 minutes.

4. Bake for 35 to 40 minutes or until light golden and firm to the touch. Let cool completely in pan on a rack, then cut into squares.

5. Store in an airtight container at room temperature for up to 3 days or individually wrapped in the freezer for up to 2 weeks.

Variation

While still warm, dust with GF confectioner's (icing) sugar. Cut into larger pieces and serve with strawberries or raspberries for dessert.

Apple Hazelnut Squares

If you love butter tart squares, just wait till you taste our apple hazelnut version!

Tip

Double the recipe and bake in a 13- by 9-inch (33 by 23 cm) baking pan. Increase the baking time in step 4 by about 5 minutes.

- Preheat oven to 350°F (180°C)
- 9-inch (23 cm) square baking pan, lightly greased, bottom and sides lined with parchment paper

Base

¼ cup	hazelnut flour	50 mL
⅔ cup	potato starch	150 mL
¼ cup	tapioca starch	50 mL
1 tsp	xanthan gum	5 mL
¼ cup	packed brown sugar	50 mL
Pinch	salt	Pinch
½ cup	cold butter, cut into 1-inch (2.5 cm) cubes	125 mL
1	egg, lightly beaten	1

Topping

2	eggs	2
⅓ cup	packed brown sugar	75 mL
¼ cup	corn syrup	50 mL
2 tbsp	amaranth flour	25 mL
2 tbsp	melted butter	25 mL
1 tbsp	brandy	15 mL
1 tsp	vanilla extract	5 mL
Pinch	ground cinnamon	Pinch
Pinch	salt	Pinch
2	apples, grated	2
1 cup	coarsely chopped hazelnuts	250 mL

1. *Base:* In a food processor, pulse hazelnut flour, potato starch, tapioca starch, xanthan gum, brown sugar and salt to combine. Add butter and pulse for 5 to 10 seconds or until mixture resembles coarse crumbs about the size of small peas. With the motor running, through the feed tube, add egg and process until dough forms a ball.

2. Spread evenly in bottom of prepared pan, smoothing with a moistened rubber spatula. Bake in preheated oven for 15 minutes or until lightly browned.

Nutritional value per serving	
Calories	218
Fat, total	14 g
Fat, saturated	5 g
Cholesterol	54 mg
Sodium	131 mg
Carbohydrate	23 g
Fiber	1 g
Protein	3 g
Calcium	28 mg
Iron	1 mg

Tips

We really like the flavor of Spartan apples, but any tart variety will do. We don't peel apples, but you can, if you like.

No food processor? Use a pastry blender or two knives to cut the butter into the dry ingredients. Add the egg and mix until a soft dough forms.

3. *Topping:* Meanwhile, in a bowl, using an electric mixer, beat eggs, brown sugar, corn syrup, amaranth flour, butter, brandy, vanilla, cinnamon and salt. Stir in apples and hazelnuts. Spread over the hot base.

4. Bake for 30 to 35 minutes or until lightly browned. Let cool completely in pan on a rack, then cut into squares.

5. Store in an airtight container at room temperature for up to 3 days or individually wrapped in the freezer for up to 2 months.

Coconut Fig Dessert Squares

**Makes 9 squares
(1 per serving)**

Perfect on a dessert tray — no one will guess that these are gluten-free.

Tips

This recipe can easily be doubled and baked in a 13- by 9-inch (33 by 23 cm) baking pan for 30 to 40 minutes.

- Preheat oven to 400°F (200°C)
- 8-inch (20 cm) square baking pan, lightly greased

Filling

1½ cups	finely snipped dried figs	375 mL
1 tbsp	grated orange zest	15 mL
¾ cup	freshly squeezed orange juice	175 mL

Crust

½ cup	sorghum flour	125 mL
⅓ cup	packed brown sugar	75 mL
¼ tsp	salt	1 mL
⅓ cup	cold butter, cut into 1-inch (2.5 cm) cubes	75 mL
¾ cup	GF rolled oats	175 mL
¾ cup	sweetened flaked coconut	175 mL

1. *Filling:* In a saucepan, combine figs, orange zest and orange juice. Bring to a boil over medium heat. Reduce heat to medium-low, cover and simmer for 10 minutes or until figs are fork-tender.

2. In a food processor, purée fig mixture until smooth, scraping sides occasionally. Transfer to a bowl and set aside. Clean the bowl of the food processor.

3. *Crust:* In the food processor, pulse sorghum flour, brown sugar and salt to combine. Add butter and pulse for 30 to 45 seconds or until crumbly. Add oats and coconut; pulse until just combined.

4. Firmly pat two-thirds of the crust mixture into bottom of prepared pan. Top with fig filling and sprinkle with the remaining crust mixture.

5. Bake in preheated oven for 20 to 25 minutes or until golden brown. Let cool completely in pan on a rack, then cut into squares.

6. Store in an airtight container at room temperature for up to 5 days or in the freezer for up to 2 months.

Variations

Omit the coconut and double the amount of oats.

Cut into smaller squares to serve along with other cookies.

Substitute amaranth, buckwheat or quinoa flakes for the oats.

Nutritional value per serving	
Calories	272
Fat, total	10 g
Fat, saturated	6 g
Cholesterol	17 mg
Sodium	152 mg
Carbohydrate	46 g
Fiber	6 g
Protein	4 g
Calcium	68 mg
Iron	3 mg

Cakes

Blueberry Swirl Cheesecake

When you only want enough cheesecake for four, this small pan makes the perfect size. If you're serving cheesecake on a buffet, make one of each: Chocolate Chunk (page 300), Maple Pecan (page 302) and this Blueberry Swirl.

Tips

If you use frozen blueberries, save any liquid that accumulates when you're thawing them to use as the blueberry juice.

If using a dark-colored springform pan, decrease the oven temperature by 25°F (10°C).

- Preheat oven to 300°F (150°C)
- 4$\frac{1}{2}$-inch (11 cm) mini springform pan
- Roasting pan

Blueberry Swirl

2 tbsp	white (granulated) sugar	25 mL
2 tsp	cornstarch	10 mL
3 tbsp	blueberry juice or water	45 mL
¾ cup	fresh or thawed frozen blueberries	175 mL
1 tsp	freshly squeezed lemon juice	5 mL

White Cake Base

½ cup	Basic White Cake crumbs (page 372)	125 mL
2 tsp	melted butter	10 mL

Cheesecake

1	package (8 oz/250 g) light or regular brick cream cheese, softened	1
2 tbsp	packed brown sugar	25 mL
½ tsp	grated lemon zest	2 mL
1 tsp	freshly squeezed lemon juice	5 mL
1	egg	1
¼ cup	GF sour cream	50 mL

1. *Blueberry swirl:* In a saucepan, combine sugar and cornstarch. Slowly add blueberry juice, stirring constantly. Add blueberries and lemon juice. Bring to a boil over medium heat, stirring constantly, until thickened. Let cool to room temperature.

2. *White cake base:* In a bowl, combine cake crumbs and butter; mix well. Press into bottom of pan.

3. *Cheesecake:* In a large bowl, using an electric mixer, beat cream cheese until smooth. Slowly beat in brown sugar, lemon zest and lemon juice until light and fluffy. Beat in egg. Stir in sour cream. Pour over the base.

4. Spoon blueberry mixture in dollops over cheesecake batter. Swirl gently with a knife.

Tips

Ultra-low-fat cream cheese or fat-free cream cheese should not be substituted for regular in baked cheesecake recipes. However, light cream cheese can be used.

Leaving the cheesecake in the oven after turning it off helps prevent large cracks.

Cheesecake can be made up to 1 month in advance. Let cool completely, then wrap whole cheesecake or individual slices tightly and freeze until ready to serve. Thaw in the refrigerator and garnish just before serving.

5. Place the springform pan in the roasting pan, and place in center of preheated oven. Pour enough hot water into the roasting pan to fill it to a depth of at least 1 inch (2.5 cm). Bake for 55 to 65 minutes or until center is just set and the blade of a knife comes out clean. Turn oven off and let cheesecake cool in oven for 1 hour (see tip, at left). Carefully remove springform pan from roasting pan. Let cool in springform pan on a rack for 30 minutes. Refrigerate until chilled, about 3 hours.

Variation

Double the recipe and bake in an 8-inch (20 cm) springform pan.

Chocolate Chunk Cheesecake

Makes 4 servings

This small pan makes the perfect size cheesecake for a dinner party of four.

Tips

If using a dark-colored springform pan, decrease the oven temperature by 25°F (10°C).

Ultra-low-fat cream cheese or fat-free cream cheese should not be substituted for regular in baked cheesecake recipes. However, light cream cheese can be used.

- Preheat oven to 300°F (150°C)
- 4½-inch (11 cm) mini springform pan
- Roasting pan

Chocolate Base

1 cup	German Chocolate Cake crumbs (page 305)	250 mL
2 tbsp	melted butter	25 mL

Cheesecake

1	package (8 oz/250 g) light or regular brick cream cheese, softened	1
2 tbsp	packed brown sugar	25 mL
1½ tsp	grated orange zest	7 mL
1 tbsp	freshly squeezed orange juice	15 mL
1	egg	1
¼ cup	plain yogurt	50 mL
2 oz	milk or semisweet chocolate, cut into small chunks	60 g

1. *Chocolate base:* In a bowl, combine cake crumbs and butter; mix well. Press into bottom of pan. Refrigerate until chilled, about 15 minutes.

2. *Cheesecake:* In a large bowl, using an electric mixer, beat cream cheese until smooth. Slowly beat in brown sugar, orange zest and orange juice until light and fluffy. Beat in egg. Stir in yogurt and chocolate chunks. Pour over the base.

3. Place the springform pan in the roasting pan, and place in center of preheated oven. Pour enough hot water into the roasting pan to fill it to a depth of at least 1 inch (2.5 cm). Bake for 60 minutes or until center is just set and the blade of a knife comes out clean. Turn oven off and let cheesecake cool in oven for 1 hour (see tip, at right). Carefully remove springform pan from roasting pan. Let cool in springform pan on a rack for 30 minutes. Refrigerate until chilled, about 3 hours.

Nutritional value per serving

Calories	373
Fat, total	23 g
Fat, saturated	14 g
Cholesterol	102 mg
Sodium	432 mg
Carbohydrate	33 g
Fiber	2 g
Protein	10 g
Calcium	157 mg
Iron	1 mg

Tips

Use the hottest tap water to fill the roasting pan.

Leaving the cheesecake in the oven after turning it off helps prevent large cracks.

Cheesecake can be made up to 1 month in advance. Let cool completely, then wrap whole cheesecake or individual slices tightly and freeze until ready to serve. Thaw in the refrigerator and garnish just before serving.

Variations

Double the recipe and bake in an 8-inch (20 cm) springform pan.

Replace the cake crumbs with Basic White Cake crumbs (page 372) or the base from Maple Pecan Cheesecake (page 302).

Maple Pecan Cheesecake

Makes 4 servings

Here's another cheesecake that's the perfect size for four.

Tips

If using a dark-colored springform pan, decrease the oven temperature by 25°F (10°C).

Ultra-low-fat cream cheese or fat-free cream cheese should not be substituted for regular in baked cheesecake recipes. However, light cream cheese can be used.

Leaving the cheesecake in the oven after turning it off helps prevent large cracks.

Cheesecake can be made up to 1 month in advance. Let cool completely, then wrap whole cheesecake or individual slices tightly and freeze until ready to serve. Thaw in the refrigerator and garnish just before serving.

Nutritional value per serving

Calories	484
Fat, total	31 g
Fat, saturated	10 g
Cholesterol	81 mg
Sodium	317 mg
Carbohydrate	42 g
Fiber	2 g
Protein	9 g
Calcium	121 mg
Iron	2 mg

- Preheat oven to 325°F (160°C)
- 4½-inch (11 cm) mini springform pan
- Roasting pan

Pecan Base

1 cup	chopped pecans	250 mL
¼ cup	packed brown sugar	50 mL
1 tbsp	butter	15 mL

Cheesecake

1	package (8 oz/250 g) light or regular brick cream cheese, softened	1
⅓ cup	pure maple syrup	75 mL
1 tsp	maple extract	5 mL
1	egg	1
2 tbsp	amaranth flour	25 mL

1. *Pecan Base:* In a food processor, process pecans, brown sugar and butter to fine crumbs. Press into bottom of pan. Bake in preheated oven for 8 to 10 minutes or until lightly toasted. Let cool to room temperature. Decrease the oven temperature to 300°F (150°C).

2. *Cheesecake:* In a bowl, using an electric mixer, beat cream cheese until smooth. Slowly beat in maple syrup and maple extract until light and fluffy. Beat in egg and amaranth flour. Pour over the base.

3. Place the springform pan in the roasting pan, and place in center of preheated oven. Pour enough hot water into the roasting pan to fill it to a depth of at least 1 inch (2.5 cm). Bake for 55 to 65 minutes or until center is just set and the blade of a knife comes out clean. Turn oven off and let cheesecake cool in oven for 1 hour (see tip, at left). Carefully remove springform pan from roasting pan. Let cool in springform pan on a rack for 30 minutes. Refrigerate until chilled, about 3 hours.

Variations

Use a 9- by 5-inch (23 by 12.5 cm) loaf pan, lined with parchment paper, and bake the crust for 8 minutes. Pour filling over cool base and bake for 35 minutes.

Recipe can be doubled and baked in an 8-inch (20 cm) springform pan.

Almond Chiffon Cake

Makes 12 to 16 servings

Chiffon cake is in the light, airy cake family, along with angel food cake and sponge cake, but it's moister than either because of the added oil.

Tips

Make sure beaters, bowl and tube pan are completely free of grease.

Eggs separate more easily when cold because the yolk is less apt to break. For information on warming egg whites to room temperature, see the Techniques Glossary, page 396.

This cake is the one your grandmother told you about: opening the oven door too often during baking or slamming the oven door can cause it to fall.

Nutritional value per serving	
Calories	192
Fat, total	8 g
Fat, saturated	1 g
Cholesterol	80 mg
Sodium	65 mg
Carbohydrate	26 g
Fiber	1 g
Protein	4 g
Calcium	27 mg
Iron	1 mg

- Preheat oven to 325°F (160°C)
- 10-inch (25 cm) tube pan, completely free of grease

½ cup	almond flour	125 mL
½ cup	amaranth flour	125 mL
¼ cup	sorghum flour	50 mL
¼ cup	tapioca starch	50 mL
1½ tsp	xanthan gum	7 mL
½ tsp	baking soda	2 mL
1⅓ cups	white (granulated) sugar	325 mL
6	egg yolks	6
½ cup	water	125 mL
⅓ cup	vegetable oil	75 mL
¼ cup	grated lemon zest	50 mL
¼ cup	freshly squeezed lemon juice	50 mL
6	egg whites, at room temperature	6
½ tsp	cream of tartar	2 mL
1½ tsp	almond extract	7 mL
2 tbsp	white (granulated) sugar	25 mL

1. In a small bowl or plastic bag, combine almond flour, amaranth flour, sorghum flour, tapioca starch, xanthan gum, baking soda and 1⅓ cups (325 mL) sugar. Mix well and set aside.

2. In a deep bowl, whisk together egg yolks, water, oil, lemon zest and lemon juice until combined. Whisk in dry ingredients until smooth. Set aside.

3. In a large bowl, using an electric mixer with wire whisk attachment, beat egg whites until foamy. Beat in cream of tartar and almond extract. Continue beating until egg whites form stiff peaks. Gradually beat in 2 tbsp (25 mL) sugar. Continue beating until mixture is very stiff and glossy but not dry. Fold in egg yolk mixture until well blended. Spoon into pan.

4. Bake in preheated oven for 45 minutes or until cake is golden, shrinks back slightly from the sides and springs back when touched. Invert cake in pan over a funnel or bottle until completely cool. Turn cake right side up. Run a spatula around the outside edges and center tube of the pan and remove cake.

Variation
Use orange zest and juice instead of the lemon.

Golden Pound Cake

Makes 9 servings

Serve this special-occasion cake at a birthday party, anniversary party or shower, with large dollops of Lemon Yogurt Cream (page 327) alongside.

Tip

Let cool completely, then wrap cake tightly and freeze cake for up to 6 weeks. Thaw in the refrigerator.

- 8-inch (20 cm) square baking pan, lightly greased and lined with parchment paper

½ cup	almond flour	125 mL
½ cup	brown rice flour	125 mL
¼ cup	low-fat soy flour	50 mL
¼ cup	tapioca starch	50 mL
1½ tsp	xanthan gum	7 mL
2 tsp	GF baking powder	10 mL
1 tsp	baking soda	5 mL
½ tsp	salt	2 mL
3	eggs	3
⅔ cup	white (granulated) sugar	150 mL
½ cup	milk	125 mL
¼ cup	vegetable oil	50 mL
1 tsp	almond extract	5 mL

1. In a small bowl or plastic bag, combine almond flour, brown rice flour, soy flour, tapioca starch, xanthan gum, baking powder, baking soda and salt. Mix well and set aside.

2. In a separate bowl, using an electric mixer, beat eggs, sugar, milk, oil and almond extract until combined. Add dry ingredients and mix until just combined.

3. Spoon batter into prepared pan. Using a moistened rubber spatula, spread to edges and smooth top. Let stand for 30 minutes. Meanwhile, preheat oven to 350°F (180°C).

4. Bake for 30 to 35 minutes or until a tester inserted in the center comes out clean. Let cool in pan on a rack for 10 minutes. Remove from pan and let cool completely on rack.

Variation

Turn this into a cottage pudding by serving it warm, smothered with Brown Sugar Sauce (page 326).

Nutritional value per serving	
Calories	232
Fat, total	11 g
Fat, saturated	1 g
Cholesterol	63 mg
Sodium	300 mg
Carbohydrate	28 g
Fiber	1 g
Protein	6 g
Calcium	73 mg
Iron	1 mg

German Chocolate Cake

Makes 9 to 12 servings

For those who enjoy a traditional, not too sweet but mild-flavored cake with a rich, dark chocolate color, this is the perfect choice!

Tips

When we have an extra moment, we like to cut parchment paper to the right size to line the bottom of our pans. Store between two pans of the same size. It's handy when you're in a hurry.

This recipe can be used as a base for Chocolate Chunk Cheesecake (page 300). It makes 6 cups (1.5 L) cake crumbs. To make crumbs, pulse pieces of cake in batches in a food processor. Store in an airtight container in the freezer for up to 3 months.

Nutritional value per serving	
Calories	158
Fat, total	5 g
Fat, saturated	3 g
Cholesterol	25 mg
Sodium	162 mg
Carbohydrate	26 g
Fiber	1 g
Protein	3 g
Calcium	88 mg
Iron	1 mg

- 9-inch (23 cm) round baking pan, lightly greased and bottom lined with parchment paper

⅔ cup	sorghum flour	150 mL
½ cup	whole bean flour	125 mL
2 tbsp	tapioca starch	25 mL
1½ tsp	xanthan gum	7 mL
1 tbsp	GF baking powder	15 mL
½ tsp	baking soda	2 mL
¼ tsp	salt	1 mL
2 oz	milk or semisweet chocolate, chopped	60 g
¼ cup	water	50 mL
1	egg	1
¾ cup	white (granulated) sugar	175 mL
1 cup	buttermilk	250 mL
¼ cup	butter, softened	50 mL
1 tsp	vanilla extract	5 mL

1. In a small bowl or plastic bag, combine sorghum flour, whole bean flour, tapioca starch, xanthan gum, baking powder, baking soda and salt. Mix well and set aside.

2. In a microwave-safe bowl, microwave chocolate and water, uncovered, on Medium (50%) for 60 to 90 seconds or until partially melted. Stir until completely melted. Let cool to room temperature.

3. In a separate bowl, using an electric mixer, beat egg, sugar, buttermilk, butter and vanilla until combined. With mixer on low speed, beat in cooled melted chocolate until combined. Add dry ingredients and mix until just combined.

4. Spoon batter into prepared pan. Using a moistened rubber spatula, spread to edges and smooth top. Let stand for 30 minutes. Meanwhile, preheat oven to 350°F (180°C).

5. Bake for 30 to 35 minutes or until a tester inserted in the center comes out clean. Let cool in pan on a rack for 10 minutes. Remove from pan and let cool completely on rack.

Best-Ever Chocolate Oat Cake

Beth Armour of Cream Hill Estates developed this recipe and has given us permission to include it in our cookbook for you. Beth tells us the original recipe came from **Eat Hearty** *(Margolese and Margolese); she modified it to make it gluten-free. It is moister than a regular chocolate cake, but has a cake-like texture.*

• 13- by 9-inch (33 by 23 cm) baking pan, lightly greased

1¼ cups	GF oat flour	300 mL
1 tsp	xanthan gum	5 mL
1½ tsp	GF baking powder	7 mL
¼ tsp	salt	1 mL
⅓ cup	unsweetened cocoa powder, sifted	75 mL
1 tsp	ground cinnamon	5 mL
3	eggs	3
1 cup	white (granulated) sugar	250 mL
¾ cup	vegetable oil	175 mL
¾ cup	milk	175 mL
1½ tsp	vanilla extract	7 mL

1. In a large bowl or plastic bag, combine oat flour, xanthan gum, baking powder, salt, cocoa and cinnamon. Mix well and set aside.

2. In a separate bowl, using an electric mixer, beat eggs, sugar, oil, milk and vanilla until combined. Add dry ingredients and mix until just combined.

3. Spoon batter into prepared pan. Using a moistened rubber spatula, spread to edges and smooth top. Let stand for 30 minutes. Meanwhile, preheat oven to 350°F (180°C).

4. Bake for 30 to 40 minutes or until a cake tester inserted in the center comes out clean. Let cool completely in pan on rack.

Variations

Add ¾ cup (175 mL) chopped nuts — try almonds, pecans or hazelnuts

Frost with your favorite chocolate frosting.

Nutritional value per serving

Calories	267
Fat, total	16 g
Fat, saturated	2 g
Cholesterol	47 mg
Sodium	72 mg
Carbohydrate	28 g
Fiber	2 g
Protein	4 g
Calcium	66 mg
Iron	2 mg

Bumbleberry Upside-Down Cake

Did you know that "bumbleberry" means a mixture of different kinds of berries? Plan to use a variety of seasonal fresh berries.

Tips

We like to use a mixture of blackberries, blueberries, strawberries and/or raspberries.

If you don't have a deep baking pan, place a baking sheet on the oven rack below, in case the berries boil over.

We tried this recipe with both high-fat and lower-fat yogurt; both worked fine. Try some of the newer flavors of yogurt, such as field berry.

Nutritional value per serving	
Calories	217
Fat, total	9 g
Fat, saturated	2 g
Cholesterol	21 mg
Sodium	144 mg
Carbohydrate	33 g
Fiber	2 g
Protein	3 g
Calcium	78 mg
Iron	1 mg

- Preheat oven to 350°F (180°C)
- 9-inch (23 cm) round, deep baking pan, lightly greased

Bumbleberry Base

3 cups	mixed berries	750 mL
1/3 cup	packed brown sugar	75 mL
2 tbsp	butter, melted	25 mL

Cake

3/4 cup	sorghum flour	175 mL
1/2 cup	pecan flour	125 mL
1/4 cup	tapioca starch	50 mL
1 1/2 tsp	xanthan gum	7 mL
2 tsp	GF baking powder	10 mL
1/2 tsp	baking soda	2 mL
1/4 tsp	salt	1 mL
1	egg	1
1/2 cup	white (granulated) sugar	125 mL
1 1/3 cups	berry-flavored yogurt	325 mL
1/3 cup	vegetable oil	75 mL
1 1/2 tsp	vanilla extract	7 mL

1. *Bumbleberry base:* In prepared pan, combine berries, brown sugar and butter. Spread evenly to edges. Set aside.

2. *Cake:* In a large bowl or plastic bag, combine sorghum flour, pecan flour, tapioca starch, xanthan gum, baking powder, baking soda and salt. Mix well and set aside.

3. In a separate bowl, using an electric mixer, beat egg, sugar, yogurt, oil and vanilla until combined. Add dry ingredients and mix until just combined. Carefully spoon over berries. Spread to edges and smooth top with a rubber spatula.

4. Bake in preheated oven for 35 to 40 minutes or until a cake tester inserted in the center comes out clean. Let cool in pan on rack for 10 minutes. Invert onto a serving plate, slice into wedges and serve warm.

Cranberry Crumble Coffee Cake

Makes 9 to 12 servings

Each slice of this beautiful cake is dotted with bright red cranberries and flavored with a hint of orange.

- 9-inch (23 cm) square baking pan, lightly greased and bottom lined with parchment paper

Pecan Topping

¾ cup	finely chopped pecans	175 mL
⅓ cup	packed brown sugar	75 mL
2 tbsp	amaranth flour	25 mL
2 tbsp	butter, melted	25 mL

Coffee Cake

1⅓ cups	sorghum flour	325 mL
⅓ cup	quinoa flour	75 mL
¼ cup	tapioca starch	50 mL
1½ tsp	xanthan gum	7 mL
1 tbsp	GF baking powder	15 mL
¼ tsp	salt	1 mL
1 tsp	ground cardamom	5 mL
1	egg	1
⅔ cup	packed brown sugar	150 mL
1 tbsp	grated orange zest	15 mL
1 cup	freshly squeezed orange juice	250 mL
¼ cup	vegetable oil	50 mL
2 cups	fresh or partially thawed frozen cranberries	500 mL

1. *Pecan topping:* In a small bowl, combine pecans, brown sugar, amaranth flour and butter. Set aside.

2. *Coffee cake:* In a large bowl or plastic bag, combine sorghum flour, quinoa flour, tapioca starch, xanthan gum, baking powder, salt and cardamom. Mix well and set aside.

3. In a separate bowl, using an electric mixer, beat egg, brown sugar, orange zest, orange juice and oil. Add dry ingredients and mix until just combined. Fold in cranberries.

Nutritional value per serving

Calories	284
Fat, total	13 g
Fat, saturated	2 g
Cholesterol	21 mg
Sodium	82 mg
Carbohydrate	41 g
Fiber	3 g
Protein	4 g
Calcium	90 mg
Iron	2 mg

Tip

To partially thaw frozen cranberries, place them in a single layer on a microwave-safe plate. Microwave on High for 2 minutes, stirring every 30 seconds.

4. Spoon batter into prepared pan. Using a moistened rubber spatula, spread to edges and smooth top. Sprinkle with topping. Let stand for 30 minutes. Meanwhile, preheat oven to 350°F (180°C).

5. Bake for 30 to 40 minutes or until a tester inserted in the center comes out clean. Let cool in pan on a rack for 10 minutes. Remove from pan and let cool completely on rack.

Variation

Replace ¼ cup (50 mL) of the orange juice with thawed frozen cranberry juice concentrate.

Banana Streusel Coffee Cake

Everyone will go bananas over this quick and easy treat.

- 9-inch (23 cm) round baking pan, lightly greased and bottom lined with parchment paper

Topping

2 tbsp	packed brown sugar	25 mL
¼ cup	almond flour	50 mL
¼ tsp	ground allspice	1 mL
1 tbsp	butter, melted	15 mL

Cake

1 cup	sorghum flour	250 mL
½ cup	amaranth flour	125 mL
2 tbsp	tapioca starch	25 mL
⅓ cup	packed brown sugar	75 mL
1½ tsp	xanthan gum	7 mL
1 tbsp	GF baking powder	15 mL
¼ tsp	salt	1 mL
½ tsp	ground allspice	2 mL
2	eggs	2
1¼ cups	mashed banana	300 mL
¼ cup	water	50 mL
3 tbsp	vegetable oil	45 mL
1 tsp	cider vinegar	5 mL
1 tsp	vanilla extract	5 mL

1. *Topping:* In a small bowl, combine brown sugar, almond flour, allspice and butter until crumbly. Set aside.

2. *Cake:* In a large bowl or plastic bag, combine sorghum flour, amaranth flour, tapioca starch, brown sugar, xanthan gum, baking powder, salt and allspice. Mix well and set aside.

3. In a separate bowl, using an electric mixer, beat eggs, banana, water, oil, vinegar and vanilla until combined. Add dry ingredients and mix until just combined.

Bake in the center of the oven.

We found that the bottom browned a lot quicker when we used a modern thin cake pan than it did with an older, heavier one.

4. Spoon batter into prepared pan. Using a moistened rubber spatula, spread to edges and smooth top. Sprinkle with topping. Let stand for 30 minutes. Meanwhile, preheat oven to 350°F (180°C).

5. Bake for 32 to 36 minutes or until a tester inserted in the center comes out clean. Let cool in pan on a rack for 10 minutes. Serve warm or at room temperature.

Variations

To make a spicier version, add $\frac{1}{2}$ tsp (2 mL) ground cinnamon, an extra $\frac{1}{4}$ tsp (1 mL) ground allspice and a pinch of ground nutmeg to the cake.

For a glaze: In a small bowl, combine $\frac{1}{2}$ cup (125 mL) sifted GF confectioner's (icing) sugar and 2 to 3 tsp (10 to 15 mL) milk to make a thin glaze. Drizzle over partially cooled coffee cake.

Pear Pecan Coffee Cake

With its delicate pear flavor, this coffee cake is a tasty way to add fiber to your diet.

- 9-inch (23 cm) round baking pan, lightly greased and bottom lined with parchment paper

Topping

1/2 cup	chopped toasted pecans	125 mL
1/4 cup	pecan meal	50 mL
2 tbsp	packed brown sugar	25 mL
1/4 tsp	ground mace	1 mL
1 tbsp	butter, melted	15 mL

Cake

1 cup	sorghum flour	250 mL
1/2 cup	whole bean flour	125 mL
1/4 cup	cornstarch	50 mL
1/3 cup	packed brown sugar	75 mL
1 1/2 tsp	xanthan gum	7 mL
1 tbsp	GF baking powder	15 mL
1/4 tsp	salt	1 mL
1/2 tsp	ground mace	2 mL
1 cup	diced drained canned pears, juice reserved	250 mL
2	eggs	2
3 tbsp	vegetable oil	45 mL
1 tsp	cider vinegar	5 mL
1 tsp	vanilla extract	5 mL
1/2 cup	chopped toasted pecans	125 mL

1. *Topping:* In a small bowl, combine pecans, pecan meal, brown sugar, mace and butter until crumbly. Set aside.

2. *Cake:* In a large bowl or plastic bag, combine sorghum flour, whole bean flour, cornstarch, brown sugar, xanthan gum, baking powder, salt and mace. Mix well and set aside.

3. Pour drained pear juice into a liquid measuring cup. Add enough water to equal 1 cup (250 mL).

4. In a separate bowl, using an electric mixer, beat pear juice, eggs, oil, vinegar and vanilla until combined. Add dry ingredients and mix until just combined. Stir in pears and pecans.

Nutritional value per serving

Calories	183
Fat, total	11 g
Fat, saturated	1 g
Cholesterol	25 mg
Sodium	56 mg
Carbohydrate	21 g
Fiber	2 g
Protein	3 g
Calcium	63 mg
Iron	1 mg

Tip

Purchase a 14-oz (398 mL) can of pears. Drain pears well to avoid adding extra liquid, which would result in a too-moist batter.

5. Spoon batter into prepared pan. Using a moistened rubber spatula, spread to edges and smooth top. Sprinkle with topping. Let stand for 30 minutes. Meanwhile, preheat oven to 350°F (180°C).

6. Bake for 40 to 45 minutes or until a tester inserted in the center comes out clean. Let cool completely in pan on a rack.

Variations

To make a spicier version, add $\frac{1}{2}$ tsp (2 mL) ground cinnamon, an extra $\frac{1}{4}$ tsp (1 mL) ground mace and a pinch of ground nutmeg to the cake.

Substitute $1\frac{1}{4}$ cups (300 mL) diced fresh pears for the canned and pear nectar for the pear juice.

Almond Fig Cake

Makes 14 to 16 servings

This Mediterranean cake uses extra virgin olive oil rather than vegetable oil.

• 9-inch (23 cm) Bundt pan, lightly greased

Topping

1/2 cup	sliced almonds	125 mL
2 tbsp	packed brown sugar	25 mL
1 tsp	ground cinnamon	5 mL
1 tbsp	butter, melted	15 mL

Cake

1 3/4 cups	diced dried figs	425 mL
2 tbsp	grated orange zest	25 mL
1 cup	freshly squeezed orange juice	250 mL
1 cup	sorghum flour	250 mL
2/3 cup	pea flour	150 mL
1/4 cup	tapioca starch	50 mL
1 1/2 tsp	xanthan gum	7 mL
2 tsp	GF baking powder	10 mL
1/2 tsp	baking soda	2 mL
1/2 tsp	salt	2 mL
2	eggs	2
1 cup	white (granulated) sugar	250 mL
1 cup	GF sour cream	250 mL
1/2 cup	extra virgin olive oil	125 mL
1 tbsp	almond extract	15 mL

1. *Topping:* In a small bowl, combine almonds, brown sugar, cinnamon and butter until crumbly. Set aside.

2. *Cake:* In a saucepan, combine figs, orange zest and orange juice. Bring to a boil over high heat. Reduce heat to medium-low and simmer for 4 to 5 minutes or until thickened and juice is almost completely absorbed. Let cool to room temperature.

3. In a large bowl or plastic bag, combine sorghum flour, pea flour, tapioca starch, xanthan gum, baking powder, baking soda and salt. Mix well and set aside.

4. In a separate bowl, using an electric mixer, beat fig mixture, eggs, sugar, sour cream, oil and almond extract until combined. Add dry ingredients and mix until just combined.

Nutritional value per serving

Calories	291
Fat, total	10 g
Fat, saturated	2 g
Cholesterol	27 mg
Sodium	144 mg
Carbohydrate	46 g
Fiber	4 g
Protein	5 g
Calcium	101 mg
Iron	1 mg

You'll need about 18 figs for 1¾ cups (425 mL) diced. Trim off the stems before dicing.

5. Spoon batter into prepared pan. Using a moistened rubber spatula, spread to edges and smooth top. Sprinkle with topping. Let stand for 30 minutes. Meanwhile, preheat oven to 350°F (180°C).

6. Bake for 35 to 40 minutes or until a tester inserted in the center comes out clean. Let cool in pan on a rack for 10 minutes. Remove from pan and let cool completely on rack.

Variations

Substitute 1¾ cups (425 mL) snipped dates for the figs. Any bean flour can be substituted for the pea flour.

Orange Almond Snacking Cake

Makes 12 servings

A CanolaInfo recipe

This moist cake is perfect to carry to a family get-together or celiac meeting. If desired, drizzle with Orange Cream Cheese Icing (page 328).

Tips

We use kitchen shears to snip whole apricots and dates into eighths, dipping the shears in hot water as they become sticky.

If you purchase chopped dates, check for wheat starch in the coating.

For information on toasting nuts, see the Techniques Glossary, page 398.

Nutritional value per serving

Calories	286
Fat, total	13 g
Fat, saturated	1 g
Cholesterol	31 mg
Sodium	220 mg
Carbohydrate	39 g
Fiber	4 g
Protein	6 g
Calcium	115 mg
Iron	3 mg

- 9-inch (23 cm) square baking pan, lightly greased and bottom lined with parchment paper

⅔ cup	sorghum flour	150 mL
½ cup	amaranth flour	125 mL
⅓ cup	almond flour	75 mL
¼ cup	tapioca starch	50 mL
1½ tsp	xanthan gum	7 mL
1 tbsp	GF baking powder	15 mL
1 tsp	baking soda	5 mL
½ tsp	salt	2 mL
2	eggs	2
½ cup	packed brown sugar	125 mL
2 tbsp	grated orange zest	25 mL
1 cup	freshly squeezed orange juice	250 mL
⅓ cup	vegetable oil	75 mL
1 tsp	almond extract	5 mL
¾ cup	slivered toasted almonds	175 mL
¾ cup	snipped dried apricots	175 mL
¾ cup	snipped dates	175 mL

1. In a large bowl or plastic bag, combine sorghum flour, amaranth flour, almond flour, tapioca starch, xanthan gum, baking powder, baking soda and salt. Mix well and set aside.

2. In a separate bowl, using an electric mixer, beat eggs, brown sugar, orange zest, orange juice, oil and almond extract until combined. Add dry ingredients and mix until just combined. Stir in almonds, apricots and dates.

3. Spoon batter into a prepared pan. Using a moistened rubber spatula, spread to edges and smooth top. Let stand for 30 minutes. Meanwhile, preheat oven to 350°F (180°C).

4. Bake for 40 to 50 minutes or until a tester inserted in the center comes out clean. Let cool completely in pan on a rack.

Lime Poppy Seed Cake

Serve this cake with fresh strawberries. It could become your new base for strawberry shortcake.

Tips

Two limes will yield about ¼ cup (50 mL) juice.

Before removing the sides of the springform pan, run a knife around the inside edge.

• 9-inch (23 cm) springform pan, lightly greased

1¼ cups	sorghum flour	300 mL
½ cup	pea flour	125 mL
¼ cup	tapioca starch	50 mL
1½ tsp	xanthan gum	7 mL
1 tbsp	GF baking powder	15 mL
½ tsp	baking soda	2 mL
¼ tsp	salt	1 mL
⅓ cup	poppy seeds	75 mL
2	eggs	2
¾ cup	white (granulated) sugar	175 mL
1 cup	plain yogurt	250 mL
⅓ cup	vegetable oil	75 mL
2 tsp	grated lime zest	10 mL
¼ cup	freshly squeezed lime juice	50 mL
1 tsp	vanilla extract	5 mL

1. In a large bowl or plastic bag, combine sorghum flour, pea flour, tapioca starch, xanthan gum, baking powder, baking soda, salt and poppy seeds. Mix well and set aside.

2. In a separate bowl, using an electric mixer, beat eggs, sugar, yogurt, oil, lime zest, lime juice and vanilla until combined. Add dry ingredients and mix until just combined.

3. Spoon batter into prepared pan. Using a moistened rubber spatula, spread to edges and smooth top. Let stand for 30 minutes. Meanwhile, preheat oven to 350°F (180°C).

4. Bake for 35 to 45 minutes or until a tester inserted in the center comes out clean. Let cool in pan on a rack for 5 minutes. Remove sides of pan, slice cake into wedges and serve warm.

Variation

Any bean flour can be substituted for the pea flour.

Nutritional value per serving

Calories	171
Fat, total	7 g
Fat, saturated	1 g
Cholesterol	24 mg
Sodium	96 mg
Carbohydrate	24 g
Fiber	2 g
Protein	4 g
Calcium	122 mg
Iron	1 mg

Lemon Ginger Almond Cake

Makes 9 to 12 servings

This ginger cake has a texture similar to that of pound cake. Served with Tangy Lemon Sauce, it makes a great dessert for company.

Tip

For information on toasting nuts, see the Techniques Glossary, page 398.

- 9-inch (23 cm) square baking pan, lightly greased and bottom lined with parchment paper

Cake

1¼ cups	sorghum flour	300 mL
⅓ cup	almond flour	75 mL
⅓ cup	tapioca starch	75 mL
1½ tsp	xanthan gum	7 mL
1 tbsp	GF baking powder	15 mL
½ tsp	baking soda	2 mL
¼ tsp	salt	1 mL
½ cup	slivered almonds, toasted	125 mL
⅓ cup	grated lemon zest	75 mL
1 tbsp	coarsely chopped gingerroot	15 mL
1	egg	1
⅔ cup	white (granulated) sugar	150 mL
1¼ cups	GF sour cream	300 mL
⅓ cup	vegetable oil	75 mL
1 tsp	almond extract	5 mL

Tangy Lemon Sauce

⅔ cup	packed brown sugar	150 mL
2 tbsp	cornstarch	25 mL
3 tbsp	butter	45 mL
½ cup	freshly squeezed lemon juice	125 mL
½ cup	slivered almonds, toasted	125 mL

1. *Cake:* In a large bowl or plastic bag, combine sorghum flour, almond flour, tapioca starch, xanthan gum, baking powder, baking soda and salt. Mix well and set aside.

2. In a food processor, pulse almonds, lemon zest and ginger until very coarsely chopped. Set aside.

3. In a separate bowl, using an electric mixer, beat egg, sugar, sour cream, oil and almond extract until combined. Add dry ingredients and almond mixture; mix until just combined.

Nutritional value per serving

Calories	364
Fat, total	17 g
Fat, saturated	3 g
Cholesterol	25 mg
Sodium	165 mg
Carbohydrate	48 g
Fiber	3 g
Protein	7 g
Calcium	146 mg
Iron	2 mg

Tips

Two lemons will yield about $\frac{1}{3}$ cup (75 mL) zest and 2 to 3 tbsp (25 to 45 mL) juice. Remove the zest when the lemon is cold, and warm the lemon before juicing.

The coarser the almond-ginger mixture, the more texture it provides for the cake.

4. Spoon batter into prepared pan. Using a moistened rubber spatula, spread to edges and smooth top. Let stand for 30 minutes. Meanwhile, preheat oven to 350°F (180°C).

5. Bake for 30 to 35 minutes or until a tester inserted in the center comes out clean. Let cool in pan on a rack for 10 minutes.

6. *Tangy Lemon Sauce:* In a small bowl, combine brown sugar and cornstarch. In a small saucepan, melt butter over medium heat. Add brown sugar mixture and lemon juice. Heat, stirring constantly, until mixture comes to a boil, becomes shiny and thickens slightly. Remove from heat.

7. Cut cake into pieces and serve warm, topped with lemon sauce and almonds.

Variations

If gingerroot is not available, substitute 3 tbsp (45 mL) crystallized or candied ginger.

Substitute buttermilk for the GF sour cream.

Orange Pumpkin Cake

Makes 9 to 12 servings

No time to make a pumpkin pie for Thanksgiving dinner? Try this cake instead. Serve topped with Orange Cream Cheese Icing (page 328).

- 9-inch (23 cm) square baking pan, lightly greased and bottom lined with parchment paper

1 cup	sorghum flour	250 mL
¾ cup	whole bean flour	175 mL
¼ cup	tapioca starch	50 mL
1½ tsp	xanthan gum	7 mL
1 tbsp	GF baking powder	15 mL
½ tsp	baking soda	2 mL
¼ tsp	salt	1 mL
1 tsp	ground cinnamon	5 mL
½ tsp	ground allspice	2 mL
½ tsp	ground nutmeg	2 mL
¼ tsp	ground cloves	1 mL
2	eggs	2
1 cup	pumpkin purée (not pie filling)	250 mL
½ cup	packed brown sugar	125 mL
2 tbsp	grated orange zest	25 mL
½ cup	freshly squeezed orange juice	125 mL
¼ cup	vegetable oil	50 mL

1. In a large bowl or plastic bag, combine sorghum flour, whole bean flour, tapioca starch, xanthan gum, baking powder, baking soda, salt, cinnamon, allspice, nutmeg and cloves. Mix well and set aside.

2. In a separate bowl, using an electric mixer, beat eggs, pumpkin purée, brown sugar, orange zest, orange juice and oil until combined. Add dry ingredients and mix until just combined.

3. Spoon batter into prepared pan. Using a moistened rubber spatula, spread to edges and smooth top. Let stand for 30 minutes. Meanwhile, preheat oven to 350°F (180°C).

Nutritional value per serving

Calories	163
Fat, total	6 g
Fat, saturated	1 g
Cholesterol	31 mg
Sodium	117 mg
Carbohydrate	26 g
Fiber	2 g
Protein	3 g
Calcium	86 mg
Iron	1 mg

Be sure to purchase pumpkin purée; pumpkin pie filling is too sweet and contains too much moisture for this snacking cake.

4. Bake for 25 to 30 minutes or until a cake tester inserted in the center comes out clean. Let cool in pan on a rack for 10 minutes. Remove from pan and let cool completely on rack.

Variations

Substitute 2 to 3 tsp (10 to 15 mL) GF pumpkin pie spice for the individual spices.

Add ¾ cup (175 mL) green pumpkin seeds or 1 cup (250 mL) snipped dates.

Chocolate Zucchini Cake

Makes 9 to 12 servings

A CanolaInfo recipe

Who would have thought that something so rich as this Chocolate Zucchini Cake could be labeled as healthy? No one will guess that there are hidden vegetables.

- 8-inch (20 cm) square baking pan, lightly greased and bottom lined with parchment paper

⅔ cup	sorghum flour	150 mL
¼ cup	quinoa flour	50 mL
2 tbsp	tapioca starch	25 mL
1½ tsp	xanthan gum	7 mL
2 tsp	GF baking powder	10 mL
½ tsp	baking soda	2 mL
¼ tsp	salt	1 mL
1 tbsp	grated orange zest	15 mL
½ tsp	ground ginger	2 mL
⅓ cup	unsweetened cocoa powder, sifted	75 mL
1	egg	1
1 cup	shredded zucchini	250 mL
¾ cup	white (granulated) sugar	175 mL
⅓ cup	vegetable oil	75 mL
¼ cup	freshly squeezed orange juice	50 mL
1 tsp	vanilla extract	5 mL
1 cup	mini semisweet chocolate chips	250 mL

1. In a large bowl or plastic bag, combine sorghum flour, quinoa flour, tapioca starch, xanthan gum, baking powder, baking soda, salt, orange zest, ginger and cocoa. Mix well and set aside.

2. In a separate bowl, using an electric mixer, beat egg, zucchini, sugar, oil, orange juice and vanilla until combined. Add dry ingredients and mix until just combined. Stir in chocolate chips.

3. Spoon batter into prepared pan. Using a moistened rubber spatula, spread to edges and smooth top. Let stand for 30 minutes. Meanwhile, preheat oven to 350°F (180°C).

Nutritional value per serving

Calories	235
Fat, total	12 g
Fat, saturated	3 g
Cholesterol	19 mg
Sodium	168 mg
Carbohydrate	33 g
Fiber	3 g
Protein	3 g
Calcium	76 mg
Iron	1 mg

Tips

To save time and add fiber to the cake, leave the zucchini peel on.

Drain any accumulated liquid from the shredded zucchini (but do not squeeze dry).

4. Bake for 35 to 45 minutes or until a tester inserted in the center comes out clean. Let cool in pan on a rack for 10 minutes. Remove from pan and let cool completely on rack.

Variation

If quinoa flour is not available, substitute an equal amount of brown rice flour.

Peanut Butter Chocolate Molten Cakes

Makes 6 servings

These individual peanut butter chocolate treats are a close relative of the molten lava cake, oozing with bittersweet chocolate and peanut butter. Serve garnished with seasonal fresh fruit.

Tips

After step 2, the cakes can be refrigerated for up to 4 hours. Let come to room temperature (about 45 minutes) before baking.

The baking time is critical; even 1 extra minute will cause the center to become solid instead of molten and the top crust to burn.

- Preheat oven to 425°F (220°C)
- Six ¾-cup (175 mL) ramekins or ceramic soufflé dishes, generously buttered

4 oz	bittersweet chocolate, chopped	125 g
½ cup	butter	125 mL
1 cup	GF confectioner's (icing) sugar, sifted	250 mL
4	eggs, at room temperature, lightly beaten	4
⅓ cup	sorghum flour	75 mL
½ tsp	xanthan gum	2 mL
⅓ cup	GF crunchy peanut butter	75 mL

1. In a large microwave-safe bowl, microwave chocolate and butter, uncovered, on Medium (50%) for 2 to 3 minutes, or until partially melted. Stir until completely melted. Add confectioner's sugar and mix well. Whisk in eggs. Stir in sorghum flour and xanthan gum.

2. Place prepared dishes on a baking sheet. Half-fill each ramekin with batter and spoon 1 tbsp (15 mL) peanut butter into the center of the batter in each cup. Cover with the remaining batter.

3. Bake in preheated oven for 12 minutes or until sides are firm but center is still soft. Let cool on a rack for 1 to 3 minutes.

4. Run a knife around the inside edge of each ramekin to loosen. Cover each ramekin with a dessert plate and invert. Carefully remove hot ramekins and serve immediately. (Or serve right in the ramekins, hot from the oven.)

Nutritional value per serving	
Calories	479
Fat, total	33 g
Fat, saturated	16 g
Cholesterol	168 mg
Sodium	202 mg
Carbohydrate	40 g
Fiber	3 g
Protein	9 g
Calcium	28 mg
Iron	1 mg

Maple Walnut Cupcakes

Makes 6 cupcakes (1 per serving)

These tasty little morsels make perfect individual servings on special occasions when a large cake is just too much. They're also great packed into your lunch for days when you deserve a treat.

Tips

Fill the muffin cups almost level with the top.

Let cupcakes cool completely, wrap individually and freeze for up to 1 month.

Recipe can be doubled.

For an extra hit of maple and walnuts, frost with Maple Buttercream Frosting (page 329), then sprinkle with chopped walnuts.

Nutritional value per serving

Calories	246
Fat, total	12 g
Fat, saturated	1 g
Cholesterol	5 mg
Sodium	229 mg
Carbohydrate	31 g
Fiber	2 g
Protein	6 g
Calcium	85 mg
Iron	2 mg

- **6-cup muffin tin, lightly greased**

½ cup	sorghum flour	125 mL
¼ cup	amaranth flour	50 mL
¼ cup	tapioca starch	50 mL
1 tsp	xanthan gum	5 mL
1 tsp	GF baking powder	5 mL
½ tsp	baking soda	2 mL
¼ tsp	salt	1 mL
¼ tsp	ground ginger	1 mL
½ cup	coarsely chopped toasted walnuts	125 mL
1	egg	1
⅓ cup	buttermilk	75 mL
⅓ cup	pure maple syrup	75 mL
2 tbsp	vegetable oil	25 mL
1½ tsp	maple extract	7 mL

1. In a large bowl or plastic bag, combine sorghum flour, amaranth flour, tapioca starch, xanthan gum, baking powder, baking soda, salt, ginger and walnuts. Mix well and set aside.

2. In a separate bowl, using an electric mixer, beat egg, buttermilk, maple syrup, oil and maple extract until combined. Add dry ingredients and mix until just combined.

3. Spoon batter evenly into prepared muffin cups. Let stand for 30 minutes. Meanwhile, preheat oven to 350°F (180°C).

4. Bake for 20 to 23 minutes or until a tester inserted in the center of a cupcake comes out clean. Let cool in pan on a rack for 5 minutes. Remove from pan and let cool completely on rack.

Variation
Substitute GF sour cream (lactose-free or regular), or a flavored yogurt (lactose-free or regular), for the buttermilk.

Brown Sugar Sauce

Egg-free
White sugar–free

**Makes 2 cups (500 mL)
(2 tbsp/25 mL per
serving)**

*Keep a Basic White
Cake (page 372) or
Golden Pound Cake
(page 304) in your
freezer for those times
when you need a
dessert in a hurry, and
smother it with this
quick and easy sauce
to make a cottage
pudding.*

Tip

Cook this sauce in a large
saucepan, as it could boil
over.

¾ cup	packed brown sugar	175 mL
3 tbsp	cornstarch	45 mL
¼ tsp	salt	1 mL
2 cups	water	500 mL
¼ cup	butter	50 mL
1 tsp	vanilla extract	5 mL

1. In a large saucepan, combine brown sugar, cornstarch
and salt. Gradually add water, stirring constantly. Bring
to a boil over medium-high heat, stirring constantly.
Boil for 3 minutes. Remove from heat. Stir in butter
and vanilla. Serve hot.

Variation

To turn this into a hot rum sauce, add 3 tbsp (45 mL) dark
rum and ¼ tsp (1 mL) ground nutmeg with the butter.

Nutritional value per serving

Calories	53
Fat, total	2 g
Fat, saturated	1 g
Cholesterol	5 mg
Sodium	52 mg
Carbohydrate	9 g
Fiber	0 g
Protein	0 g
Calcium	8 mg
Iron	0 mg

Lemon Yogurt Cream

Egg-free

**Makes 1¼ cups
(300 mL)
(¼ cup/50 mL per
serving)**

*Enjoy this low-calorie
sauce over our Golden
Pound Cake (page
304) as a change from
the sweeter Brown
Sugar Sauce (page
326).*

Tips

To drain yogurt, place
2 cups (500 mL) yogurt in
a cheesecloth-lined sieve
set over a bowl. Refrigerate
for 3 hours or overnight,
until reduced to 1 cup
(250 mL).

Balkan-style, no-gelatin or
plain yogurt work well.

1 cup	drained plain yogurt (see tip, at left)	250 mL
⅓ cup	white (granulated) sugar	75 mL
2 tbsp	grated lemon zest	25 mL
1 tbsp	freshly squeezed lemon juice	15 mL

1. In a small bowl, combine yogurt, sugar, lemon zest and
   lemon juice, stirring well.
2. Cover and refrigerate for at least 1 hour, until chilled,
   or for up to 3 days.

Variation
Fold in fresh or thawed frozen raspberries just before
serving.

Nutritional value per serving

Calories	85
Fat, total	1 g
Fat, saturated	1 g
Cholesterol	3 mg
Sodium	35 mg
Carbohydrate	17 g
Fiber	0 g
Protein	3 g
Calcium	93 mg
Iron	0 mg

Orange Cream Cheese Icing

Makes 9 to 12 servings, or enough to frost one 9-inch (23 cm) cake

Spread this icing on Orange Pumpkin Cake (page 320) or Orange Almond Snacking Cake (page 316).

Tips

To soften an 8-oz (250 g) package of cream cheese quickly, cut it into 1-inch (2.5 cm) cubes, arrange them in a circle on a microwave-safe plate and microwave on High for 1 minute.

Make sure your cake has cooled completely before spreading icing on it.

1	package (8 oz/250 g) light or regular brick cream cheese, softened	1
½ cup	sifted GF confectioner's (icing) sugar	125 mL
2 tbsp	grated orange zest	25 mL
2 tbsp	freshly squeezed orange juice	25 mL

1. In a small bowl, using an electric mixer, beat cream cheese, confectioner's sugar, orange zest and orange juice until light and fluffy.

Variations

For a stronger orange flavor, substitute thawed frozen orange juice concentrate for the freshly squeezed orange juice.

Nutritional value per serving	
Calories	89
Fat, total	7 g
Fat, saturated	4 g
Cholesterol	20 mg
Sodium	61 mg
Carbohydrate	6 g
Fiber	0 g
Protein	1 g
Calcium	2 mg
Iron	0 mg

Maple Buttercream Frosting

*Top each Maple Walnut
Cupcake (page 325)
with a dollop of this
frosting.*

Tips

Sifting the confectioner's
(icing) sugar before
measuring helps prevent
lumps in the frosting.

Check to make sure your
confectioner's (icing)
sugar is gluten-free. It can
contain up to 5% starch,
which could be from
wheat.

Make sure your cake or
cupcakes have cooled
completely before
spreading frosting on
them.

Double or triple the recipe
to frost a layer cake.

1 cup	sifted GF confectioner's (icing) sugar	250 mL
¼ cup	butter, softened	50 mL
2 tbsp	pure maple syrup	25 mL
½ tsp	maple extract	2 mL

1. In a bowl, using an electric mixer, beat confectioner's
sugar, butter, maple syrup and maple extract until
smooth and creamy.

Variation
For a lighter frosting, fold in 1 cup (250 mL) whipped cream.

Nutritional value per serving	
Calories	91
Fat, total	4 g
Fat, saturated	2 g
Cholesterol	10 mg
Sodium	39 mg
Carbohydrate	15 g
Fiber	0 g
Protein	0 g
Calcium	4 mg
Iron	0 mg

White Chocolate Lime Glaze

*Drizzle this glaze over
slices of Lime Poppy
Seed Cake (page 317),
a chocolate fudge cake
or fresh fruit.*

Tips

This glaze can be
made up to 1 day in
advance and stored in an
airtight container in the
refrigerator. Bring it to
room temperature, or heat
gently on Low (10%) in the
microwave, before serving.

We keep extra lime zest
and juice in the freezer, so
it is handy for occasions
when we need only a small
amount.

½ cup	whipping (35%) cream	125 mL
4 oz	white chocolate, finely chopped	125 g
½ tsp	ground ginger	2 mL
1 tsp	finely grated lime zest	5 mL
1 tsp	freshly squeezed lime juice	5 mL

1. Place cream in a microwave-safe bowl and microwave
   on High for 1 to 2 minutes or until tiny bubbles form
   around the edge. Stir in white chocolate, ginger, lime
   zest and lime juice until well combined. Serve warm
   or let cool to room temperature.

Nutritional value per serving	
Calories	271
Fat, total	19 g
Fat, saturated	12 g
Cholesterol	33 mg
Sodium	41 mg
Carbohydrate	24 g
Fiber	0 g
Protein	3 g
Calcium	89 mg
Iron	0 mg

Pies and Other Desserts

Peach Pecan Pie with Raspberry Glaze

- Preheat oven to 350°F (180°C)
- 9-inch (23 cm) tart pan with removable bottom, lightly greased

Raspberry Glaze

2 cups	raspberries, mashed	500 mL
1/2 cup	white (granulated) sugar	125 mL
3 tbsp	cornstarch	45 mL
1/4 cup	water	50 mL

Pecan Crust

3/4 cup	pecan flour	175 mL
1/2 cup	brown rice flour	125 mL
1/4 cup	tapioca starch	50 mL
1/2 tsp	xanthan gum	2 mL
1/4 tsp	salt	1 mL
1/3 cup	white (granulated) sugar	75 mL
1/3 cup	cold butter, cut into 1-inch (2.5 cm) pieces	75 mL
2	egg yolks, lightly beaten	2

Peach Filling

1	package (8 oz/250 g) light or regular brick cream cheese, softened	1
4 cups	sliced peaches	1 L

1. *Raspberry glaze:* In a saucepan, combine berries, sugar and cornstarch. Stir in water. Cook over medium heat, stirring constantly, until mixture comes to a boil, thickens and becomes shiny. Let cool to room temperature.

2. *Pecan crust:* In a food processor, pulse pecan flour, brown rice flour, tapioca starch, xanthan gum, salt and sugar 3 or 4 times to combine. Add butter and pulse for 5 to 10 seconds or until mixture resembles coarse crumbs about the size of small peas. Add egg yolks and pulse until the dough holds together.

Nutritional value per serving	
Calories	210
Fat, total	9 g
Fat, saturated	5 g
Cholesterol	57 mg
Sodium	188 mg
Carbohydrate	29 g
Fiber	2 g
Protein	4 g
Calcium	36 mg
Iron	1 mg

Tips

1 liter, or 1 quart, of fresh raspberries yields 4 cups. A 6-oz (170 g) package yields about 1 cup (250 mL).

Remove the pan sides, place 1 tsp (5 mL) GF confectioners' (icing) sugar in a fine sieve and dust the tart just before serving.

3. Press dough into bottom and $\frac{1}{2}$ inch (1 cm) up sides of prepared pan.

4. Bake in preheated oven for 10 to 12 minutes or until lightly browned. Let cool to room temperature.

5. *Peach filling:* In a small bowl, beat cream cheese until smooth. Spread over cooled crust and top with peach slices. Drizzle with glaze. Cover with waxed or parchment paper and refrigerate for at least 3 hours, until chilled, or for up to 24 hours.

Raspberry Almond Crumb Tart

Makes 8 servings

We can't wait for summer, and raspberry season, to make this delicious dessert. Don't delay, as the season is a short one.

Tip

A 6-oz (170 g) package of raspberries yields about 1 cup (250 mL).

- Preheat oven to 350°F (180°C)
- 9-inch (23 cm) tart pan with removable bottom, lightly greased

Almond Topping

1/3 cup	almond flour	75 mL
2 tbsp	white (granulated) sugar	25 mL

Almond Crust

2	egg yolks	2
1 tsp	almond extract	5 mL
3/4 cup	almond flour	175 mL
1/2 cup	brown rice flour	125 mL
1/4 cup	tapioca starch	50 mL
1/2 tsp	xanthan gum	2 mL
1/4 tsp	salt	1 mL
1/3 cup	white (granulated) sugar	75 mL
1/3 cup	cold butter, cut into 1-inch (2.5 cm) pieces	75 mL

Raspberry Filling

4 cups	raspberries	1 L
2 tbsp	amaranth flour	25 mL

1. *Almond topping:* In a small bowl, combine almond flour and sugar. Set aside.

2. *Almond crust:* In another small bowl, whisk together egg yolks and almond extract. Set aside.

3. In a food processor, pulse almond flour, brown rice flour, tapioca starch, xanthan gum, salt and sugar 3 or 4 times to combine. Add butter and pulse for 5 to 10 seconds or until mixture resembles coarse crumbs about the size of small peas. Add egg yolk mixture and pulse until the dough holds together.

4. Press dough into bottom and 1/2 inch (1 cm) up the sides of prepared pan.

Tips

If you don't have a tart pan, you can use a springform pan.

Remove the pan sides, place 1 tsp (5 mL) GF confectioners' (icing) sugar in a fine sieve and dust the tart just before serving.

5. *Raspberry filling:* In a bowl, gently toss together raspberries and amaranth flour. Spoon evenly into crust and sprinkle with topping.

6. Bake in preheated oven for 12 to 15 minutes. Reduce temperature to 325°F (170°C) and bake for 15 to 20 minutes or until crust is golden brown. Let cool in pan on a rack for about 30 minutes. Serve warm or at room temperature.

Variation
Substitute blueberries or sliced peaches for the raspberries.

Pecan Tart Pastry

**Makes 6 tart shells
(1 per serving)**

A CanolaInfo recipe

You can use this recipe to make any tart, but we developed it especially for Pecan Butter Tarts (page 338).

Tips

Due to the small quantity of ingredients, it is critical to measure accurately.

Refrigerate the dough for a few minutes if it becomes sticky.

- Preheat oven to 375°F (190°C) (optional)
- Parchment paper
- 4-inch (10 cm) round cookie cutter
- 6-cup muffin or tart tin

1/2 cup	sorghum flour	125 mL
1/4 cup	pecan flour	50 mL
1/2 cup	cornstarch	125 mL
1/4 cup	tapioca starch	50 mL
1 tsp	white (granulated) sugar	5 mL
1 tsp	GF baking powder	5 mL
1/2 tsp	salt	2 mL
1	egg yolk	1
1/4 cup	ice water	50 mL
3 tbsp	vegetable oil	45 mL
2 tsp	cider vinegar	10 mL

1. In a food processor, pulse sorghum flour, pecan flour, cornstarch, tapioca starch, sugar, baking powder and salt until mixed. Set aside.

2. In a small bowl, whisk together egg yolk, ice water, oil and vinegar.

3. With the food processor running, through the feed tube, add egg mixture in a slow, steady stream. Process until dough just holds together. Do not let it form a ball.

4. Gently gather into a ball and flatten into a disc. Place the pastry disc between two sheets of parchment paper. Using quick, firm strokes of the rolling pin, roll out the dough into an 11-inch (28 cm) circle about 1/8 to 1/4 inch (0.25 to 0.5 cm) thick.

5. Carefully remove the top sheet of parchment paper and cut out 6 tart shells using the cookie cutter, rerolling scraps as necessary. Ease each shell into a cup in the muffin tin.

Tips

If the pastry cracks while you're handling it, don't worry: just use the excess to patch.

Don't worry about rerolling the pastry scraps; they'll be just as tender the third or fourth time as the first.

6. Use unbaked as directed in recipe. Or, to prevent pastry from shrinking or puffing up, prick bottom and sides with a fork. Bake in preheated oven for 13 to 15 minutes or until golden. Let cool completely before filling.

Variations

Fill cooled baked tart shells with raspberry jam or lemon meringue.

Double the ingredients to line a 9-inch (23 cm) pie plate. If prebaking, bake at 425°F (220°C) for 18 to 20 minutes.

Pecan Butter Tarts

**Makes 6 tarts
(1 per serving)**

A CanolaInfo recipe

There is nothing more Canadian than butter tarts. We know you'll love ours.

Tip
To prevent butter tarts from bubbling over, stir the filling as little as possible.

- Preheat oven to 375°F (190°C)
- 6-cup muffin or tart tin

1/3 cup	packed brown sugar	75 mL
1/4 cup	coarsely chopped pecans	50 mL
1/4 cup	corn syrup	50 mL
2 tbsp	butter, melted	25 mL
2 tbsp	vegetable oil	25 mL
1/4 tsp	vanilla extract	1 mL
1	egg, lightly beaten	1
1	recipe Pecan Tart Pastry (page 336), unbaked	1

1. In a bowl, combine brown sugar, pecans, corn syrup, butter, oil and vanilla. Mix gently. Add egg and mix until just blended.
2. Spoon filling into unbaked pastry shells, filling shells two-thirds full.
3. Bake in preheated oven for 15 to 20 minutes or until filling is golden brown. Let cool completely in pan on a rack.

Variation
Substitute raisins for the pecans.

For a creamier filling, omit the pecans.

Nutritional value per serving

Calories	379
Fat, total	20 g
Fat, saturated	4 g
Cholesterol	75 mg
Sodium	264 mg
Carbohydrate	48 g
Fiber	1 g
Protein	4 g
Calcium	66 mg
Iron	1 mg

Apple Raisin Custard Crumble

Makes 4 to 6 servings

When you want true comfort food, here's an updated apple crisp.

Tips

To increase the fiber in this dish, leave the peel on the apples.

Use your favorite baking apple variety. We like Spartan, Cortland, Crispin (Mutsu), Golden Delicious, Granny Smith, Ida Red, Jonagold, Northern Spy or Braeburn.

- Preheat oven to 325°F (160°C)
- 8-cup (2 L) baking dish, lightly greased

4 cups	sliced apples	1 L
½ cup	raisins	125 mL
2	eggs	2
1 cup	milk	250 mL
1 tbsp	grated lemon zest	15 mL
1 tsp	vanilla extract	5 mL
2 tbsp	packed brown sugar	25 mL
2 tbsp	amaranth flour	25 mL
Crumble		
1⅓ cups	GF oats	325 mL
½ cup	packed brown sugar	125 mL
½ cup	amaranth flour	125 mL
1 tbsp	ground cinnamon	15 mL
½ cup	butter, melted	125 mL

1. Place apples and raisins in the prepared baking dish. Set aside.

2. In a small bowl, whisk together eggs, milk, lemon zest and vanilla. Set aside.

3. In a separate bowl, combine brown sugar and amaranth flour. Whisk in egg mixture. Pour over apple mixture and spread evenly to cover apples.

4. *Crumble:* In another bowl, combine oats, brown sugar, amaranth flour, cinnamon and butter until crumbly. Sprinkle over apple mixture.

5. Bake in preheated oven for 30 to 35 minutes or until apples are tender, custard is thickened and topping is golden.

Variations

Substitute ½ cup (125 mL) dried mango pieces or dried papaya for the raisins.

Add ⅓ cup (75 mL) unsweetened shredded coconut to the crumble.

Nutritional value per serving

Calories	494
Fat, total	20 g
Fat, saturated	11 g
Cholesterol	107 mg
Sodium	211 mg
Carbohydrate	71 g
Fiber	6 g
Protein	9 g
Calcium	139 mg
Iron	6 mg

Plum, Apricot and Plumcot Crisp

Makes 4 servings

When plums, apricots and plumcots are in season, this is the first of many ways we like to use them. Make several crisps when the fruit is plentiful, and freeze to enjoy in late fall.

Tips

To store, let cool completely, wrap airtight and freeze for up to 3 months.

See the Ingredients Glossary, page 393, for information on plumcots.

If plumcots aren't available, add 3 more apricots.

There's no need to peel the fresh fruit.

If baked in a smaller or deeper casserole dish, the baking time may be up to twice as long.

Nutritional value per serving

Calories	517
Fat, total	23 g
Fat, saturated	7 g
Cholesterol	26 mg
Sodium	107 mg
Carbohydrate	69 g
Fiber	7 g
Protein	11 g
Calcium	96 mg
Iron	4 mg

- Preheat oven to 350°F (180°C)
- 8-cup (2 L) shallow casserole dish, lightly greased

Base

6	large plums, each cut into 8 wedges	6
3	large apricots, each cut into 8 wedges	3
3	plumcots, each cut into 8 wedges	3
3 tbsp	cornstarch	45 mL
2 tbsp	liquid honey	25 mL

Topping

1½ cups	GF oats	375 mL
⅓ cup	almond flour	75 mL
⅓ cup	slivered or sliced almonds	75 mL
3 tbsp	packed brown sugar	45 mL
½ tsp	ground nutmeg	2 mL
¼ cup	butter, melted	50 mL

1. *Base:* In prepared casserole dish, combine plums, apricots, plumcots, cornstarch and honey. Set aside.

2. *Topping:* In a bowl, combine oats, almond flour, almonds, brown sugar and nutmeg. Drizzle with butter and mix until crumbly. Sprinkle over the fruit. Do not pack.

3. Bake in preheated oven for 25 to 30 minutes or until fruit is fork-tender and bubbly around the edges and topping is browned. Serve warm.

Variations

Recipe can be divided in half and baked in a lightly greased 9- by 5-inch (23 by 12.5 cm) glass loaf pan.

Instead of baking, microwave, uncovered, on High for 4 minutes. Turn dish a quarter-turn and microwave on High for 3 to 4 minutes or until fruit is tender. Let stand for 5 minutes.

To make this nut-free, substitute amaranth flour for the almond flour and omit the almonds.

Summer Fruit Crisp

Makes 6 to 8 servings

A fruit crisp is one of our favorite ways to use up an abundance of seasonal fruits. Make several crisps when the fruit is plentiful, and freeze to enjoy in late fall.

Tips

To store, let cool completely, wrap airtight and freeze for up to 3 months.

If baked in a smaller or deeper casserole dish, the baking time may be up to twice as long.

- Preheat oven to 350°F (180°C)
- 8-cup (2 L) shallow casserole dish, lightly greased

Base

4	large peaches, cut into wedges	4
5	plums, cut into wedges	5
1 cup	blueberries	250 mL
3 tbsp	amaranth flour	45 mL
2 tbsp	packed brown sugar	25 mL

Topping

1½ cups	GF oats	375 mL
⅓ cup	amaranth flour	75 mL
¼ cup	packed brown sugar	50 mL
½ tsp	ground mace	2 mL
¼ cup	butter, melted	50 mL

1. *Base:* In prepared casserole dish, gently combine peaches, plums, blueberries, amaranth flour and brown sugar. Set aside.

2. *Topping:* In a bowl, combine oats, amaranth flour, brown sugar and mace. Drizzle with butter and mix just until crumbly. Sprinkle over the fruit. Do not pack.

3. Bake in preheated oven for 20 to 25 minutes or until fruit is bubbly around the edges and fork-tender, and topping is browned. Serve warm.

Variations

Recipe can be divided in half and baked in a lightly greased 9- by 5-inch (23 by 12.5 cm) glass loaf pan.

Substitute sorghum flour for the amaranth flour in both the base and the topping.

Instead of baking, microwave, uncovered, on High for 4 minutes. Turn dish a quarter-turn and microwave on High for 3 to 4 minutes or until fruit is tender. Let stand for 5 minutes.

Nutritional value per serving

Calories	238
Fat, total	7 g
Fat, saturated	3 g
Cholesterol	13 mg
Sodium	54 mg
Carbohydrate	40 g
Fiber	4 g
Protein	5 g
Calcium	37 mg
Iron	4 mg

Apricot Fool

As you enjoy this light British dessert, the crunchy pieces of meringue, surrounded by apricots, will melt in your mouth.

Tips

The meringue can be wrapped tightly and stored at room temperature for up to 2 days.

For information on warming eggs, see the Techniques Glossary, page 396.

To get the most volume from the whipping cream, chill the bowl and beaters for at least 1 hour first.

If you're not serving the whole dessert at once, wait to add the meringue to the leftover portion until just before you serve it.

Nutritional value per serving	
Calories	216
Fat, total	9 g
Fat, saturated	5 g
Cholesterol	29 mg
Sodium	28 mg
Carbohydrate	34 g
Fiber	1 g
Protein	2 g
Calcium	26 mg
Iron	0 mg

- Preheat oven to 250°F (120°C)
- Baking sheet, lined with parchment paper

Meringue

2	egg whites, at room temperature	2
1/2 tsp	white vinegar	2 mL
1/2 cup	white (granulated) sugar	125 mL
2 tbsp	almond flour	25 mL

Apricot Filling

6	fresh apricots, each cut into 8 wedges	6
1/3 cup	white (granulated) sugar	75 mL
1/3 cup	apricot jam	75 mL
1 tsp	almond extract	5 mL
1 1/2 cups	cold whipping (35%) cream	375 mL

1. *Meringue:* In a large bowl, using an electric mixer with wire whisk attachment, beat egg whites and vinegar until soft peaks form. Gradually beat in sugar. Continue beating until mixture is stiff and glossy but not dry. Fold in almond flour.

2. Spread meringue on prepared baking sheet and bake in preheated oven for 45 minutes or until dry. Let cool completely.

3. *Apricot filling:* In a saucepan, combine apricots, sugar and jam. Bring to a boil over medium heat. Reduce heat to low and simmer for 10 minutes or until apricots are tender. Remove from heat and add almond extract. Let cool completely.

4. Just before serving, break meringue into pieces. Set aside.

5. In a bowl, using an electric mixer with wire whisk attachment, beat cream until soft peaks form. Fold in apricot mixture and meringue pieces. Spoon into serving dishes. Serve immediately.

Variation

Instead of making the apricot filling in step 3, you can simply stir 1 tsp (5 mL) almond extract into 1/3 cup (75 mL) apricot purée baby food.

Strawberry Rhubarb Fool

Makes 6 servings

Sweet strawberries combine with tart rhubarb in our modern version of this classic British dessert.

Tips

Balkan-style, no-gelatin or plain yogurt work equally well.

Drained yogurt can be stored in an airtight container in the refrigerator for up to 3 days.

Use drained yogurt as a lower-fat substitute in any dip recipe that calls for sour cream.

2 cups	plain yogurt	500 mL
4 cups	chopped rhubarb (1/2-inch/1 cm pieces)	1 L
1/3 cup	liquid honey	75 mL
2 tbsp	freshly squeezed orange juice	25 mL
2/3 cup	coarsely chopped strawberries	150 mL
3/4 tsp	vanilla extract	4 mL

1. Line a large sieve with a double layer of cheesecloth and set it over a large bowl. Place yogurt in sieve and refrigerate for 8 hours or overnight, until reduced to about 1 cup (250 mL). Discard liquid.

2. In a large saucepan, bring rhubarb, honey and orange juice to a simmer over medium-low heat. Simmer, stirring frequently, for 7 to 8 minutes or until very tender. Stir in strawberries and simmer, stirring once or twice, for 2 to 3 minutes or until strawberries are soft. Remove from heat and stir in vanilla. Let cool completely.

3. Gently fold drained yogurt into rhubarb mixture until marbled. Spoon into serving dishes.

Variations

For a classic fool, fold fruit into 2 cups (500 mL) whipped cream instead of yogurt.

Layer cooled cooked fruit and drained yogurt in parfait glasses. Garnish with Heather's Granola (page 50).

Nutritional value per serving	
Calories	135
Fat, total	2 g
Fat, saturated	1 g
Cholesterol	5 mg
Sodium	62 mg
Carbohydrate	27 g
Fiber	2 g
Protein	5 g
Calcium	223 mg
Iron	0 mg

Poached Pears
with Cranberry Sauce

Makes 4 servings

When the whole basket of pears ripens overnight, use up some of them in this delicious dessert!

Tips

For the orange-flavored liqueur, choose from Grand Marnier, Triple Sec or Cointreau.

Choose firm pears that hold up well in cooking, such as Bosc or Bartlett.

Place pears in a paper bag at room temperature to ripen. To test pears for ripeness, press lightly at the stem end. It should give slightly.

2 cups	unsweetened apple cider or apple juice	500 mL
½ cup	dried cranberries	125 mL
¼ cup	packed brown sugar	50 mL
2 tsp	grated orange zest	10 mL
1 tsp	ground cardamom	5 mL
4	pears, peeled and halved lengthwise	4
2 tbsp	orange-flavored liqueur	25 mL

1. In a saucepan, combine apple cider, cranberries, brown sugar, orange zest and cardamom. Bring to a boil over medium-high heat. Reduce heat to low and simmer for 15 minutes. Add pears and simmer for 5 minutes or until tender. Remove from heat and stir in liqueur. Serve warm or chilled.

Variation

Substitute thawed frozen orange juice concentrate for the liqueur.

Nutritional value per serving	
Calories	284
Fat, total	1 g
Fat, saturated	0 g
Cholesterol	0 mg
Sodium	15 mg
Carbohydrate	68 g
Fiber	6 g
Protein	1 g
Calcium	41 mg
Iron	1 mg

Apple Berry Clafouti

Easier than apple pie (and lighter too), this custard-based dessert or brunch dish perfectly balances the sweetness of apples with the tang of cranberries. It is equally delicious served hot, warm or cold.

Tip

Use your favorite baking apple variety. We like Spartan, Cortland, Crispin (Mutsu), Golden Delicious, Granny Smith, Ida Red, Jonagold, Northern Spy and Braeburn.

- Preheat oven to 400°F (200°C)
- 8-cup (2 L) oval or square baking dish, lightly greased

4 cups	thinly sliced apples	1 L
1 cup	fresh or partially thawed frozen cranberries	250 mL
1/4 cup	packed brown sugar	50 mL
1/3 cup	sorghum flour	75 mL
2 tbsp	tapioca starch	25 mL
1/2 tsp	xanthan gum	2 mL
1/2 tsp	ground cardamom	2 mL
Pinch	salt	Pinch
1 cup	milk	250 mL
1 tbsp	butter	15 mL
2	eggs	2
1/3 cup	white (granulated) sugar	75 mL
1/2 tsp	vanilla extract	2 mL

1. In prepared baking dish, combine apples, cranberries and brown sugar. Set aside.

2. In a small bowl or plastic bag, combine sorghum flour, tapioca starch, xanthan gum, cardamom and salt. Mix well and set aside.

3. In a microwave-safe bowl, microwave milk and butter on High for 2 to 3 minutes or until tiny bubbles form around the edge. Mix well and set aside.

4. In a large bowl, using an electric mixer with wire whisk attachment, beat eggs and sugar until light and fluffy. Add dry ingredients and mix until just combined. Add milk mixture and vanilla; mix until smooth. Pour over fruit.

5. Bake in preheated oven for 35 to 40 minutes or until puffy and slightly golden, custard is just set and a tester inserted in the center comes out clean.

Variations

Substitute raspberries for the cranberries.

In the summer, at the height of the fresh fruit season, use any fresh fruit, or a combination, and omit the sugar. We've used a combination of peaches, blackberries, raspberries and strawberries.

Nutritional value per serving

Calories	223
Fat, total	4 g
Fat, saturated	2 g
Cholesterol	69 mg
Sodium	111 mg
Carbohydrate	44 g
Fiber	3 g
Protein	4 g
Calcium	75 mg
Iron	1 mg

Winter Fruit Clafouti

This custardy fruit pudding is a favorite of both adults and children when fresh fruit is not available. It is equally delicious served hot, warm or cold.

Tips

We used a combination of frozen peaches, blackberries, raspberries and strawberries.

Look for frozen fruit mixtures, such as bumbleberry or peach mango mixture.

- Preheat oven to 400°F (200°C)
- 8-cup (2 L) oval or square baking dish, lightly greased

4 cups	frozen mixed fruit, thawed and drained	1 L
¼ cup	liquid honey	50 mL
⅓ cup	low-fat soy flour	75 mL
2 tbsp	tapioca starch	25 mL
½ tsp	xanthan gum	2 mL
Pinch	salt	Pinch
1 cup	milk	250 mL
1 tbsp	butter	15 mL
2	eggs	2
⅓ cup	white (granulated) sugar	75 mL
½ tsp	almond extract	2 mL

1. In prepared baking dish, combine fruit and honey. Set aside.

2. In a small bowl or plastic bag, combine soy flour, tapioca starch, xanthan gum and salt. Mix well and set aside.

3. In a microwave-safe bowl, microwave milk and butter on High for 2 to 3 minutes or until tiny bubbles form around the edge. Mix well and set aside.

4. In a large bowl, using an electric mixer with wire whisk attachment, beat eggs and sugar until light and fluffy. Add dry ingredients and mix until just combined. Add milk mixture and almond extract; mix until smooth. Pour over fruit.

5. Bake in preheated oven for 30 to 35 minutes or until puffy and slightly golden, custard is just set and a tester inserted in the center comes out clean.

Variation

In the summer, at the height of the fresh fruit season, use any fresh fruit, or a combination, and omit the honey.

If you can't tolerate soy flour, use the custard topping from the Apple Berry Clafouti recipe (page 345) instead of making the one in this recipe.

Nutritional value per serving	
Calories	335
Fat, total	4 g
Fat, saturated	2 g
Cholesterol	69 mg
Sodium	114 mg
Carbohydrate	70 g
Fiber	3 g
Protein	8 g
Calcium	84 mg
Iron	1 mg

Ginger Pear Pudding

Makes 12 servings

This dessert gives you a delicious way to add fiber and fruit servings to your diet.

Tips

On average, pears purchased in a grocery store will require from 4 to 7 days to ripen completely. Ripen in a paper bag at room temperature. When the stem end yields to gentle pressure, the pear is ripe.

Anjou pears hold their shape well when baked.

Nutritional value per serving

Calories	243
Fat, total	10 g
Fat, saturated	1 g
Cholesterol	16 mg
Sodium	66 mg
Carbohydrate	39 g
Fiber	3 g
Protein	2 g
Calcium	42 mg
Iron	1 mg

- Preheat oven to 350°F (180°C)
- 9-inch (23 cm) square baking pan, lightly greased

6	pears, peeled and cubed	6
2 tbsp	liquid honey	25 mL
¼ cup	minced crystallized ginger	50 mL
½ cup	sorghum flour	125 mL
¼ cup	yellow pea flour	50 mL
½ cup	packed brown sugar	125 mL
½ tsp	xanthan gum	2 mL
½ tsp	baking soda	2 mL
2 tsp	ground ginger	10 mL
1	egg	1
¾ cup	hot water	175 mL
½ cup	vegetable oil	125 mL
¼ cup	light (fancy) molasses	50 mL

1. Spread pears in prepared baking pan. Top with honey and crystallized ginger.

2. In a bowl or plastic bag, combine sorghum flour, pea flour, brown sugar, xanthan gum, baking soda and ginger. Mix well and set aside.

3. In a separate bowl, using an electric mixer, beat egg, water, oil and molasses until combined. Add dry ingredients and mix until just combined. Pour over pears. Using a moistened rubber spatula, spread to edges and smooth top.

4. Bake in preheated oven for 35 to 40 minutes or until a tester inserted in the center comes out clean. Serve warm.

Variations

Use canned pears and omit the honey.

Substitute 4 cups (1 L) chopped peaches, or a combination of peaches and plums, for the pears.

For a milder flavor, omit the crystallized ginger.

Serve with a lemon sauce.

Substitute any bean flour for the pea.

Mango Sponge Pudding

Makes 3 servings

This soufflé-like pudding has a delicious mango custard sauce, and is just enough for three.

Tips

For information on warming eggs, see the Techniques Glossary, page 396.

Use a small handheld or immersion mixer to beat the egg white.

To safely remove ramekins from the boiling water, slide a spatula under each. Lift gently and, once clear of the water, support the ramekin with an oven mitt–covered hand.

This recipe can be doubled or tripled.

- Preheat oven to 350°F (180°C)
- Three ¾-cup (175 mL) ramekins
- 8-inch (20 cm) square baking pan

¼ cup	white (granulated) sugar	50 mL
2 tbsp	almond flour	25 mL
Pinch	salt	pinch
1	egg yolk	1
⅓ cup	milk	75 mL
⅓ cup	Mango Purée (see recipe, opposite)	75 mL
1	egg white, at room temperature	1
	Boiling water	

1. In a large bowl, whisk together sugar, almond flour and salt. Whisk in egg yolk, milk and Mango Purée. Set aside.

2. In a separate bowl, using an electric mixer, beat egg white until stiff peaks form. Gently stir in mango mixture.

3. Pour into ramekins. Set ramekins in baking pan and pour in enough boiling water to come halfway up sides of ramekins.

4. Bake in preheated oven for about 20 minutes or until tops are lightly browned and set. Remove ramekins from baking pan and let cool on a rack for about 30 minutes. Serve warm or let cool completely.

Variations

If you can't tolerate nuts, use brown rice flour instead of the almond flour.

Dollop 1 tbsp (15 mL) extra Mango Purée on the center of each pudding just before baking.

Nutritional value per serving

Calories	149
Fat, total	4 g
Fat, saturated	1 g
Cholesterol	72 mg
Sodium	133 mg
Carbohydrate	25 g
Fiber	1 g
Protein	4 g
Calcium	57 mg
Iron	0 mg

**Makes 2 cups (500 mL)
(1/3 cup/75 mL per
serving)**

*The rich flavor and
color of mangos takes
a dessert from simple
to exotic. Drizzle purée
over GF ice cream or
use it to make Mango
Sponge Pudding
(opposite).*

Tip

For information on
working with mangos, see
the Techniques Glossary,
page 397.

Mango Purée

2	very ripe large mangos, peeled and cut into cubes	2
1 cup	water	250 mL
3 tbsp	white (granulated) sugar	45 mL
2 tsp	freshly squeezed lime juice	10 mL

1. In a large saucepan, combine mangos, water, sugar and lime juice. Bring to a boil over medium-high heat, stirring often. Reduce heat to medium-low and simmer, stirring often, for 15 to 20 minutes or until mangos are soft.

2. Transfer to a blender or food processor and purée until smooth.

3. Store in an airtight container in the refrigerator for up to 2 days.

Variations

Substitute 4 large peaches for the mangos and lemon juice for the lime juice.

Add 2 tbsp (25 mL) white rum to the purée just before serving.

Nutritional value per serving	
Calories	70
Fat, total	0 g
Fat, saturated	0 g
Cholesterol	0 mg
Sodium	3 mg
Carbohydrate	18 g
Fiber	1 g
Protein	0 g
Calcium	8 mg
Iron	0 mg

Rice Pudding Brûlée

Egg-Free

Makes 8 servings

If you enjoy crème brûlée, you'll love this take on it! We like to make it for company, as it can be prepared ahead and finished at the last minute.

Tip

Balkan-style, no-gelatin or plain yogurt work equally well. Store drained yogurt in the refrigerator for up to 3 days.

- Eight ¾-cup (175 mL) ramekins or ceramic soufflé dishes

1 cup	plain yogurt	250 mL
4½ cups	milk	1.125 L
¾ cup	short-grain white rice, such as Arborio	175 mL
¼ cup	white (granulated) sugar	50 mL
2 tbsp	butter	25 mL
1 tsp	grated orange zest	5 mL
½ tsp	vanilla extract	2 mL
Topping		
1 cup	white (granulated) sugar	250 mL
1 tsp	ground cinnamon	5 mL

1. Line a large sieve with a double layer of cheesecloth and set it over a large bowl. Place yogurt in sieve and refrigerate for 8 hours or overnight, until reduced to about ½ cup (125 mL). Discard liquid.

2. In a heavy saucepan, combine milk, rice, sugar, butter and orange zest. Heat over medium heat, stirring frequently, until tiny bubbles form around the edge. Reduce heat to low and simmer, stirring frequently, for 45 to 50 minutes or until rice is tender and most of the milk is absorbed. Fold in drained yogurt and vanilla.

3. Spoon hot rice pudding into ramekins. Cover with plastic wrap and refrigerate for at least 3 hours, until chilled, or for up to 2 days.

4. Preheat broiler.

5. *Topping:* In a small bowl, combine sugar and cinnamon. Sprinkle over rice puddings.

Nutritional value per serving	
Calories	292
Fat, total	5 g
Fat, saturated	3 g
Cholesterol	15 mg
Sodium	120 mg
Carbohydrate	55 g
Fiber	0 g
Protein	7 g
Calcium	230 mg
Iron	0 mg

Tips

Arborio rice absorbs large quantities of liquid and develops a creamy texture.

Stir frequently enough that rice doesn't stick to the saucepan, particularly in the last 10 minutes.

Wipe the rim of each ramekin after filling it with pudding; any pudding left on the rim will burn under the broiler.

6. Broil for 7 to 9 minutes or until tops are glossy and brown and large bubbles have mostly disappeared. Let cool for 8 to 10 minutes or until caramel is hardened.

Variations

Instead of broiling the puddings, use a kitchen torch to caramelize the topping, gently sweeping the flame across the surface.

You can omit the 1 cup (250 mL) sugar in the topping and steps 4 to 6, simply stirring in cinnamon and adding 1 cup (250 mL) raisins with the yogurt and vanilla.

Orange Soufflé

Don't let this dessert fool you — it's not low-cal. But, we would like to emphasize, it's worth it.

Tips

This recipe contains raw egg whites. If the food safety of raw eggs is a concern for you, use ¼ cup (50 mL) pasteurized liquid egg whites instead.

For information on warming egg whites, see the Techniques Glossary, page 396.

Don't overbeat the cream, or you'll end up with butter. If this happens, start over with a fresh supply of cream.

If you add sugar too soon or too quickly to the beaten egg whites, the mixture becomes thin and shiny.

- Six ¾-cup (175 mL) ramekins or ceramic soufflé dishes

¼ cup	amaranth flour	50 mL
⅓ cup	white (granulated) sugar	75 mL
1½ tsp	unflavored gelatin powder	7 mL
¼ tsp	salt	1 mL
2	egg yolks	2
¾ cup	frozen orange juice concentrate, thawed	175 mL
2	egg whites, at room temperature	2
Pinch	cream of tartar	Pinch
¼ cup	white (granulated) sugar	50 mL
¾ cup	whipping (35%) cream	175 mL

1. In a saucepan, combine amaranth flour, sugar, gelatin and salt. Stir in egg yolks and orange juice concentrate. Heat over medium heat, stirring constantly, for 3 to 5 minutes or until mixture just comes to a boil. Remove from heat. Let cool to room temperature.

2. In a large bowl, using an electric mixer with wire whisk attachment, beat egg whites and cream of tartar until foamy. Gradually beat in sugar. Continue beating until mixture is stiff and glossy but not dry. Fold in orange juice mixture.

3. In a small bowl, using an electric mixer with clean wire whisk attachment, beat cream until soft peaks form. Fold into egg white mixture.

4. Spoon into ramekins. Cover and refrigerate for 3 to 4 hours or until firm.

Variations

To make this in one container, use a 6-cup (1.5 L) soufflé dish that is at least 3 inches (7.5 cm) deep.

Feel free to substitute packed brown sugar for the white sugar.

Nutritional value per serving

Calories	224
Fat, total	7 g
Fat, saturated	4 g
Cholesterol	90 mg
Sodium	124 mg
Carbohydrate	37 g
Fiber	1 g
Protein	4 g
Calcium	36 mg
Iron	2 mg

Pumpkin Thanksgiving Dessert

Makes 12 large squares (1 per serving)

Hate making pastry? Try this for your Thanksgiving dessert.

Tips

This recipe can be halved and baked in an 8-inch (20 cm) square baking pan. Bake for 20 to 25 minutes in step 3.

For information on making your own pecan flour, see the Techniques Glossary, page 398.

These bars can be stored in an airtight container in the refrigerator for up to 2 days.

- Preheat oven to 350°F (180°C)
- 13- by 9-inch (33 by 23 cm) baking pan, ungreased

Crust

1 cup	pecan flour	250 mL
½ cup	sorghum flour	125 mL
1½ cups	GF oats	375 mL
⅔ cup	packed brown sugar	150 mL
½ cup	butter, melted	125 mL

Filling

3	eggs	3
1	can (28 oz/796 mL) pumpkin purée (not pie filling)	1
⅔ cup	packed brown sugar	150 mL
1	can (12 oz or 370 mL) evaporated milk	1
1 tsp	ground cinnamon	5 mL
1 tsp	ground ginger	5 mL

1. *Crust:* In a large bowl, combine pecan flour, sorghum flour, oats, brown sugar and butter. Mix well and firmly pat into pan. Bake in preheated oven for 15 minutes. Let cool on a rack for 10 minutes.

2. *Filling:* Meanwhile, in a bowl, using an electric mixer, beat eggs, pumpkin purée, brown sugar, milk, cinnamon and ginger until smooth. Pour over warm crust.

3. Bake for 20 to 30 minutes or until a tester inserted in the center comes out clean. Let cool completely in pan on rack, then cut into squares.

Variations

Substitute ½ cup (125 mL) freshly squeezed orange juice for half the evaporated milk.

For a crunchier base, use GF large-flake rolled oats, if available, and add ½ cup (125 mL) coarsely chopped pecans.

Nutritional value per serving

Calories	315
Fat, total	10 g
Fat, saturated	6 g
Cholesterol	69 mg
Sodium	143 mg
Carbohydrate	48 g
Fiber	3 g
Protein	9 g
Calcium	148 mg
Iron	3 mg

Jelly Roll with Lotsa Lime Filling

Makes 8 to 10 servings

This recipe is a little bit fiddly, so take your time and handle the cake with care as you roll it.

Tips

See the Techniques Glossary, page 396, for information on warming egg whites.

For better volume when beating egg whites, make sure the bowl and beaters are completely free of grease and egg yolk. Wash them right before using them.

Wrapped airtight, the jelly roll can be frozen for up to 1 month. Thaw, wrapped, in the refrigerator.

Nutritional value per serving	
Calories	222
Fat, total	9 g
Fat, saturated	3 g
Cholesterol	137 mg
Sodium	93 mg
Carbohydrate	31 g
Fiber	1 g
Protein	4 g
Calcium	31 mg
Iron	1 mg

- Preheat oven to 375°F (190°C)
- 15- by 10-inch (40 by 25 cm) jelly roll pan, lined with parchment paper

½ cup	almond flour	125 mL
2 tbsp	cornstarch	25 mL
1½ tsp	xanthan gum	7 mL
4	egg whites, at room temperature	4
¼ tsp	cream of tartar	1 mL
¾ cup	white (granulated) sugar, divided	175 mL
4	egg yolks	4
Pinch	salt	Pinch
½ tsp	almond extract	2 mL
	GF confectioner's (icing) sugar	
1½ cups	Lotsa Lime Filling (see recipe, opposite)	375 mL

1. In a small bowl, combine almond flour, cornstarch and xanthan gum. Mix well and set aside.

2. In a large bowl, using an electric mixer with wire whisk attachment, beat egg whites until foamy. Beat in cream of tartar. Continue beating until egg whites are stiff. Gradually beat in ¼ cup (50 mL) of the white sugar. Continue beating until mixture is very stiff and glossy but not dry. Set aside.

3. In a small bowl, using an electric mixer, beat egg yolks, the remaining ½ cup (125 mL) white sugar, salt and almond extract for about 5 minutes or until thick and lemon-colored.

4. Fold egg yolk mixture into egg white mixture. Sprinkle with half the dry ingredients and fold in gently. Repeat with the remaining half. Spoon into prepared pan and carefully spread to the edges.

5. Bake in preheated oven for 10 to 12 minutes or until top springs back when lightly touched. Let cool in pan on a rack for 5 minutes.

6. Loosen edges of cake with a knife. Dust cake lightly with confectioner's sugar. Turn out onto a clean, lint-free tea towel set on a rack and carefully remove parchment paper. Starting at a long end, roll up cake in the towel. Let cool on rack for 20 minutes.

7. Gently unroll cake, being careful not to flatten it. Spread with Lotsa Lime Filling. Roll up again and place seam side down on a serving platter. Cover and refrigerate for 30 to 60 minutes, until chilled, or for up to 1 day.

Variation

Fill with raspberry jam instead of Lotsa Lime Filling.

Lotsa Lime Filling

½ cup	white (granulated) sugar	125 mL
3 tbsp	cornstarch	45 mL
1 cup	water	250 mL
2 tsp	grated lime zest	10 mL
⅓ cup	freshly squeezed lime juice	75 mL
3 tbsp	butter	45 mL
2	egg yolks, lightly beaten	2

Microwave Method

1. In a microwave-safe bowl, combine sugar and cornstarch. Add water, lime zest, lime juice and butter. Microwave on High, stopping to stir occasionally, for 3 to 5 minutes or until mixture boils and thickens.

2. Add a small amount of the hot mixture to the egg yolks, stirring constantly. Add the egg yolk mixture to the rest of the hot mixture, stirring constantly. Let cool completely before using.

Stovetop Method

1. In a saucepan, combine sugar and cornstarch. Add water, lime zest, lime juice and butter. Heat over medium heat, stirring constantly, for 5 to 8 minutes or until mixture boils and thickens.

2. Add a small amount of the hot mixture to the egg yolks, stirring constantly. Add the egg yolk mixture to the rest of the hot mixture, stirring constantly. Let cool completely before using.

Coconut Mango Sorbet

**Makes 2 cups (500 mL)
(½ cup/125 mL per
serving)**

*This frozen dessert is
refreshing on a hot
summer day.*

Tips

Select the coconut milk
according to the amount
of fat you desire. Be sure
to shake the can well
before using.

If freezing fresh mangos,
arrange the pieces in a
single layer so they do not
stick together in one large
piece when frozen.

1 cup	canned coconut milk	250 mL
1 cup	frozen mango pieces	250 mL
½ cup	crushed ice	125 mL
	Fresh mint leaves	

1. In a blender or food processor, purée coconut milk, mango and ice until smooth. Freeze for at least 2 hours or for up to 2 weeks.

2. Let stand at room temperature until soft enough to serve. Garnish with mint leaves.

Variations

Add 2 tbsp (25 mL) freshly squeezed lime juice.

Thin with extra coconut milk for a smoothie.

Nutritional value per serving	
Calories	138
Fat, total	12 g
Fat, saturated	11 g
Cholesterol	0 mg
Sodium	8 mg
Carbohydrate	9 g
Fiber	1 g
Protein	1 g
Calcium	14 mg
Iron	2 mg

Favorites By Request

Blue Cheese Walnut Ciabatta

We've had many requests for ciabatta with this flavor combination. Right from the oven, this quick and easy flatbread with a tangy crunch complements soup, salad or stew.

Tip

To ensure success, see page 178 for extra information on using your bread machine, and page 214 for extra information on mixer-method bread baking.

Nutritional value per serving

Calories	224
Fat, total	13 g
Fat, saturated	3 g
Cholesterol	55 mg
Sodium	319 mg
Carbohydrate	20 g
Fiber	2 g
Protein	9 g
Calcium	95 mg
Iron	3 mg

- 8-inch (20 cm) round baking pan, lightly greased and floured with sweet rice flour

¾ cup	whole bean flour	175 mL
½ cup	amaranth flour	125 mL
¼ cup	tapioca starch	50 mL
2 tbsp	white (granulated) sugar	25 mL
2 tsp	xanthan gum	10 mL
1 tbsp	bread machine or instant yeast	15 mL
2 tbsp	chopped fresh marjoram	25 mL
½ tsp	salt	2 mL
½ tsp	freshly ground black pepper	2 mL
½ cup	chopped walnuts	125 mL
¾ cup	water	175 mL
2 tbsp	vegetable oil	25 mL
1 tsp	cider vinegar	5 mL
2	eggs, lightly beaten	2
⅔ cup	cubed GF blue cheese (½-inch/1 cm cubes)	150 mL
2 to 3 tbsp	sweet rice flour	25 to 45 mL

Bread Machine Method

1. In a large bowl or plastic bag, combine whole bean flour, amaranth flour, tapioca starch, sugar, xanthan gum, yeast, marjoram, salt, pepper and walnuts. Mix well and set aside.

2. Pour water, oil and vinegar into the bread machine baking pan. Add eggs. Select the **Dough Cycle**. As the bread machine is mixing, gradually add the dry ingredients, scraping bottom and sides of pan with a rubber spatula. Try to incorporate all the dry ingredients within 1 to 2 minutes. Stop bread machine as soon as the kneading portion of the cycle is complete. Do not let bread machine finish the cycle. Remove baking pan from the bread machine. Fold in blue cheese.

Tips

This dough is thicker than most gluten-free doughs. Resist the temptation to add extra liquid.

When dusting with sweet rice flour, use a flour sifter for a light, even sprinkle.

Mixer Method

1. In a large bowl or plastic bag, combine whole bean flour, amaranth flour, tapioca starch, sugar, xanthan gum, yeast, marjoram, salt, pepper and walnuts. Mix well and set aside.

2. In a separate bowl, using a heavy-duty electric mixer with paddle attachment, combine water, oil, vinegar and eggs until well blended. With the mixer on its lowest speed, slowly add the dry ingredients until combined. Stop the machine and scrape the bottom and sides of the bowl with a rubber spatula. With the mixer on medium speed, beat for 4 minutes. Fold in blue cheese.

For Both Methods

3. Gently transfer dough to prepared pan and spread evenly to the edges, leaving the top rough and uneven. Generously dust top with sweet rice flour. With well-floured fingers, make deep indents all over the dough, pressing all the way down to the pan. Let rise, uncovered, in a warm, draft-free place for 60 to 75 minutes or until almost doubled in volume. Meanwhile, preheat oven to 400°F (200°C).

4. Bake for 20 to 25 minutes or until top is golden. Remove from pan immediately. Cut into 8 wedges and serve warm.

Variations

Dust with either brown rice flour or whole bean flour instead of the sweet rice flour.

Substitute GF Stilton for the blue cheese.

Oat Pizza Crust

Makes 8 servings

Beth Armour of Cream Hill Estates adapted this recipe from our original pizza crust (found in Complete Gluten-Free Cookbook*) and has given us permission to include it in our newest cookbook, so you can enjoy it too.*

Tip

To ensure success, see page 178 for extra information on using your bread machine, and page 214 for extra information on mixer-method bread baking.

Nutritional value per serving

Calories	114
Fat, total	3 g
Fat, saturated	0 g
Cholesterol	0 mg
Sodium	223 mg
Carbohydrate	19 g
Fiber	3 g
Protein	3 g
Calcium	15 mg
Iron	1 mg

- Preheat oven to 400°F (200°C)
- 12-inch (30 cm) pizza pan, lightly greased

1¼ cups	GF oat flour	300 mL
¼ cup	potato flour (not potato starch)	50 mL
¼ cup	tapioca starch	50 mL
1 tsp	white (granulated) sugar	5 mL
2 tsp	xanthan gum	10 mL
1 tbsp	bread machine or instant yeast	15 mL
¾ tsp	salt	4 mL
1¼ cups	water	300 mL
1 tbsp	extra virgin olive oil	15 mL
1 tsp	cider vinegar	5 mL

Bread Machine Method

1. In a large bowl or plastic bag, combine oat flour, potato flour, tapioca starch, sugar, xanthan gum, yeast and salt. Mix well and set aside.

2. Pour water, oil and vinegar into the bread machine baking pan. Select the **Dough Cycle**. Allow the liquids to mix until combined. As the machine is mixing, gradually add the dry ingredients, scraping bottom and sides of pan with a rubber spatula. Try to incorporate all the dry ingredients within 1 to 2 minutes. Stop bread machine as soon as the kneading portion of the cycle is complete. Do not let bread machine finish cycle.

Mixer Method

1. In a large bowl or plastic bag, combine oat flour, potato flour, tapioca starch, sugar, xanthan gum, yeast and salt. Mix well and set aside.

2. In a separate bowl, using a heavy-duty electric mixer with paddle attachment, combine water, oil and vinegar until well blended. With the mixer on its lowest speed, slowly add the dry ingredients until combined. Stop the machine and scrape the bottom and sides of the bowl with a rubber spatula. With the mixer on medium speed, beat for 4 minutes.

Tips

To make pizza, add your favorite topping ingredients and bake until crust is brown and crisp and top is bubbly.

Potato flour and potato starch are two completely different ingredients and cannot be substituted for one another.

You may need to dust your hands with potato flour if the dough is a little sticky.

Partially baked pizza crust can be wrapped airtight and frozen for up to 4 weeks. Thaw in the refrigerator overnight before using to make pizza.

For Both Methods

3. Gently transfer dough to prepared pan and, using a moistened rubber spatula, spread evenly to the edges. Do not smooth top.

4. Bake in preheated oven for 12 minutes or until bottom is golden and crust is partially baked.

Variation

Add 2 tsp (10 mL) dried oregano with the dry ingredients.

Banana Raisin Sticky Buns

*This recipe was
requested by several
folks who enjoy our
Cinnamon Buns
(Complete Gluten-
Free Cookbook, page
228). It is a bit tricky,
so don't try it first if
you've never baked
gluten-free before.
However, the results
are worth the effort
and time it takes.*

Tips

To ensure success, see page
178 for extra information
on using your bread
machine, and page 214
for extra information on
mixer-method baking.

This dough is thicker than
that of most gluten-free
breads; in fact, we were
able to use the mixer's
dough hook attachment.

Nutritional value per serving	
Calories	354
Fat, total	13 g
Fat, saturated	4 g
Cholesterol	62 mg
Sodium	277 mg
Carbohydrate	57 g
Fiber	3 g
Protein	6 g
Calcium	45 mg
Iron	2 mg

- 9-inch (23 cm) round silicone baking pan with 2-inch (5 cm) sides

1¼ cups	sorghum flour	300 mL
⅓ cup	whole bean flour	75 mL
¼ cup	almond flour	50 mL
½ cup	tapioca starch	125 mL
⅓ cup	cornstarch	75 mL
2 tbsp	potato flour (not potato starch)	25 mL
¼ cup	packed brown sugar	50 mL
1 tbsp	xanthan gum	15 mL
2 tbsp	bread machine or instant yeast	25 mL
1 tsp	salt	5 mL
⅓ cup	water	75 mL
¼ cup	vegetable oil	50 mL
1 tsp	cider vinegar	5 mL
1 cup	mashed ripe bananas	250 mL
3	eggs, lightly beaten	3
⅓ to ½ cup	sweet rice flour	75 to 125 mL

Pan Glaze

⅓ cup	packed brown sugar	75 mL
¼ cup	butter, melted	50 mL

Filling

1⅔ cups	raisins	400 mL
¼ cup	packed brown sugar	50 mL
½ tsp	ground cinnamon	2 mL
2 tbsp	butter, melted	25 mL

Bread Machine Method

1. In a large bowl or plastic bag, combine sorghum flour, whole bean flour, almond flour, tapioca starch, cornstarch, potato flour, brown sugar, xanthan gum, yeast and salt. Mix well and set aside.

2. Pour water, oil and vinegar into the bread machine baking pan. Add bananas and eggs. Select the **Dough Cycle.** As the bread machine is mixing, gradually add the dry ingredients, scraping bottom and sides of pan with a rubber spatula. Try to incorporate all the dry ingredients within 1 to 2 minutes. Stop bread machine as soon as the kneading portion of the cycle is complete. Do not let bread machine finish the cycle.

Tips

We don't recommend using a springform pan unless you want to clean your oven and test your smoke alarm battery — ours leaked!

Be sure to prepare both the pan glaze and the filling before removing the first square of dough from the refrigerator. Work quickly when rolling out the dough and assembling the buns. Return the dough to the refrigerator for a few minutes if it becomes sticky.

We prefer to cut the dough into buns with a pizza wheel; however, kitchen shears or a sharp knife work well too. You may have to dip the cutter in hot water between cuts.

This dough takes longer to rise than most, because it is cold.

Mixer Method

1. In a large bowl or plastic bag, combine sorghum flour, whole bean flour, almond flour, tapioca starch, cornstarch, potato flour, brown sugar, xanthan gum, yeast and salt. Mix well and set aside.

2. In a separate bowl, using a heavy-duty electric mixer with dough hook attachment, combine water, oil, vinegar, bananas and eggs until well blended. With the mixer on its lowest speed, slowly add the dry ingredients until combined. Stop the machine and scrape the bottom and sides of the bowl with a rubber spatula. With the mixer on medium speed, beat for 4 minutes.

For Both Methods

3. Generously coat two large sheets of plastic wrap with some of the sweet rice flour. Divide dough in half and place each half on a sheet of plastic wrap. Generously dust each with sweet rice flour. Top with another sheet of plastic wrap and pat out to a square about $1/2$ inch (1 cm) thick. Wrap airtight and refrigerate for at least 2 hours, until chilled, or overnight.

4. *Pan glaze:* In baking pan, combine brown sugar and butter; spread evenly over bottom of pan. Set aside.

5. *Filling:* In a bowl, combine raisins, brown sugar, cinnamon and butter. Set aside.

6. Remove one square of dough from the refrigerator. Place on a sheet of parchment paper generously dusted with sweet rice flour. Generously dust dough with sweet rice flour and cover with another sheet of parchment paper. Lightly roll out to a 9-inch (23 cm) square, about $1/4$ inch (0.5 cm) thick. Remove top sheet of parchment paper. With your fingers or a pastry brush, brush off excess flour.

7. Sprinkle half the filling over the dough. Roll up dough like a jelly roll, lifting the parchment paper to help the dough form a roll. Using a pizza wheel dipped in hot water, cut into 6 equal pieces. Place cut side up, fairly close together, in prepared pan. Repeat with the remaining dough and filling. Let rise in a warm, draft-free place for $1\frac{1}{2}$ to 2 hours or until doubled in volume. Meanwhile, preheat oven to 350°F (180°C).

continued...

Banana Raisin Sticky Buns, continued...

Tips

To safely turn a silicone baking pan upside down, first place it on a cooling rack, then, using the ends of the rack as handles, invert it over a serving platter.

The wrapped squares of dough can be frozen for up to 1 month. Defrost overnight in the refrigerator.

Baked sticky buns can be frozen, individually wrapped, for up to 2 weeks. Defrost in the microwave.

8. Bake for 25 minutes. Tent with foil and bake for 15 to 20 minutes or until internal temperature of buns registers 200°F (100°C) on an instant-read thermometer. Immediately invert onto a serving platter. Let stand for 5 minutes before removing pan. Serve warm.

Variation

Divide pan glaze evenly among the cups of a lightly greased 12-cup muffin tin. Place a bun, cut side up, in each cup. Reduce the baking time to 20 to 25 minutes.

Savory Rosemary Currant Biscotti

**Makes 24 biscotti
(1 per serving)**

These savory biscotti go well with roast pork or a luncheon salad.

Tip

Biscotti will be medium-firm and crunchy. For softer, chewier biscotti, bake for only 10 minutes in step 6; for very firm biscotti, bake for 20 minutes.

Nutritional value per serving	
Calories	61
Fat, total	1 g
Fat, saturated	0 g
Cholesterol	16 mg
Sodium	18 mg
Carbohydrate	13 g
Fiber	1 g
Protein	1 g
Calcium	12 mg
Iron	1 mg

- Preheat oven to 325°F (160°C)
- 8-inch (20 cm) square baking pan, lightly greased
- Baking sheets, ungreased

¾ cup	sorghum flour	175 mL
¼ cup	brown rice flour	50 mL
3 tbsp	tapioca starch	45 mL
2 tbsp	potato starch	25 mL
¾ tsp	xanthan gum	4 mL
½ tsp	GF baking powder	2 mL
Pinch	salt	Pinch
½ cup	dried currants	125 mL
¼ cup	snipped fresh rosemary	50 mL
2	eggs	2
¼ cup	white (granulated) sugar	50 mL

1. In a large bowl or plastic bag, combine sorghum flour, brown rice flour, tapioca starch, potato starch, xanthan gum, baking powder, salt, currants and rosemary. Mix well and set aside.

2. In a separate bowl, using an electric mixer, beat eggs and sugar until combined. Slowly beat in dry ingredients until just combined.

3. Spoon batter into prepared pan. Using a moistened rubber spatula, spread to edges and smooth top.

4. Bake in preheated oven for 20 to 25 minutes or until firm to the touch and top is just turning golden. Let cool in pan for 5 minutes. Remove from pan and let cool on a cutting board for 5 minutes. Reduce oven temperature to 300°F (150°C).

5. Using a very sharp knife, carefully cut into quarters, then cut each quarter into 6 slices. Arrange slices upright (with both cut sides exposed) at least ½ inch (1 cm) apart on baking sheets.

6. Bake for 10 to 15 minutes or until dry and crisp. Transfer to a rack and let cool completely.

7. Store in an airtight container at room temperature for up to 3 weeks or in the freezer for up to 2 months.

Variation
Substitute your favorite herb for the rosemary.

Lemon Pepper Biscotti

Makes 24 biscotti
(1 per serving)

Serve these savory biscotti with appetizers, soups or salads.

- Preheat oven to 325°F (160°C)
- 8-inch (20 cm) square baking pan, lightly greased
- Baking sheets, ungreased

½ cup	brown rice flour	125 mL
½ cup	low-fat soy flour	125 mL
3 tbsp	tapioca starch	45 mL
2 tbsp	potato starch	25 mL
¾ tsp	xanthan gum	4 mL
½ tsp	GF baking powder	2 mL
Pinch	salt	Pinch
½ tsp	freshly cracked black pepper	2 mL
2 tbsp	grated lemon zest	25 mL
2	eggs	2
2 tbsp	white (granulated) sugar	25 mL
¼ cup	freshly squeezed lemon juice	50 mL

1. In a large bowl or plastic bag, combine brown rice flour, soy flour, tapioca starch, potato starch, xanthan gum, baking powder, salt, pepper and lemon zest. Mix well and set aside.

2. In a separate bowl, using an electric mixer, beat eggs, sugar and lemon juice until combined. Slowly beat in dry ingredients until just combined.

3. Spoon batter into prepared pan. Using a moistened rubber spatula, spread to edges and smooth top.

4. Bake in preheated oven for 15 to 20 minutes or until firm to the touch and top is just turning golden. Let cool in pan for 5 minutes. Remove from pan and let cool on a cutting board for 5 minutes. Reduce oven temperature to 300°F (150°C).

5. Using a very sharp knife, carefully cut into quarters, then cut each quarter into 6 slices. Arrange slices upright (with both cut sides exposed) at least ½ inch (1 cm) apart on baking sheets.

Nutritional value per serving

Calories	35
Fat, total	1 g
Fat, saturated	0 g
Cholesterol	16 mg
Sodium	18 mg
Carbohydrate	6 g
Fiber	0 g
Protein	2 g
Calcium	13 mg
Iron	0 mg

Tips

Use a clean coffee grinder or pepper mill to crack the peppercorns.

Biscotti will be medium-firm and crunchy. For softer, chewier biscotti, bake for only 10 minutes in step 6; for very firm biscotti, bake for 20 minutes.

6. Bake for 15 to 20 minutes or until dry and crisp. Transfer to a rack and let cool completely.

7. Store in an airtight container at room temperature for up to 3 weeks or in the freezer for up to 2 months.

Variation

For a slightly milder lemon flavor, substitute water for half the lemon juice.

Gingerbread Cookies

Joan Segee, a Moncton, New Brunswick, celiac has baked gingerbread cookies for Christmas since 1977, and asked us to convert her original recipe to one that is gluten-free. Here you go, Joan!

Tips

This recipe can be doubled.

To soften ½ cup (125 mL) of butter without melting, cut into ½-inch (1 cm) pieces and microwave on 20% power for 20 to 30 seconds.

- 2-inch (5 cm) cookie cutter
- Baking sheets, lightly greased

1½ cups	sorghum flour	375 mL
⅔ cup	pea flour	150 mL
⅓ cup	tapioca starch	75 mL
1 tsp	xanthan gum	5 mL
¾ tsp	baking soda	4 mL
¼ tsp	salt	1 mL
1 tsp	ground cinnamon	5 mL
1 tsp	ground ginger	5 mL
½ tsp	ground cloves	2 mL
½ cup	white (granulated) sugar	125 mL
½ cup	butter, softened	125 mL
½ cup	light (fancy) molasses	125 mL
1 tbsp	cider vinegar	15 mL
1	egg	1

1. In a large bowl or plastic bag, combine sorghum flour, pea flour, tapioca starch, xanthan gum, baking soda, salt, cinnamon, ginger and cloves. Mix well and set aside.

2. In a separate bowl, using an electric mixer, cream sugar, butter, molasses, vinegar and egg. Slowly beat in dry ingredients until just combined.

3. Divide dough into thirds. Wrap each in plastic wrap. Flatten slightly into a disc and refrigerate overnight.

4. Preheat oven to 350°F (180°C).

5. Remove one disc of dough from the refrigerator. Discard plastic wrap. Place on a sheet of parchment paper and cover with another sheet of parchment paper. Roll out to just under ¼-inch (0.5 cm) thickness. Cut out circles with the cookie cutter, rerolling scraps as necessary. Repeat with the remaining dough. Place cookies 1 inch (2.5 cm) apart on prepared baking sheets.

Nutritional value per serving	
Calories	72
Fat, total	3 g
Fat, saturated	2 g
Cholesterol	12 mg
Sodium	72 mg
Carbohydrate	11 g
Fiber	0 g
Protein	1 g
Calcium	14 mg
Iron	1 mg

Tips

If you prefer to roll out the dough on a board, be sure to flour the board and rolling pin, using extra sorghum flour.

If the dough sticks to the cookie cutter, dip the cutter in a saucer of sweet rice flour or return the dough to the refrigerator until thoroughly chilled.

Watch carefully while the cookies are baking, as a couple of extra minutes can cause them to burn on the bottom.

6. Bake one sheet at a time in the top third of the oven for 10 to 12 minutes or until set. Let cool on pans on racks for 1 minute. Transfer to racks and let cool completely.

7. Store in an airtight container at room temperature for up to 5 days or in the freezer for up to 2 months.

Variations

Substitute any bean flour for the pea flour.

Joan decorates her cookies with hard icing.

Welsh Cakes

**Makes 18 cakes
(1 per serving)**

In Welsh, the name of this recipe is pice ar y maen *meaning "cakes on the stone."*

Tips

If using the food processor, pulse just enough to mix in raisins or they will break up.

Make sure dough is rolled out no thicker than ¼ inch (0.5 cm) or the outside of the cakes will burn before the center cooks.

- 2½-inch (6 cm) cookie cutter
- 10-inch (25 cm) cast-iron skillet or griddle, lightly greased

1	egg	1
¼ cup	milk	50 mL
¾ cup	amaranth flour	175 mL
¼ cup	sorghum flour	50 mL
¼ cup	cornstarch	50 mL
1 tbsp	potato flour (not potato starch)	15 mL
½ cup	white (granulated) sugar	125 mL
1½ tsp	xanthan gum	7 mL
1 tsp	GF baking powder	5 mL
⅛ tsp	salt	0.5 mL
⅛ tsp	ground nutmeg	0.5 mL
¼ cup	cold butter, cut into 1-inch (2.5 cm) cubes	50 mL
½ cup	sultana raisins	125 mL
1 to 2 tbsp	sweet rice flour	15 to 25 mL

Food Processor Method

1. In a small bowl, combine egg and milk. Set aside.

2. In a food processor, pulse amaranth flour, sorghum flour, cornstarch, potato flour, sugar, xanthan gum, baking powder, salt and nutmeg 3 or 4 times to combine. Add butter and pulse for 3 to 5 seconds or until mixture resembles coarse crumbs about the size of small peas. Add egg mixture all at once; process until dough begins to hold together, scraping sides and bottom occasionally. Add raisins and pulse until just combined.

Traditional Method

1. In a small bowl, combine egg and milk. Set aside.

2. In a large bowl combine amaranth flour, sorghum flour, cornstarch, potato flour, sugar, xanthan gum, baking powder, salt and nutmeg. Using a pastry blender or two knives, cut in butter until mixture resembles coarse crumbs about the size of small peas. Add egg mixture all at once, stirring with a fork to make a thick dough. Stir in raisins until just combined.

Nutritional value per serving

Calories	97
Fat, total	3 g
Fat, saturated	1 g
Cholesterol	16 mg
Sodium	44 mg
Carbohydrate	17 g
Fiber	1 g
Protein	2 g
Calcium	28 mg
Iron	2 mg

Tips

If the dough becomes too soft to handle while you're cutting it out, place it in the refrigerator for 10 to 15 minutes.

For information on cleaning and seasoning a cast-iron skillet, see the Techniques Glossary, page 395.

To prevent a cast-iron skillet from rusting, set it on a warm stove element to dry completely before storing. Be careful: the handle gets hot.

For Both Methods

3. Sprinkle 2 sheets of plastic wrap with sweet rice flour. Divide dough in half and place each half on a sheet of plastic wrap. Dust each with sweet rice flour. Top with another sheet of plastic wrap and pat out to a disc about $\frac{1}{2}$ inch (1 cm) thick. Wrap airtight and refrigerate for at least 1 hour, until chilled, or overnight.

4. Remove one disc of dough from the refrigerator. Place between two clean sheets of plastic wrap. Roll out to $\frac{1}{4}$-inch (0.5 cm) thickness. Cut out circles with the cookie cutter, rerolling scraps as necessary. If dough sticks to cutter, dip the cutter into sweet rice flour. Repeat with the remaining dough.

5. Preheat prepared skillet over medium-low heat. Working in batches, cook Welsh cakes for 2 minutes or until bottoms are golden. Turn and cook for 1 minute or until bottoms are golden. Leave cooked cakes on the skillet for a minute to dry slightly. Serve immediately.

Variations

Substitute dried currants for the raisins.

For sweeter Welsh cakes, sprinkle with white (granulated) sugar while still warm.

Sheila Green of London, Ontario, asked us to develop the recipe for these teacakes, which she remembers her Nan making for her in Swansea, Wales. She brought the wheat variety to a conference, so we could taste the originals. Today, the Welsh treasure these on St. David's Day, the 1st of March. When we sent the recipe to Sheila, she said, "It was wonderful to smell the comforting aroma while they were cooking — it always evokes such warm memories of my Nan. You have formulated a recipe that is so close to the original, which makes me *very happy*."

Basic White Cake

You asked for a plain white cake without butter or shortening. Here it is.

Tips

To remove the cake from the pan, run a metal spatula or knife around the edge of the pan. Turn the cake out onto the rack and let it cool completely before frosting.

This recipe makes 10 cups (2.5 L) cake crumbs, which you can use to make Blueberry Swirl Cheesecake (page 298). Pulse in batches in the food processor and store in an airtight container in the freezer for up to 3 months.

- 8-inch (20 cm) square baking pan, lightly greased and lined with parchment paper

1¾ cups	brown rice flour	425 mL
½ cup	tapioca starch	125 mL
¼ cup	cornstarch	50 mL
1 tsp	xanthan gum	5 mL
2 tsp	GF baking powder	10 mL
½ tsp	salt	2 mL
3	eggs	3
1 cup	white (granulated) sugar	250 mL
¾ cup	milk	175 mL
⅓ cup	vegetable oil	75 mL
1 tsp	vanilla extract	5 mL
1 tsp	cider vinegar	5 mL

1. In a large bowl or plastic bag, combine brown rice flour, tapioca starch, cornstarch, xanthan gum, baking powder and salt. Mix well and set aside.

2. In a separate bowl, using an electric mixer, beat eggs, sugar, milk, oil, vanilla and vinegar until combined. Add dry ingredients and mix until just combined.

3. Spoon batter into prepared pan. Using a moistened rubber spatula, spread to edges and smooth top. Let stand for 30 minutes. Meanwhile, preheat oven to 350°F (180°C).

4. Bake for 40 minutes or until a tester inserted in the center comes out clean. Let cool in pan on a rack for 10 minutes. Remove from pan and let cool completely on rack.

Variation

Make 12 cupcakes in a lightly greased 12-cup muffin tin. Decrease the baking time to 20 to 25 minutes.

Nutritional value per serving

Calories	341
Fat, total	11 g
Fat, saturated	1 g
Cholesterol	63 mg
Sodium	162 mg
Carbohydrate	57 g
Fiber	2 g
Protein	5 g
Calcium	85 mg
Iron	1 mg

Sponge Cake

Makes 12 to 16 servings

Adele Simonetta of Richmond Hill, Ontario, sent us a special request: for her celiac daughter's bridal shower, she wanted to make a white sponge cake and a chocolate sponge cake, both gluten-free. We were more than happy to develop the recipes for her. Here's the white sponge cake; the chocolate one is on page 374.

Tips

Substitute 1¼ cups (300 mL) liquid egg whites for the 12 egg whites.

Make sure the mixer bowl and beaters are completely free of grease before beating whites.

Use this sponge cake to make strawberry shortcake.

Nutritional value per serving

Calories	104
Fat, total	2 g
Fat, saturated	1 g
Cholesterol	67 mg
Sodium	80 mg
Carbohydrate	17 g
Fiber	1 g
Protein	4 g
Calcium	17 mg
Iron	2 mg

- Preheat oven to 350°F (180°C)
- 13- by 9-inch (33 by 23 cm) baking pan, bottom lined with parchment paper

¾ cup	amaranth flour	175 mL
½ cup	tapioca starch	125 mL
1½ tsp	xanthan gum	7 mL
12	egg whites, at room temperature	12
1 tbsp	freshly squeezed lemon juice	15 mL
1½ tsp	vanilla extract	7 mL
½ tsp	cream of tartar	2 mL
¼ tsp	salt	1 mL
¾ cup	white (granulated) sugar, divided	175 mL
5	egg yolks, at room temperature	5

1. In a small bowl or plastic bag, combine amaranth flour, tapioca starch and xanthan gum. Mix well and set aside.

2. In a large bowl, using an electric mixer with wire whisk attachment, beat egg whites until foamy. Beat in lemon juice, vanilla, cream of tartar and salt. Continue beating until egg whites form stiff peaks. Gradually beat in ½ cup (125 mL) of the sugar. Continue beating until mixture is very stiff and glossy but not dry.

3. In a deep bowl, using an electric mixer, beat egg yolks and the remaining ¼ cup (50 mL) sugar for about 5 minutes or until thick and lemon-colored.

4. Fold egg yolk mixture into egg white mixture. Sift in dry ingredients, one-third at a time, gently folding in each addition until well blended. Spoon into prepared pan and carefully spread to the edges.

5. Bake in preheated oven for 30 to 35 minutes or until cake is golden and springs back when lightly touched. Invert cake onto a rack, leaving the pan on top, and let cool completely. Using a spatula, loosen the edges of the pan and remove.

Variation

Turn this into a Daffodil Cake by folding in 2 tbsp (25 mL) grated lime zest and 1 tbsp (15 mL) grated orange zest with the dry ingredients. Drizzle wedges of cake with Lotsa Lime Filling (page 355).

Chocolate Sponge Cake

Makes 12 to 16 servings

Tips

This is the ideal time to use liquid egg whites. Substitute 1¼ cups (300 mL) for the 12 egg whites.

Make sure the mixer bowl and beaters are completely free of grease before beating whites.

For the best volume when whipping egg whites, be sure they are warmed to room temperature. See the Techniques Glossary, page 396.

To slice the cake without squishing it, use dental floss or a knife with a serrated edge, such as an electric knife.

Use this sponge cake to make strawberry shortcake. Drizzle with chocolate sauce.

- Preheat oven to 350°F (180°C)
- 13- by 9-inch (33 by 23 cm) baking pan, bottom lined with parchment paper

⅔ cup	amaranth flour	150 mL
⅓ cup	tapioca starch	75 mL
1½ tsp	xanthan gum	7 mL
¼ cup	unsweetened cocoa powder, sifted	50 mL
12	egg whites, at room temperature	12
1 tbsp	freshly squeezed lemon juice	15 mL
1½ tsp	vanilla extract	7 mL
½ tsp	cream of tartar	2 mL
¼ tsp	salt	1 mL
1 cup	white (granulated) sugar, divided	250 mL
4	egg yolks, at room temperature	4

1. In a small bowl or plastic bag, combine amaranth flour, tapioca starch, xanthan gum and cocoa. Mix well and set aside.

2. In a large bowl, using an electric mixer with wire whisk attachment, beat egg whites until foamy. Beat in lemon juice, vanilla, cream of tartar and salt. Continue beating until egg whites form stiff peaks. Gradually beat in ¾ cup (175 mL) of the sugar. Continue beating until mixture is very stiff and glossy but not dry.

3. In a deep bowl, using an electric mixer, beat egg yolks and the remaining ¼ cup (50 mL) sugar for about 5 minutes or until thick and lemon-colored.

4. Fold egg yolk mixture into egg white mixture. Sift in dry ingredients, one-third at a time, gently folding in each addition until well blended. Spoon into prepared pan and carefully spread to the edges.

5. Bake in preheated oven for 30 to 35 minutes or until cake is golden brown and springs back when lightly touched. Invert cake onto a rack, leaving the pan on top, and let cool completely. Using a spatula, loosen the edges of the pan and remove.

Nutritional value per serving

Calories	109
Fat, total	2 g
Fat, saturated	1 g
Cholesterol	53 mg
Sodium	80 mg
Carbohydrate	19 g
Fiber	1 g
Protein	4 g
Calcium	16 mg
Iron	2 mg

Soy-Free Pineapple Carrot Cake

White sugar–free

Makes 9 servings

We created this recipe after a special request from Anna Denti, who can't tolerate soy and loves carrot cake. Frost it with our Orange Cream Cheese Icing (page 328).

Tip

Wrap cake airtight (before icing) and store in the freezer for up to 6 weeks. Thaw, wrapped, in the refrigerator.

- **8-inch (20 cm) square baking pan, lightly greased and lined with parchment paper**

¾ cup	brown rice flour	175 mL
½ cup	amaranth flour	125 mL
¼ cup	quinoa flour	50 mL
¼ cup	tapioca starch	50 mL
1½ tsp	xanthan gum	7 mL
2 tsp	GF baking powder	10 mL
1 tsp	baking soda	5 mL
½ tsp	salt	2 mL
1 tsp	ground cinnamon	5 mL
½ tsp	ground nutmeg	2 mL
2	eggs	2
⅔ cup	packed brown sugar	150 mL
½ cup	GF sour cream	125 mL
½ cup	canned crushed pineapple, including juice	125 mL
1½ cups	shredded carrots	375 mL
½ cup	chopped walnuts	125 mL

1. In a large bowl or plastic bag, combine brown rice flour, amaranth flour, quinoa flour, tapioca starch, xanthan gum, baking powder, baking soda, salt, cinnamon and nutmeg. Mix well and set aside.

2. In a separate bowl, using an electric mixer, beat eggs, brown sugar, sour cream and pineapple until combined. Add dry ingredients and mix until just combined. Stir in carrots and walnuts.

3. Spoon batter into prepared pan. Using a moistened rubber spatula, spread to edges and smooth top. Let stand for 30 minutes. Meanwhile, preheat oven to 350°F (180°C).

4. Bake for 45 minutes or until a tester inserted in the center comes out clean. Let cool in pan on a rack for 10 minutes. Remove from pan and let cool completely on rack.

Variations

Double the recipe and bake it in a 13- by 9-inch (33 by 23 cm) baking pan for 40 to 45 minutes.

To make this cake nut-free, substitute raisins or dried cranberries for the walnuts.

Nutritional value per serving

Calories	252
Fat, total	7 g
Fat, saturated	2 g
Cholesterol	46 mg
Sodium	313 mg
Carbohydrate	43 g
Fiber	3 g
Protein	5 g
Calcium	113 mg
Iron	3 mg

Spicy Marble Cake

Joan Segee of Moncton, New Brunswick, asked us to develop a gluten-free version of a recipe she first baked when she was 12. It was her father's favorite, as he didn't like a marble cake made with chocolate.

- 10-inch (25 cm) Bundt pan, lightly greased

Spicy Cake

1/2 cup	butter	125 mL
1 cup	boiling water	250 mL
3/4 cup	sorghum flour	175 mL
3/4 cup	whole bean flour	175 mL
1/4 cup	tapioca starch	50 mL
1 tsp	xanthan gum	5 mL
1/2 tsp	GF baking powder	2 mL
1/4 tsp	baking soda	1 mL
1/4 tsp	salt	1 mL
1 1/2 tsp	ground cinnamon	7 mL
3/4 tsp	ground cloves	4 mL
2	eggs	2
2/3 cup	packed brown sugar	150 mL
2/3 cup	light (fancy) molasses	150 mL

White Cake

2/3 cup	brown rice flour	150 mL
1/2 cup	tapioca starch	125 mL
1/3 cup	cornstarch	75 mL
3/4 tsp	xanthan gum	4 mL
1 1/2 tsp	GF baking powder	7 mL
1/2 tsp	salt	2 mL
3/4 cup	white (granulated) sugar	175 mL
1/2 cup	butter, softened	125 mL
3	eggs	3
1/2 cup	milk	125 mL
1 tsp	cider vinegar	5 mL
3/4 tsp	vanilla extract	4 mL

1. *Spicy cake:* Place butter in a small bowl and pour boiling water over top. Set aside to melt and cool slightly.

2. In a large bowl or plastic bag, combine sorghum flour, whole bean flour, tapioca starch, xanthan gum, baking powder, baking soda, salt, cinnamon and cloves.

3. In a separate bowl, using an electric mixer, beat eggs, brown sugar and molasses until combined. Add butter mixture and beat until smooth. Add dry ingredients and mix until just combined. Spoon batter into prepared pan.

Nutritional value per serving	
Calories	426
Fat, total	18 g
Fat, saturated	10 g
Cholesterol	119 mg
Sodium	369 mg
Carbohydrate	64 g
Fiber	2 g
Protein	5 g
Calcium	123 mg
Iron	2 mg

Tips
Don't swirl the batters too much: you want large pockets of each color.

Letting the batter stand for 30 minutes results in a more tender cake.

4. *White cake:* In a large bowl, sift together brown rice flour, tapioca starch, cornstarch, xanthan gum, baking powder and salt. Set aside.

5. In a separate bowl, using an electric mixer, beat sugar and butter until light and fluffy. Beat in eggs, milk, vinegar and vanilla until smooth. Add dry ingredients and mix until just combined.

6. With a large spoon, dollop half of the white cake batter on top of the spicy cake layer. Swirl the batters by lifting some of the spicy layer up through the white layer. Spoon on the remaining white batter and swirl again. Avoid overmixing. Let stand for 30 minutes. Meanwhile, preheat oven to 325°F (160°C).

7. Bake for 60 minutes or until a tester inserted in the center comes out clean. Let cool in pan on a rack for 10 minutes. Remove from pan and let cool completely on rack.

Variation
Substitute any bean or pea flour for the whole bean flour.

Donna and Heather's White Fruitcake

*Bake lots of this
fruitcake, as it is moist
and holds together
well from the time
it is cool enough to
cut. There is more
fruit than cake —
how delightful! It's
perfect for a wedding,
a christening or
Christmas.*

Tip

You'll need about 2 lbs
(1 kg) candied citron,
10 oz (300 g) golden raisins,
1 lb (500 g) glacé cherries,
8 oz (250 g) slivered
almonds and 12 oz (375 g)
candied pineapple.

- Three 9- by 5-inch (23 by 12.5 cm) loaf pans
- Shallow 13- by 9-inch (33 by 23 cm) baking pan

4 cups	mixed candied citron	1 L
2 cups	seedless golden raisins	500 mL
2 cups	green and red glacé cherries, halved	500 mL
1½ cups	slivered almonds	375 mL
1½ cups	candied pineapple, coarsely chopped	375 mL
¾ cup	white rum	175 mL
1½ cups	amaranth flour	375 mL
½ cup	almond flour	125 mL
½ cup	tapioca starch	125 mL
1½ tsp	xanthan gum	7 mL
½ tsp	baking soda	2 mL
¼ tsp	salt	1 mL
1 cup	white (granulated) sugar	250 mL
½ cup	butter, softened	125 mL
3	eggs	3
1 cup	canned crushed pineapple, including juice	250 mL
1 tsp	almond extract	5 mL

1. In a large bowl, combine citron, raisins, cherries, almonds, candied pineapple and rum; cover and let stand overnight, stirring when convenient.

2. Line the bottom and sides of each loaf pan with a double layer of heavy brown paper and one layer of parchment paper.

3. Position the oven racks to divide the oven into thirds. Fill the baking pan with 1 inch (2.5 cm) of hot water and place on the bottom shelf. Preheat oven to 250°F (120°C).

4. In a large bowl or plastic bag, combine amaranth flour, almond flour, tapioca starch, xanthan gum, baking soda and salt. Mix well and set aside.

5. In a very large bowl, using a heavy-duty electric mixer, cream sugar and butter until light and fluffy. Add eggs, one at a time, beating well after each addition. Stir in crushed pineapple and almond extract. Gradually beat in dry ingredients until smooth. Stir in dried fruit mixture.

Nutritional value per serving	
Calories	117
Fat, total	3 g
Fat, saturated	1 g
Cholesterol	9 mg
Sodium	58 mg
Carbohydrate	21 g
Fiber	1 g
Protein	1 g
Calcium	23 mg
Iron	1 mg

Tips

You will need a very large mixing bowl. If you don't have one large enough for the whole recipe, use your roasting pan or divide the batter in half before stirring in the dried fruit.

Always slice fruitcake cold from the refrigerator. Use a very sharp knife and wipe the blade with a damp cloth between slices.

6. Spoon batter evenly into prepared loaf pans. Using a moistened rubber spatula, spread into the corners and smooth tops.

7. Bake cakes on the top rack of the oven for $2\frac{1}{2}$ to 3 hours or until internal temperature registers 200°F (100°C) on an instant-read thermometer. Do not overbake. Let cool in pans on racks for 10 minutes. Remove cakes from pans and let cool completely on racks.

8. Wrap cakes airtight and store in the refrigerator for up to 2 months or in the freezer for up to 1 year.

Variations

Top the cooled cakes with a thick layer of GF marzipan.

Substitute unsweetened apple juice for the rum.

Substitute mixed candied peel for the mixed candied citron.

Red Velvet Cupcakes

**Makes 12 cupcakes
(1 per serving)**

We received a special request for this recipe via email from a celiac living in the Deep South who fondly remembers these from her childhood. Traditionally, red velvet cakes are iced with Red Velvet Cake Frosting (page 381), but you can use your favorite cream cheese frosting recipe instead.

Tips

Fill the muffin cups almost level with the top.

Let cupcakes cool completely, wrap individually and freeze for up to 1 month.

Nutritional value per serving	
Calories	186
Fat, total	7 g
Fat, saturated	1 g
Cholesterol	32 mg
Sodium	345 mg
Carbohydrate	28 g
Fiber	1 g
Protein	4 g
Calcium	41 mg
Iron	1 mg

• 12-cup muffin tin, lightly greased

⅔ cup	sorghum flour	150 mL
⅔ cup	whole bean flour	150 mL
3 tbsp	tapioca starch	45 mL
1 cup	white (granulated) sugar	250 mL
1 tsp	xanthan gum	5 mL
2 tsp	baking soda	10 mL
½ tsp	salt	2 mL
2 tbsp	unsweetened cocoa powder, sifted	25 mL
2	eggs	2
1¼ cups	buttermilk	300 mL
⅓ cup	vegetable oil	75 mL
2 tbsp	GF red food coloring	25 mL
2 tsp	cider vinegar	10 mL

1. In a large bowl or plastic bag, combine sorghum flour, whole bean flour, tapioca starch, sugar, xanthan gum, baking soda, salt and cocoa. Mix well and set aside.

2. In a separate bowl, using an electric mixer, beat eggs, buttermilk, oil, food coloring and vinegar until combined. Add dry ingredients and mix until just combined.

3. Spoon batter evenly into prepared muffin cups. Let stand for 30 minutes. Meanwhile, preheat oven to 350°F (180°C).

4. Bake for 20 to 25 minutes or until a tester inserted in the center of a cupcake comes out clean. Let cool in pan on a rack for 5 minutes. Remove from pan and let cool completely on rack.

Variations

Sprinkle iced cakes with coconut.

Bake as a cake in a lightly greased 8-inch (20 cm) square baking pan. Increase the baking time to 35 to 45 minutes.

Red Velvet Cake Frosting

Makes 1½ cups (375 mL), enough to frost 12 cupcakes (2 tbsp/25 mL per serving)

Here is our version of the traditional frosting for Red Velvet Cupcakes (page 380).

Tip

This frosting will have the consistency of whipped cream.

2 tbsp	amaranth flour	25 mL
½ cup	milk	125 mL
½ cup	white (granulated) sugar	125 mL
½ cup	butter, softened	125 mL
½ tsp	vanilla extract	2 mL

1. In a small microwave-safe bowl, combine amaranth flour and milk. Microwave on High for 2 minutes, stopping to stir occasionally, until boiling and thickened. Let cool completely.

2. In a small bowl, cream sugar, butter and vanilla until light and fluffy. Beat in flour mixture until light and fluffy.

Nutritional value per serving

Calories	109
Fat, total	8 g
Fat, saturated	5 g
Cholesterol	21 mg
Sodium	82 mg
Carbohydrate	10 g
Fiber	0 g
Protein	1 g
Calcium	17 mg
Iron	0 mg

Ruth's Chocolate Fudge Pie

Makes 8 servings

Ellie Steele told us about a chocolate pie that has become a favorite over the years, originally made for her son by an elderly neighbor, Ruth, who served it to him when he delivered her newspaper.

Tips

We have pie crust recipes in our earlier gluten-free cookbooks. The one in *125 Best Gluten-Free Recipes* (page 136) uses rice flour with shortening; the one in *The Best Gluten-Free Family Cookbook* (page 152) uses sorghum flour with vegetable oil. Both books have lots of tips on making a pie crust.

When preparing the filling, be sure to stir all the way to the bottom, as it can easily thicken and stick to the pan.

Nutritional value per serving	
Calories	276
Fat, total	13 g
Fat, saturated	6 g
Cholesterol	56 mg
Sodium	171 mg
Carbohydrate	38 g
Fiber	2 g
Protein	6 g
Calcium	102 mg
Iron	3 mg

2	egg yolks, lightly beaten	2
1 tsp	vanilla extract	5 mL
½ cup	amaranth flour	125 mL
2 tbsp	cornstarch	25 mL
⅔ cup	white (granulated) sugar	150 mL
Pinch	salt	Pinch
2 cups	milk	500 mL
3 oz	unsweetened chocolate, coarsely chopped	90 g
1	9-inch (23 cm) single-crust pie shell, baked and cooled (see tip, at left)	1

1. In a small bowl, whisk together egg yolks and vanilla. Set aside.

2. In a heavy saucepan, combine amaranth flour, cornstarch, sugar and salt. Gradually stir in milk and chocolate. Heat over medium heat, stirring constantly, for 7 minutes or until mixture comes to a boil and thickens.

3. Gradually whisk ½ cup (125 mL) of the hot milk mixture into the egg yolk mixture. Add the egg yolk mixture to the rest of the hot milk mixture, stirring constantly. Cook for 1 to 2 minutes or until thickened. Let cool for 5 minutes.

4. Pour into pie shell. Place plastic wrap directly on surface of filling. Refrigerate for 3 to 4 hours, until chilled, or overnight.

Variations

Substitute bittersweet chocolate for the unsweetened.

The filling can be prepared in the top of a double boiler over hot water. It will take longer, but it doesn't need to be stirred constantly this way.

Stewed Rhubarb with Strawberries

Makes 6 servings

This recipe was a special request from a celiac who remembered her grandmother serving this to her in early spring.

Tip

If you use the oven method, the juice will become a deep rosy red.

4 cups	chopped rhubarb (1/2-inch/1 cm pieces)	1 L
2 cups	coarsely chopped strawberries	500 mL
3/4 cup	liquid honey	175 mL

Oven Method

1. Preheat oven to 350°F (180°C). In an 8-cup (2 L) baking dish, combine rhubarb, strawberries and honey. Cover and bake for 30 to 40 minutes or until fruit is tender.

Stovetop Method

1. In a large saucepan, bring rhubarb, strawberries and honey to a simmer over medium-low heat. Simmer, stirring frequently, for 7 to 8 minutes or until fruit is tender.

Variation

Use this recipe as the base for a rhubarb crisp (see Summer Fruit Crisp, page 341, for topping and method).

Nutritional value per serving	
Calories	163
Fat, total	0 g
Fat, saturated	0 g
Cholesterol	0 mg
Sodium	6 mg
Carbohydrate	42 g
Fiber	1 g
Protein	1 g
Calcium	80 mg
Iron	1 mg

Cream Puffs

*Many seasoned bakers
have asked us to
develop this recipe, as
they missed making
one of their favorite
desserts.*

Tips

Liquid whole eggs are
perfect for this recipe;
you'll need about ½ cup
(125 mL).

If puffs have become soft
before you're ready to fill
them, heat them in the
oven for 5 minutes.

- Preheat oven to 375°F (190°C)
- Baking sheet, lightly greased and lined with parchment paper

⅓ cup	sorghum flour	75 mL
2 tbsp	potato starch	25 mL
1 tbsp	white (granulated) sugar	15 mL
Pinch	salt	Pinch
½ cup	water	125 mL
3 tbsp	butter	45 mL
2	eggs	2
2 cups	Lemon Filling (page 385)	500 mL

1. In a small bowl, combine sorghum flour, potato starch, sugar and salt. Mix well and set aside.

2. In a saucepan, bring water and butter to a boil over medium-high heat. Add dry ingredients all at once and cook, stirring constantly, until mixture pulls away from the sides of the pan. Let cool slightly.

3. Add eggs, one at a time, beating vigorously with a wooden spoon after each addition. Return to low heat and beat for 2 minutes. The mixture will be very thick and rough in texture. Drop by large spoonfuls 2 inches (5 cm) apart on prepared baking sheet.

4. Bake in preheated oven for 35 to 40 minutes or until deep golden brown. Remove from oven and immediately cut a 1-inch (2.5 cm) horizontal slit in the side of each puff. Return to the oven and bake for 5 minutes. Remove from pan to a rack and let cool completely.

5. Slice off the top third of each puff. Using your fingers, remove and discard any moist, uncooked dough from the center of the puff, leaving a hollow shell. Fill puffs with Lemon Filling and replace tops.

Variation

Make 10 small puffs, bake for 30 to 35 minutes, fill and serve as a starter.

Nutritional value per serving

Calories	451
Fat, total	24 g
Fat, saturated	13 g
Cholesterol	261 mg
Sodium	188 mg
Carbohydrate	55 g
Fiber	1 g
Protein	6 g
Calcium	52 mg
Iron	1 mg

Lemon Filling

**Makes 2 cups (500 mL)
(½ cup/125 mL per
serving)**

*We developed this
versatile filling recipe
to use with our Cream
Puffs (page 384), but
you will think of many
other uses for it.*

Tips

To get the most volume out
of your whipped cream,
chill the bowl and beaters
for at least 1 hour.

Serve this as a lemon
pudding, with fresh fruit.

⅔ cup	white (granulated) sugar	150 mL
2 tbsp	cornstarch	25 mL
½ cup	water	125 mL
1 tbsp	grated lemon zest	15 mL
⅓ cup	freshly squeezed lemon juice	75 mL
2	egg yolks	2
1 cup	whipping (35%) cream	250 mL

1. In a small saucepan, combine sugar and cornstarch. Slowly whisk in water until smooth. Stir in lemon zest, lemon juice and egg yolks. Cook over medium heat, stirring constantly, for about 7 minutes or until mixture comes to a boil. Boil, stirring constantly, for 1 minute. Remove from heat.

2. Transfer to a bowl. Cover surface with plastic wrap and refrigerate for 1 hour, until chilled, or for up 2 days.

3. In a large bowl, using an electric mixer with wire whisk attachment, whip cream until stiff peaks form. Fold in lemon mixture.

Variation
For a stronger lemon flavor, omit the cream.

Nutritional value per serving

Calories	277
Fat, total	13 g
Fat, saturated	7 g
Cholesterol	145 mg
Sodium	15 mg
Carbohydrate	40 g
Fiber	0 g
Protein	2 g
Calcium	35 mg
Iron	0 mg

Evelyn's Play Dough

A CanolaInfo recipe

Mothers of young children have asked us for a play dough recipe that is soft and pliable. Heather's friend Evelyn gave us the original wheat-based recipe, and we adapted it to make it gluten-free.

Tips

Use a large, firm spoon to stir the dough, as it forms a solid yet pliable ball very quickly.

Store in an airtight container in the refrigerator. So far, we have had ours for 3 months, and it is still soft, pliable and great to play with. Ours is in a plastic bag. Your children or grandchildren will let you know when it becomes too dry to play with.

½ cup	whole bean flour	125 mL
½ cup	cornstarch	125 mL
½ cup	salt	125 mL
1 cup	water	250 mL
1 tbsp	vegetable oil	15 mL
2 tsp	cream of tartar	10 mL
2 to 3	drops food coloring	2 to 3

1. In a large saucepan, combine whole bean flour, cornstarch, salt, water, oil, cream of tartar and food coloring. Heat over medium heat, stirring constantly, for 2 to 3 minutes or until dough forms a ball.

2. Let cool long enough for young hands to handle.

Variations

Any type of bean or pea flour can be used.

Omit the food coloring, divide the dough into small amounts and work a few drops of food coloring into each portion; that way, you can offer the kids several different color options.

Equipment Glossary

Colander. A bowl-shaped utensil with many holes, used to drain liquids from solids.

Cooling rack. Parallel and perpendicular thin bars of metal at right angles, with feet attached, used to hold hot baking off the surface to allow cooling air to circulate.

Griddle. A flat metal surface on which food is cooked. Can be built into a stove or stand-alone.

Grill. Heavy rack set over a heat source, used to cook food, usually on a propane, natural gas or charcoal barbecue.

Instant-read thermometer. See page 45.

Jelly roll pan. A rectangular baking pan, 15 by 10 by 1 inch (40 by 25 by 2.5 cm), used for baking thin cakes.

Kitchen torch. A small handheld torch used to blacken the skin of peppers and caramelize sugar. Many use butane or propane and have an adjustable flame.

Loaf pan. Container used for baking loaves. Common pan sizes are 9 by 5 inches (23 by 12.5 cm) and 8 by 4 inches (20 by 10 cm).

Mezzaluna. A two-handled knife with one or more thick, crescent-shaped blades (*mezzaluna* is Italian for "half moon"). Used to chop or mince herbs and vegetables. Also known as a mincing knife.

OXO angled measuring cups. Made to give an accurate measure while set on the counter. There's no need to hold the measuring cup at eye level — you can look straight down as you fill it, and the angled insert lets you know when it is full enough. These cups are dishwasher-safe, but not microwaveable. Sizes available include $\frac{1}{4}$ cup (50 mL), 1 cup (250 mL), 2 cups (500 mL) and 4 cups (1 L). All sizes indicate metric and imperial amounts.

Parchment paper. Heat-resistant paper similar to waxed paper, usually coated with silicon on one side; used with or as an alternative to other methods (such as applying vegetable oil or spray) to prevent baked goods from sticking to the baking pan. Sometimes labeled "baking paper."

Pastry blender. Used to cut solid fat into flour, it consists of five or six metal blades or wires held together by a handle.

Pastry brush. Small brush with nylon or natural bristles used to apply glazes or egg washes to dough. Wash thoroughly after each use. To store, lay flat or hang on a hook through the hole in the handle.

Pizza wheel. A sharp-edged wheel (without serrations) anchored to a handle.

Portion scoop. A utensil similar to an ice cream scoop, used to measure equal amounts of batter. Cookie scoops come in different sizes, for 2-inch (5 cm), $2\frac{1}{2}$-inch (6 cm) and $3\frac{1}{4}$-inch (8 cm) cookies. Muffin scoops have a $\frac{1}{4}$-cup (50 mL) capacity.

Ramekins. Usually sold as a set of small, deep, straight-sided ceramic soufflé dishes also known as mini bakers. Used to bake individual servings of a pudding, cobbler or custard. Capacity ranges from 4 oz, or $\frac{1}{2}$ cup (125 mL), to 8 oz, or 1 cup (250 mL).

Rolling pin. A smooth cylinder of wood, marble, plastic or metal; used to roll out dough.

Sieve. A bowl-shaped utensil with many holes, used to drain liquids from solids.

Soufflé dish. A round porcelain dish with a ridged exterior and a straight, smooth interior.

Spatula. A utensil with a handle and a blade that can be long or short, narrow or wide, flexible or inflexible. It is used to spread, lift, turn, mix or smooth foods. Spatulas are made of metal, rubber, plastic or silicone.

Springform pan. A circular baking pan, available in a range of sizes, with a separable bottom and side. The side is removed by releasing a clamp, making the contents easy to serve.

Tart pan. A shallow baking pan with a removable bottom. The sides are frequently fluted.

Tester. A thin, long wooden or metal stick or wire attached to a handle, used for baked products to test for doneness.

Thermometers.

- *Candy/fat thermometer.* Used to test the temperature of candy syrup or hot oil. Temperatures range from 75°F (25°C) to 400°F (200°C). A metal clip fastens to the side of the cooking pot, holding the tip of the thermometer off the bottom.

- *Instant-read thermometer.* See page 45.

- *Meat thermometer.* Used to read internal temperature of meat. Temperatures range from 120°F to 200°F (60°C to 100°C). Before placing meat in the oven, insert the thermometer into the thickest part, avoiding the bone and gristle. (If using an instant-read thermometer, remove meat from oven and test with thermometer. For more information, see Digital instant-read thermometer in the Techniques Glossary, page 396.)

- *Oven thermometer.* Used to measure temperatures from 200°F to 500°F (100°C to 260°C). It either stands on or hangs from an oven rack.

Wok. A metal cooking pan with a rounded bottom and curved sides. It is frequently used for deep-frying or stir-frying.

Zester. A tool used to cut very thin strips of outer peel from citrus fruits. One type has a short, flat blade tipped with five small holes with sharp edges. Another style of zester that is popular is made of stainless steel and looks like a tool used for planing wood in a workshop.

Ingredient Glossary

Almond flour (almond meal). See page 32.

Almonds. An ivory-colored nut with a pointed oval shape and a smooth texture. Almonds have a thin, medium-brown skin that adheres to the nut. Sweet almonds have a delicate taste that is delicious in breads, cookies, cakes, fillings and candies. Blanched (skin off) and natural (skin on) almonds are interchangeable in recipes. Almonds are available whole, sliced, slivered or ground.

Amaranth flour. See page 17.

Apricots. A small stone fruit with a thin, pale yellow to orange skin and meaty orange flesh. Dried unpeeled apricot halves are used in baking.

Arborio rice. See page 22.

Arrowroot. See page 33.

Asiago cheese. A pungent grayish-white hard cheese from northern Italy. Cured for more than 6 months, its texture is ideal for grating.

Baking chips. Similar in consistency to chocolate chips, but with different flavors, such as butterscotch, peanut butter, cinnamon and lemon. Check to make sure they are gluten-free and lactose-free.

Baking powder. A chemical leavener, containing an alkali (baking soda) and an acid (cream of tartar), that gives off carbon dioxide gas under certain conditions. Select gluten-free baking powder.

Baking soda (sodium bicarbonate). A chemical leavener that gives off carbon dioxide gas in the presence of moisture — particularly acids such as lemon juice, buttermilk and sour cream. It is also one of the components of baking powder.

Balsamic vinegar. A dark Italian vinegar made from grape juice that has been cooked until the water content is reduced by half, then aged for several years in wooden barrels. It has a pungent sweetness and can be used to make salad dressings and marinades or drizzled over roasted or grilled vegetables.

Bean flours. See page 31.

Bell peppers. The sweet-flavored members of the capsicum family (which includes chiles and other hot peppers), these peppers have a hollow interior lined with white ribs and seeds attached at the stem end. They are most commonly green, red, orange or yellow, but can also be white or purple.

Blueberries. Wild low-bush berries are smaller than the cultivated variety and more time-consuming to pick, but their flavor makes every minute of picking time worthwhile. Readily available year-round in the frozen fruit section of most grocery stores.

Bocconcini. Italian for "mouthful," bocconcini is fresh mozzarella cheese shaped into small balls about 1 inch (2.5 cm) in diameter. Soft, unripened buffalo-style mozzarella is another fresh mozzarella.

Brown rice flour. See page 24.

Brown sugar. See page 36.

Buckwheat. See page 18.

Butter. A spread produced from dairy fat and milk solids, butter is interchangeable with shortening, oil or margarine in most recipes. See also Lactose Intolerance, page 42.

Capers. A pickled bud of the caper bush, grown in Mediterranean countries. Purchase in grocery stores in 2- to 3-oz (60 to 90 g) glass jars to use in sauces and salads and to enhance the flavor of smoked salmon.

Cardamom. This popular spice is a member of the ginger family. A long green or brown pod contains the strong, spicy, lemon-flavored seed. Although native to India, cardamom is used in Middle Eastern, Indian and Scandinavian cooking — in the latter case, particularly for seasonal baked goods.

Cassava. The plant from which tapioca comes.

Celery seeds. Small, light brown to khaki-colored seeds with an aroma similar to celery stalks. Their flavor is strong and bitter, and lingers on the palate.

Chickpea (garbanzo bean) flour. See page 31.

Cilantro. See Coriander.

Coconut. The fruit of a tropical palm tree, with a hard woody shell that is lined with a hard white flesh. There are three dried forms available, which can be sweetened or not: flaked, shredded and the smallest, desiccated (thoroughly dried).

Coconut milk. A white liquid made by pouring boiling water over shredded coconut; the mixture is then cooled and strained.

Confectioner's (icing) sugar. See page 35.

Coriander. These tiny, yellow-ridged seeds taste of cardamom, cloves, white pepper and orange. Coriander leaves (also known as cilantro) have a flavor reminiscent of lemon, sage and caraway. To increase flavor in a recipe, substitute cilantro for parsley.

Corn flour. See page 19.

Cornmeal. See page 19.

Cornstarch. See page 33.

Corn syrup. See page 37.

Cranberries. Grown in bogs on low vines, these sweet-tart berries are available fresh, frozen and dried. Fresh cranberries are available only in season — typically from mid-October until January, depending on your location — but can be frozen right in the bag. Substitute dried cranberries for sour cherries, raisins or currants.

Cream of tartar. Used to give volume and stability to beaten egg whites, cream of tartar is also an acidic component of baking powder. Tartaric acid is a fine white crystalline powder that forms naturally on the inside of wine barrels during the fermentation of grape juice.

Currants. Similar in appearance to small dark raisins, currants are made by drying a special seedless variety of grape. Not the same as a type of berry that goes by the same name.

Dates. The fruit of the date palm tree, dates are long and oval in shape, with a paper-thin skin that turns from green to dark brown when ripe. Eaten fresh or dried, dates have a very sweet, light brown flesh around a long, narrow seed.

Demerara sugar. See page 36.

Egg replacer. See Egg-Free Baking, page 44.

Eggs. Liquid egg products, such as Naturegg Simply Whites, Break-Free and Omega Pro liquid eggs and Just Whites, are available in the United States and Canada. Powdered egg whites, such as Just Whites, can be used by reconstituting with warm water or as a powder. A similar product is called meringue powder in Canada. Substitute 2 tbsp (25 mL) liquid egg product for each white of a large egg.

Fava bean flour. See page 31.

Feta cheese. A crumbly white Greek-style cheese with a salty, tangy flavor. Store in the refrigerator, in its brine, and drain well before using. Traditionally made with sheep's or goat's milk in Greece and usually with cow's milk in Canada and the U.S. A lactose-free flavored soy product is also available.

Fig. A pear-shaped fruit with a thick, soft skin, available in green and purple. Eaten fresh or dried, the tan-colored sweet flesh contains many tiny edible seeds.

Flaxseed. See page 30.

Fruit sugar. See page 35.

Garbanzo bean flour. See page 31.

Garfava flour. See page 31.

Garlic. An edible bulb composed of several sections (cloves), each covered with a papery skin. An essential ingredient in many styles of cooking.

Gelatin, unflavored. A colorless, odorless, flavorless powder used as a thickener. When dissolved in hot liquid and then cooled, it forms a jelly-like substance.

Gingerroot. A bumpy rhizome, ivory to greenish yellow in color, with a tan skin. Fresh gingerroot has a peppery, slightly sweet flavor, similar to lemon and rosemary, and a pungent aroma. Ground ginger is made from dried gingerroot. It is spicier and not as sweet or as fresh. Crystallized, or candied, ginger is made from pieces of fresh gingerroot that have been cooked in sugar syrup and coated with sugar.

Gluten. A natural protein in wheat flour that becomes elastic with the addition of moisture and kneading. Gluten traps gases produced by leaveners inside the dough and causes it to rise.

Glutinous rice flour. See Sweet rice flour, page 24.

Golden raisins. See Raisins.

Granulated sugar. See page 35.

Guar gum. A white, flour-like substance made from an East Indian seed high in fiber, this vegetable substance contains no gluten. It may have a laxative effect for some people. It can be substituted for xanthan gum.

Hazelnut flour (hazelnut meal). See page 32.

Hazelnut liqueur. The best known is Frangelico, a hazelnut-flavored liqueur made in Italy.

Hazelnuts. Slightly larger than filberts, hazelnuts have a weaker flavor. Both nuts have a round, smooth shell and look like small brown marbles. They have a sweet, rich flavor and are interchangeable in recipes.

Herbs. Plants whose stems, leaves or flowers are used as a flavoring, either dried or fresh. To substitute fresh herbs for dried, a good rule of thumb is to use three times the amount of fresh as dried. Taste and adjust the amount to suit your preference.

Honey. See page 37.

Italian eggplant. A miniature variety shaped like a large, plump pear, with shiny black-purple skin. Also known as baby eggplant.

Jalapeño peppers. Named for the Mexican city of Jalapa, these short, tapered chile peppers have a thick flesh, are moderately hot and are dark green in color.

Kalamata olives. See Olives, kalamata.

Kasha. See page 18.

Linseed. See Flaxseed, page 30.

Mangos. Mangos can be as small as an egg or as heavy as 5 pounds (2.3 kg), and can be oval, round or kidney-shaped. They have a large, tongue-shaped pit surrounded by flesh that ranges in color from yellow to red. Mangos are picked unripe and should be firm, with green skin and no blemishes. When ripe, they are completely colored with areas of green, yellow and red and should be quite firm to the touch, with a sweet, fruity smell.

Maple syrup. See page 37.

Margarine. A solid fat derived from one or more types of vegetable oil. Do not use lower-fat margarines in baking, as they contain too much added water. See also Lactose Intolerance, page 42.

Mesclun. A mixture of small, young, tender salad greens such as spinach, frisée, arugula, oak leaf and radicchio. Also known as salad mix, spring mix or baby greens and sold prepackaged or in bulk in the grocery produce section.

Millet. See page 19.

Mixed candied citron. See Mixed glazed fruit.

Mixed glazed fruit. A mixture of dried candied orange and lemon peel, citron and glazed cherries. Citron, which can be expensive, is often replaced in the mix by candied rutabaga.

Molasses. See page 36.

Montina™. See page 20.

Muscovado sugar. See page 36.

Nut flour (nut meal). See page 32.

Oats, pure uncontaminated. See page 20.

Oat flour, pure uncontaminated. See page 21.

Olive oil. Produced from pressing tree-ripened olives. Extra virgin oil is taken from the first cold pressing; it is the finest and fruitiest, pale straw to pale green in color, with the least amount of acid, usually less than 1%. Virgin oil is taken from a subsequent pressing; it contains 2% acid and is pale yellow. Light oil comes from the last pressing; it has a mild flavor, light color and up to 3% acid. It also has a higher smoke point. Product sold as "pure olive oil" has been cleaned and filtered; it is very mild-flavored and has up to 3% acid.

Olives, kalamata. A large, flavorful variety of Greek olive, typically dark purple in color and pointed at one end.

Parsley. A biennial herb with dark green curly or flat leaves used fresh as a flavoring or garnish. It is also used dried in soups and other mixes. Substitute parsley for half the amount of a strong-flavored herb such as basil.

Pea fiber. See page 31.

Pea flour. See page 31.

Pecan flour (pecan meal). See page 33.

Pecans. This sweet, mellow nut is smooth and oval, golden brown on the outside and tan on the inside. You can purchase pecans whole, halved, chopped or in chips.

Peel (mixed, candied or glacé). This type of peel is crystallized in sugar.

Peppers. See Bell peppers; Jalapeño peppers.

Plumcot. This new hybrid, also called a pluot, is a cross between a plum and an apricot, with speckled skin. Plumcots are available in various colors and sizes.

Poppy seeds. These tiny, kidney-shaped seeds have a mild, sweet, nutty, dusty flavor. They are available whole or ground. They are most flavorful when roasted and crushed.

Potato flour. See page 33.

Potato starch (potato starch flour). See page 33.

Pumpkin seeds. Available roasted or raw, salted or unsalted, and with or without hulls. Raw pumpkin seeds without hulls — often known as pepitas ("little seeds" in Spanish) — are a dull, dark olive green. Roasted pumpkin seeds have a rich, almost peanuty flavor.

Quinoa. See page 21.

Raisins. Dark raisins are sun-dried Thompson seedless grapes. Golden raisins are treated with sulfur dioxide and dried artificially, yielding a moister, plumper product.

Raw sugars. See page 36.

Rhubarb. A perennial plant with long, thin red- to pink-colored stalks resembling celery, and large green leaves. Only the tart-flavored stalks are used for cooking, as the leaves are poisonous. For 2 cups (500 mL) cooked rhubarb, you will need 3 cups (750 mL) chopped fresh, about 1 lb (500 g).

Rice bran. See page 24.

Rice flours. See page 24.

Rice polish. See page 24.

Salba®. See page 45.

Sanding sugar. See page 35.

Sesame seeds. These flat oval seeds, which can be ivory, red, brown, pale gold or black, have a nutty, slightly sweet flavor. Black sesame seeds have a more pungent flavor and bitter taste than white or natural sesame seeds.

Shortening. A solid, white flavorless fat made from vegetable sources.

Slurry. A mixture of a raw starch and cold liquid used for thickening.

Snow peas. An edible-pod pea with a bright green pod and small pale green seeds. Also known as Chinese snow peas and sugar peas.

Sorghum. See page 25.

Sour cream. A thick, smooth, tangy product made by adding bacterial cultures to pasteurized, homogenized cream containing varying amounts of butterfat. Check the label: some lower-fat and fat-free brands may contain gluten.

Sour cream, lactose-free. See Lactose Intolerance, page 42.

Soy beverage, fortified. See Lactose Intolerance, page 42.

Soy flour. See page 32.

Squash. An edible fruit of the gourd family; varieties are divided into winter squash and summer squash, which are not interchangeable in recipes. Winter squash has a hard shell that isn't eaten. The flesh is sweeter and stronger in flavor than that of summer squash.

Starch. See page 33.

Sun-dried tomatoes. Available either dry or packed in oil, sun-dried tomatoes have a dark red color, a soft chewy texture and a strong tomato flavor. Use dry, not oil-packed, sun-dried tomatoes in recipes. Use scissors to snip. Oil-packed and dry are not interchangeable in recipes.

Sunflower seeds. These plump, nutlike kernels grow in teardrop shapes within gray-and-white shells. They are sold raw or roasted, and salted, seasoned or plain. Shelled sunflower seeds are sometimes labeled "sunflower kernels" or "nutmeats." When buying seeds in shell, look for clean, unbroken shells.

Superfine sugar. See page 35.

Sweet peppers. See Bell peppers.

Sweet potato. A tuber with orange flesh that stays moist when cooked. Not the same as a yam, although yams can substitute for sweet potatoes in recipes.

Sweet rice flour. See page 24.

Tapioca starch. See page 34.

Tarragon. An herb with narrow, pointed, dark green leaves and a distinctive anise-like flavor with undertones of sage. Use fresh or dried.

Teff. See page 26.

Treacle. See page 37.

Turbinado sugar. See page 36.

Vegetable oil. Common oils used are canola, corn, sunflower, safflower, olive, peanut, soy and walnut.

Walnuts. Inside a tough shell, a walnut's curly nutmeat halves offer a rich, sweet flavor, and the edible, papery skin adds a hint of bitterness to baked goods. Walnuts are available whole (shelled and unshelled), halved and chopped.

White (granulated) sugar. See page 35.

Whole bean flour. See page 31.

Wild rice. See page 24.

Xanthan gum. See page 37.

Yeast. A tiny, single-celled organism that, given moisture, food and warmth, creates gas that is trapped in bread dough, causing it to rise. Bread machine yeast (instant yeast) is added directly to the dry ingredients of bread. We use this yeast rather than active dry as it does not need to be activated in water before using. Store in the freezer in an airtight container for up to 2 years. To test for freshness, see the Techniques Glossary, page 399.

Yogurt. Made by fermenting cow's milk using a bacteria culture. Plain yogurt is gluten-free, but not all flavored yogurt is.

Yogurt, lactose-free. See Lactose Intolerance, page 42.

Zest. Strips from the outer layer of rind (colored part only) of citrus fruit. Avoid the bitter part underneath. Used for its intense flavor.

Techniques Glossary

Almonds. *To blanch:* Cover almonds with boiling water and let stand, covered, for 3 to 5 minutes. Drain. Grasp the almond at one end, pressing between your thumb and index finger, and the nut will pop out of the skin. Nuts are more easily chopped or slivered while still warm from blanching. *To toast:* see Nuts.

Almond flour (almond meal). *To make:* See Nut flour. *To toast:* Spread in a 9-inch (23 cm) baking pan and bake at 350°F (180°C), stirring occasionally, for 8 minutes or until light golden.

Baking pan. *To prepare, or to grease:* Either spray the bottom and sides of the baking pan with nonstick cooking spray or brush with a pastry brush or a crumpled-up piece of waxed paper dipped in vegetable oil or shortening.

Bananas. *To mash and freeze:* Select overripe fruit, mash and package in 1-cup (250 mL) amounts in freezer containers. Freeze for up to 6 months. Defrost and warm to room temperature before using. About 2 to 3 medium bananas yield 1 cup (250 mL) mashed.

Beat. To stir vigorously to incorporate air, using a spoon, whisk, handheld beater or electric mixer.

Blanch. To completely immerse food in boiling water and then quickly in cold water, to loosen and easily remove skin, for example.

Blend. To mix two or more ingredients together thoroughly, with a spoon or using the low speed of an electric mixer.

Blueberries, frozen. *To partially defrost:* Place 1 cup (250 mL) frozen blueberries in a single layer on a microwave-safe plate and microwave on High for 80 seconds.

Bread crumbs. *To make fresh:* For best results, the GF bread should be at least 1 day old. Using the pulsing operation of a food processor or blender, process until crumbs are of the desired consistency. *To make dry:* Spread bread crumbs in a single layer on a baking sheet and bake at 350°F (180°C) for 6 to 8 minutes, shaking pan frequently, until lightly browned, crisp and dry. (Or microwave, uncovered, on High for 1 to 2 minutes, stirring every 30 seconds.) *To store:* Package in airtight containers and freeze for up to 3 months.

Cake crumbs. See Bread crumbs.

Cast-iron skillet. *To clean:* Add 2 tbsp (25 mL) salt to a dry cast-iron skillet. Rub with an old toothbrush. Keep replacing salt until it remains white. This usually requires two to three applications of salt and about 5 minutes. *To season:* Coat bottom and sides evenly with vegetable oil. Place in a 400°F (200°C) oven for 30 minutes. Turn oven off and let pan cool completely. Using a paper towel, wipe off any remaining oil.

Combine. To stir two or more ingredients together for a consistent mixture.

Cream. To combine softened fat and sugar by beating to a soft, smooth creamy consistency while trying to incorporate as much air as possible.

Cut in. To combine solid fat and flour until the fat is the size required (for example, the size of small peas or meal). Use either two knives or a pastry blender.

Digital instant-read thermometer. *To test meat for doneness:* Insert the metal stem of the thermometer at least 2 inches (5 cm) into the thickest part of cooked chicken, fish, pork, beef, etc. For thin cuts, it may be necessary to insert the thermometer horizontally. Meatballs can be stacked. *To test baked goods for doneness:* Insert the metal stem of the thermometer at least 2 inches (5 cm) into the thickest part of baked good. Temperature should register 200°F (100°C).

Drizzle. To slowly spoon or pour a liquid (such as frosting or melted butter) in a very fine stream over the surface of food.

Drugstore fold. *To make:* Bring the sides of parchment or foil up to meet in the center, fold over the edges, then fold the edges of the ends together. Allow room for the packets to expand, then crimp the edges.

Dust. To coat by sprinkling GF confectioner's (icing) sugar, unsweetened cocoa powder or any GF flour lightly over food or a utensil.

Eggs. *To warm to room temperature:* Place eggs in the shell from the refrigerator in a bowl of hot water and let stand for 5 minutes.

Egg whites. *To warm to room temperature:* Separate eggs while cold. Place bowl of egg whites in a larger bowl of hot water and let stand for 5 minutes. *To whip to soft peaks:* Beat to a thickness that comes up as the beaters are lifted and folds over at the tips. *To whip to stiff peaks:* Beat past soft peaks until the peaks remain upright when the beaters are lifted.

Egg yolks. *To warm to room temperature:* Separate eggs while cold. Place bowl of egg yolks in a larger bowl of hot water and let stand for 5 minutes.

Flaxseed. *To grind:* Place whole seeds in a coffee grinder or blender. Grind only the amount required. If necessary, store extra ground flaxseed in the refrigerator. *To crack:* Pulse in a coffee grinder, blender or food processor just long enough to break the seed coat but not long enough to grind completely.

Fold in. To combine two mixtures of different weights and textures (for example, gluten-free flours into stiffly beaten egg whites) in a way that doesn't deflate the batter. Place the lighter mixture on top of the heavier one. Use a large rubber spatula to gently cut down through the two mixtures on one side of the bowl, then gently move the spatula up the opposite side. Rotate the bowl a quarter-turn and repeat until the mixtures are thoroughly combined.

Garlic. *To peel:* Use the flat side of a sharp knife to flatten the clove of garlic. Skin can then be easily removed. *To roast:* Cut off top of head to expose clove tips. Drizzle with $\frac{1}{4}$ tsp (1 mL) olive oil and microwave on High for 70 seconds, until fork-tender. Or bake in a pie plate or baking dish at 375°F (190°C) for 15 to 20 minutes, or until fork-tender. Let cool slightly, then squeeze cloves from skins.

Glaze. To apply a thin, shiny coating to the outside of a baked, sweet or savory food to enhance the appearance and flavor.

Grease pan. See Baking pan.

Griddle. *To test for the correct temperature:* Sprinkle a few drops of water on the surface. If the water bounces and dances across the pan, it is ready to use.

Hazelnuts. *To remove skins:* Place hazelnuts in a 350°F (180°C) oven for 15 to 20 minutes. Immediately place in a clean, dry kitchen towel. With your hands, rub the nuts against the towel. Skins will be left in the towel. Be careful: hazelnuts will be very hot.

Hazelnut flour (hazelnut meal). *To make:* See Nut flour. *To toast:* Spread in a 9-inch (23 cm) baking pan and bake at 350°F (180°C), stirring occasionally, for 8 minutes or until light golden. Let cool before using.

Herbs. *To store full stems:* Fresh-picked herbs can be stored for up to 1 week with stems standing in water. (Keep leaves out of water.) *To remove leaves:* Remove small leaves from stem by holding the top and running fingers down the stem in the opposite direction of growth. Larger leaves should be snipped off the stem using scissors. *To clean and store fresh leaves:* Rinse under cold running water and spin-dry in a lettuce spinner. If necessary, dry between layers of paper towels. Place a dry paper towel along with the clean herbs in a plastic bag in the refrigerator. Use within 2 to 3 days. Freeze or dry for longer storage. *To measure:* Pack leaves tightly into correct measure. *To snip:* After measuring, transfer to a small glass and cut using the tips of sharp kitchen shears/scissors to avoid bruising the tender leaves. *To dry:* Tie fresh-picked herbs together in small bunches and hang upside down in a well-ventilated location with low humidity and out of sunlight until the leaves are brittle and fully dry. If they turn brown (rather than stay green), the air is too hot. Once fully dried, strip leaves off the stems for storage. Store whole herbs in an airtight container in a cool, dark place for up to 1 year and crushed herbs for up to 6 months. (Dried herbs are

stored in the dark to prevent the color from fading.) Before using, check herbs and discard any that have faded, lost flavor or smell old and musty. *To dry using a microwave:* Place $\frac{1}{2}$ to 1 cup (125 to 250 mL) herbs between layers of paper towels. Microwave on High for 3 minutes, checking often to be sure they are not scorched. Then microwave for 10-second periods until leaves are brittle and can be pulled from stems easily. *To freeze:* Lay whole herbs in a single layer on a flat surface in the freezer for 2 to 4 hours. Leave whole and pack in plastic bags. Herbs will keep in the freezer for 2 to 3 months. Crumble frozen leaves directly into the dish. Herb leaves are also easier to chop when frozen. Use frozen leaves only for flavoring and not for garnishing, as they lose their crispness when thawed. Some herbs, such as chives, have a very weak flavor when dried, and do not freeze well, but they do grow well inside on a windowsill.

Leeks. *To clean:* Trim roots and wilted green ends. Peel off tough outer layer. Cut leeks in half lengthwise and rinse under cold running water, separating the leaves so the water gets between the layers. Trim individual leaves at the point where they start to become dark in color and coarse in texture — this will be higher up on the plant the closer you get to the center.

Mango. *To ripen:* Place mangos in a paper bag at room temperature for 3 to 5 days. Once ripe, they can be refrigerated in a plastic bag for up to 1 week. *To pit:* Lay mango narrow side up on a cutting board. Cut flesh from each side of the pit and discard pit, then slice flesh lengthwise. You can also try using a mango splitter, a tool similar in appearance to an apple corer. Its sharp, elliptical, centered metal blade slides down around the pit, slicing the fruit in half at the same time. Two handles, opposite each other, prevent your hands from slipping. It works best on large mangos. *To cube:* After pitting, cut a grid pattern in the flesh, down to (but not through) the skin. Gently push skin to turn inside out; cut off flesh.

Mix. To combine two or more ingredients uniformly by stirring or using an electric mixer on a low speed.

Nut flour (nut meal). *To make:* Toast nuts (see Nuts), cool to room temperature and grind in a food processor or blender to desired consistency. *To make using ground nuts:* Bake at 350°F (180°C) for 6 to 8 minutes, cool to room temperature and grind finer.

Nuts. *To toast:* Spread nuts in a single layer on a baking sheet and bake at 350°F (180°C) for 6 to 8 minutes, shaking the pan frequently, until fragrant and lightly browned. (Or microwave, uncovered, on High for 1 to 2 minutes, stirring every 30 seconds.) Nuts will darken upon cooling.

Oat flour. *To make:* In a food processor or blender, pulse oats until finely ground, or to desired consistency.

Olives. *To pit:* Place olives under the flat side of a large knife; push down on knife until pit pops out.

Onions. *To caramelize:* In a nonstick frying pan, heat 1 tbsp (15 mL) oil over medium heat. Add 2 cups (500 mL) sliced or chopped onions; cook slowly until soft and caramel-colored. If necessary, add 1 tbsp (15 mL) water or white wine to prevent sticking while cooking.

Peaches. *To blanch:* See Blanch.

Pecan flour (pecan meal). *To make:* See Nut flour.

Pork tenderloin. *To roast:* Bake in a preheated 400°F (200°C) oven for 20 to 25 minutes or until it reaches an internal temperature of 155°F (68°C).

Pumpkin seeds. *To toast:* See Seeds.

Quinoa grain. *To prepare:* Before cooking, quinoa seeds may need to be rinsed to remove their bitter resin-like coating, called saponin. Quinoa is often rinsed before it is sold, but rinse it again to remove any soapy residue that remains. The presence of saponin is obvious by the appearance of soapy-looking "suds" when the seeds are swished in water. Place quinoa seeds in a fine-mesh strainer and rinse thoroughly with water. *To toast:* Spread in a single layer in a large skillet and toast over medium heat for 3 to 4 minutes or until quinoa is golden. Quinoa will darken upon cooling. *To cook:* For 1 cup (250 mL) cooked quinoa, bring to a boil $\frac{1}{4}$ cup (50 mL) quinoa and $\frac{3}{4}$ cup (175 mL) water. Reduce heat to low; cover and simmer for 18 to 20 minutes. Remove from heat. Let stand, covered, for 5 to 10 minutes or until water is absorbed, quinoa grains have turned from white to transparent and the tiny spiral-like germ is separated.

Red bell pepper. *To roast:* Place whole peppers on a baking sheet, piercing each near the stem with a knife. Bake at 425°F (220°C) for 18 minutes. Turn and bake for 15 minutes or until the skins blister. (Or roast on the barbecue, turning frequently, until skin is completely charred.) Place in a paper or plastic bag. Seal and let cool for 10 minutes or until skin is loose. Peel and discard seeds.

Rice. *To cook:* See Cooking Rice, page 23.

Sauté. To cook quickly at high temperature in a small amount of fat.

Seeds. *To toast:* There are three methods you could use: 1) Spread seeds in a single layer on a baking sheet and bake at 350°F (180°C) for 6 to 10 minutes, shaking the pan frequently, until aromatic and lightly browned; 2) Spread seeds in a single layer in a large skillet and toast over medium heat for 5 to 8 minutes, shaking pan frequently; or 3) Microwave seeds, uncovered, on High for 1 to 2 minutes, stirring every 30 seconds. Seeds will darken upon cooling.

Sesame seeds. *To toast:* See Seeds.

Skillet. *To test for correct temperature:* Sprinkle a few drops of water on the surface. If the water bounces and dances across the pan, it is ready to use. If the drops of water evaporate, it is too hot.

Sunflower seeds. *To toast:* See Seeds.

Tomatoes. *To peel:* See Blanch. *To seed:* Cut fresh tomatoes in half crosswise. Squeeze to remove seeds.

Wild rice. *To cook:* See Cooking Rice, page 23.

Yeast. *To test for freshness:* Dissolve 1 tsp (5 mL) granulated sugar in $\frac{1}{2}$ cup (125 mL) lukewarm water. Add 2 tsp (10 mL) yeast and stir gently. In 10 minutes, the mixture should have a strong yeasty smell and be foamy. If it doesn't, the yeast is too old — time to buy new yeast!

Yogurt. *To drain:* Place 2 cups (500 mL) yogurt in a cheesecloth-lined sieve set over a bowl. Refrigerate for 3 hours or overnight, until reduced to 1 cup (250 mL).

Zest. *To zest:* Use a zester, the fine side of a box grater or a small sharp knife to peel off thin strips of the colored part of the skin of citrus fruits. Be sure not to remove the bitter white pith below.

About the Nutrient Analysis

The nutrient analysis done on the recipes in this book was derived from The Food Processor Nutrition Analysis Software, version 7.71, ESHA Research (2001).

Where necessary, data was supplemented using the following references:

1. Shelley Case, *Gluten-Free Diet: A Comprehensive Resource Guide*, Expanded Edition (Regina, SK: Case Nutrition Consulting, 2006).

2. Bob's Red Mill Natural Foods. Nutritional information product search. Retrieved April 15, 2009, from www.bobsredmill.com/catalog/index.php?action=search.

3. Gluten-free oats and oat flour from Cream Hill Estates (www.creamhillestates.com). Certificate of Analysis of Pure Oats (Lasalle, QC: Silliker Canada Co., 2005). Certificate of Analysis of Oat Flour (Lasalle, QC: Silliker Canada Co., 2006).

4. Flax Council of Canada. Nutritional information product search. Retrieved April 15, 2009, from www.flaxcouncil.ca.

Recipes were evaluated as follows:

- The larger number of servings was used where there is a range.
- Where alternatives are given, the first ingredient and amount listed were used.
- Optional ingredients and ingredients that are not quantified were not included.
- Calculations were based on imperial measures and weights.
- Nutrient values were rounded to the nearest whole number.
- Defatted soy flour, 25% reduced-sodium broth and brown rice flour were used, including where these ingredients are listed as soy flour, stock and rice flour.
- Calculations involving meat and poultry used lean portions without skin.
- Canola oil was used where the type of fat was not specified.
- Recipes were analyzed prior to cooking.

It is important to note that the cooking method used to prepare the recipe may alter the nutrient content per serving, as may ingredient substitutions and differences among brand-name products.

Library and Archives Canada Cataloguing in Publication

Washburn, Donna
    250 gluten-free favorites : includes dairy-free, egg-free and white sugar–free recipes /
Donna Washburn & Heather Butt.

Includes index.
ISBN 978-0-7788-0225-9

    1. Gluten-free diet--Recipes. 2. Milk-free diet--Recipes. 3. Egg-free diet--Recipes.
4. Sugar-free diet--Recipes.
I. Butt, Heather II. Title. III. Title: Two hundred fifty gluten-free favorites.

RM237.86.W383 2009   641.5'638   C2009-902264-8

Index

More Great Books
from Robert Rose

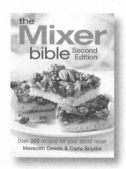

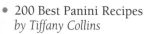

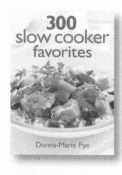

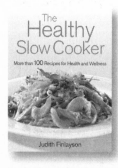

Appliance Cooking

- The Mixer Bible Second Edition
  by Meredith Deeds and Carla Snyder
- The Dehydrator Bible
  by Jennifer MacKenzie, Jay Nutt & Don Mercer
- The Juicing Bible Second Edition
  by Pat Crocker
- 200 Best Panini Recipes
  by Tiffany Collins
- 200 Best Pressure Cooker Recipes
  by Cinda Chavich
- 300 Slow Cooker Favorites
  by Donna-Marie Pye
- The 150 Best Slow Cooker Recipes
  by Judith Finlayson
- Delicious & Dependable Slow Cooker Recipes
  by Judith Finlayson
- 125 Best Vegetarian Slow Cooker Recipes
  by Judith Finlayson
- The Healthy Slow Cooker
  by Judith Finlayson
- The Best Convection Oven Cookbook
  by Linda Stephen
- 250 Best American Bread Machine Baking Recipes
  by Donna Washburn and Heather Butt
- 250 Best Canadian Bread Machine Baking Recipes
  by Donna Washburn and Heather Butt

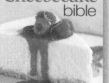

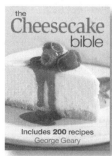

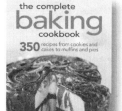

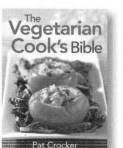

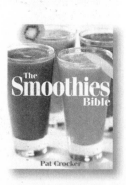

Baking

- The Cheesecake Bible
  by George Geary
- 1500 Best Bars, Cookies, Muffins, Cakes & More
  by Esther Brody
- The Complete Book of Baking
  by George Geary
- The Complete Book of Bars & Squares
  by Jill Snider
- The Complete Book of Pies
  by Julie Hasson
- 125 Best Chocolate Recipes
  by Julie Hasson
- 125 Best Cupcake Recipes
  by Julie Hasson
- Complete Cake Mix Magic
  by Jill Snider

Healthy Cooking

- The Vegetarian Cook's Bible
  by Pat Crocker
- The Vegan Cook's Bible
  by Pat Crocker
- 125 Best Vegetarian Recipes
  by Byron Ayanoglu with contributions from Algis Kemezys
- The Smoothies Bible
  by Pat Crocker
- 125 Best Vegan Recipes
  by Maxine Effenson Chuck and Beth Gurney

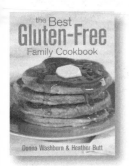

- 200 Best Lactose-Free Recipes
  by Jan Main
- 500 Best Healthy Recipes
  Edited by Lynn Roblin, RD
- Complete Gluten-Free Cookbook
  by Donna Washburn and Heather Butt
- The Best Gluten-Free Family Cookbook
  by Donna Washburn and Heather Butt
- 125 Best Gluten-Free Recipes
  by Donna Washburn and Heather Butt

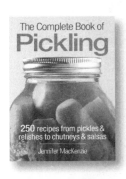

- Diabetes Meals for Good Health
  by Karen Graham, RD
- Canada's Diabetes Meals for Good Health
  by Karen Graham, RD
- America's Complete Diabetes Cookbook
  Edited by Katherine E. Younker, MBA, RD
- Canada's Complete Diabetes Cookbook
  Edited by Katherine E. Younker, MBA, RD

Recent Bestsellers

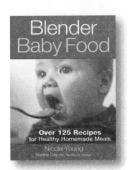

- The Complete Book of Pickling
  by Jennifer MacKenzie
- Baby Blender Food
  by Nicole Young
- 125 Best Ice Cream Recipes
  by Marilyn Linton and Tanya Linton

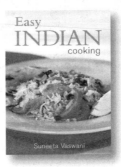

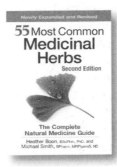

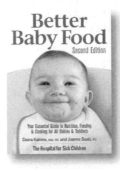

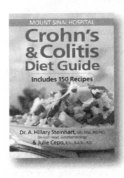

- The Convenience Cook
  by Judith Finlayson
- Easy Indian Cooking
  by Suneeta Vaswani
- Simply Thai Cooking
  by Wandee Young and Byron Ayanoglu

Health

- 55 Most Common Medicinal Herbs Second Edition
  by Dr. Heather Boon, B.Sc.Phm., Ph.D. and Michael Smith, B.Pharm, M.R.Pharm.S., ND
- Canada's Baby Care Book
  by Dr. Jeremy Friedman MBChB, FRCP(C), FAAP, and Dr. Norman Saunders MD, FRCP(C)
- The Baby Care Book
  by Dr. Jeremy Friedman MBChB, FRCP(C), FAAP, and Dr. Norman Saunders MD, FRCP(C)
- Better Baby Food Second Edition
  by Daina Kalnins, MSc, RD, and Joanne Saab, RD
- Better Food for Pregnancy
  by Daina Kalnins, MSc, RD, and Joanne Saab, RD
- Crohn's & Colitis
  by Dr. A. Hillary Steinhart, MD, MSc, FRCP(C)
- Crohn's & Colitis Diet Guide
  by Dr. A. Hillary Steinhart, MD, MSc, FRCP(C), and Julie Cepo, BSc, BASc, RD

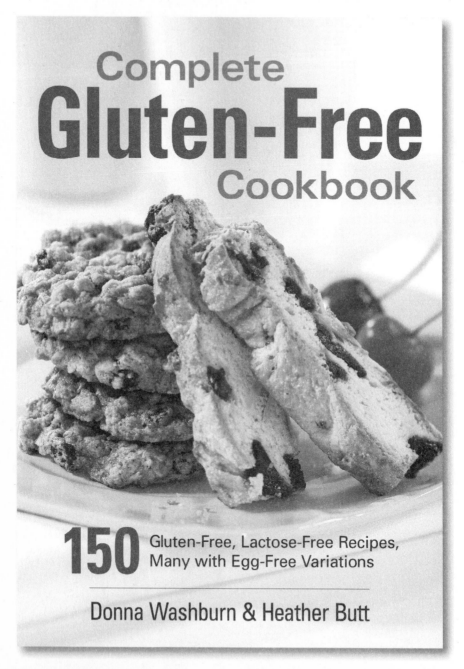